Women's Health

Women's Health

The Commonwealth Fund Survey

Edited by

MARILYN M. FALIK, PH.D.

and

KAREN SCOTT COLLINS, M.D., M.P.H.

The Johns Hopkins University Press

Baltimore and London

The Johns Hopkins University Press
2715 North Charles Street
Baltimore, Maryland 21218-4319
The Johns Hopkins Press Ltd., London

Library of Congress Cataloging-in-Publication Data
will be found at the end of this book.
A catalog record for this book is available from the British Library.

ISBN 0-8018-5353-2
ISBN 0-8018-5354-0 (pbk)

Contents

Foreword

The Commonwealth Fund's 1993 groundbreaking national survey revealed disquieting facts about American women's health and refuted the assumption that women live longer because they enjoy good health. Findings showed that many women are living severely impaired lives and are even dying from health conditions that can be prevented through early detection and treatment or through changes in health behavior.

- Thirteen percent of women did not get the medical care they needed in the past year, compared with 9 percent of men. Uninsured women were even more markedly affected: more than one-third did not receive needed care in the previous 12 months.
- More than one-third of women did not have basic preventive services in the past year: a Pap smear, a clinical breast exam, a pelvic exam, or a complete physical exam.
- Physicians often fail women when help is needed. Forty-one percent of women have changed physicians because they are dissatisfied, compared with 27 percent of men. Many women found physicians condescending or dismissive, and one in ten women would not discuss problems with physicians because they were uncomfortable.

Alarmed by these initial findings, The Commonwealth Fund's Commission on Women's Health brought together a panel of expert health researchers to further analyze the data. Its aim was to understand in greater detail the barriers that women face in providing for their own health. This volume, the product of that endeavor, raises important questions—for policy makers at a time of great change in the nation's health care system, for women as aging Baby Boomers comprise the largest group of midlife women in the history of this country, and for health care professionals for whom women's health must become far more than reproductive health.

Throughout its history, The Commonwealth Fund has been concerned with the health of women. Commonwealth Fund support was instrumental in the development of state maternal and child health programs in the 1920s and in the development of the Pap smear in the 1940s. Today The Commonwealth Fund's Commission on Women's Health is charged with identifying key issues in women's health and making targeted recommendations for social change. Under the leadership of Ellen Futter, chair of the commission, and Joan Leiman, executive director, the commission seeks to raise women's awareness of what they can do to prevent disease; help physicians counsel women patients about health risks; identify barriers minority, low-income, and other disadvantaged women encounter in obtaining care; conduct research on important and neglected women's health issues; and identify public policies to improve women's health. This book is an important contribution to that effort, and the authors of each of the chapters are to be congratulated. I also want to commend co-editors Marilyn Falik and Karen Scott Collins for their outstanding work in shaping this compelling profile of the issues that women face in taking their own health in hand.

Karen Davis
President
The Commonwealth Fund

Acknowledgments

We begin by expressing our sincere appreciation to all our contributors. They gave generously of their expertise, time, and talent in developing this multidisciplinary volume.

We express our indebtedness and deep appreciation to The Commonwealth Fund, especially Karen Davis, for assuming a leadership role in recognizing the need for research on women's health. Importantly, The Commonwealth Fund proceeded to develop opportunities to explore women's health issues and to build a foundation for enhancing women's health and well-being. The Commonwealth Fund's financial support for the 1993 survey on women's health and this resulting volume begin to give voice and meaning to women's experiences. We also acknowledge the considerable contribution of Louis Harris and Associates in conducting the 1993 survey and providing technical assistance, as requested, by our contributors. This volume would not have been possible nor as valuable without their respective commitment and continuing support.

We wish to extend our sincere appreciation to the "outside reviewer" selected by the Johns Hopkins University Press, who continues to be unknown to us. He/she provided valuable comments and suggestions, and importantly, was very supportive of our efforts and approach. We also wish to acknowledge the reviewers of early draft chapters, especially Deborah Lewis-Idema, Edna Jonas, and Cheryl Ulmer, MDS Associates, and Mary Lou Russell, Director of Communications, The Commonwealth Fund, for their valuable comments and support along the way. We acknowledge Jane Stein and her staff for valuable editorial assistance on earlier drafts, and David C. denBoer and Maria denBoer for their timely and professional editorial assistance on the final manuscript.

We are especially indebted to and acknowledge Wendy Harris, our wondrous editor at the Johns Hopkins University Press. From the outset, she was enthusiastic and highly supportive; she also provided collegial assistance and counsel beyond measure.

Contributors

JANICE BOWIE, M.P.H., Department of Health Policy and Management, Johns Hopkins University School of Hygiene and Public Health, Baltimore, Maryland

E. RICHARD BROWN, Ph.D., Professor of Public Health, School of Public Health, University of California, Los Angeles, California

KAREN SCOTT COLLINS, M.D., M.P.H., Assistant Vice President, The Commonwealth Fund, New York, New York

KIMBERLY A. DUKES, M.A., statistician, Primary Care Outcomes Research Institute, New England Medical Center, Boston, Massachusetts

MARILYN M. FALIK, Ph.D., Vice President, MDS Associates, Wheaton, Maryland

LINDA M. FRIED, M.D., M.P.H., Associate Professor of Medicine and Epidemiology, Johns Hopkins Medical Institutions, Baltimore, Maryland

SHELDON GREENFIELD, M.D., Director, Primary Care Outcomes Research Institute, New England Medical Center, Boston, Massachusetts

HEIDI I. HARTMANN, Ph.D., Director, Institute for Women's Policy Research, Washington, D.C.

SHERRIE H. KAPLAN, Ph.D., M.P.H., Senior Scientist and Co-Director, Primary Care Outcomes Research Institute, New England Medical Center, Boston, Massachusetts

AMINA KHAN, M.A., statistician, Primary Care Outcomes Research Institute, New England Medical Center, Boston, Massachusetts

JOAN A. KURIANSKY, J.D., M.A., Director, S.T.O.P. Violence Against Women, Technical Assistance Project, Washington, D.C.

JOAN M. LEIMAN, Ph.D., Executive Deputy Vice President for Health Sciences, Columbia University, College of Physicians and Surgeons, New York, New York

MARY CLARE LENNON, Ph.D., M.S., Assistant Professor, School of Public Health, Columbia University, New York, New York

MARSHA LILLIE-BLANTON, Dr.P.H., Assistant Professor, Department of Health Policy and Management, Johns Hopkins University School of Hygiene and Public Health, Baltimore, Maryland

BARBARA LYONS, M.H.S., Program Officer, Henry J. Kaiser Family Foundation, and Associate Director, Kaiser Commission on the Future of Medicaid, Washington, D.C.

CHRISTINE L. OWENS, J.D., Executive Director, Pay Discrimination Institute, Washington, D.C.

STACEY B. PLICHTA, Sc.D., Assistant Professor, Old Dominion University, College of Health Sciences, Norfolk, Virginia

ANNETTE B. RAMÍREZ DE ARELLANO, Dr.P.H., Executive Director, Hispanic AIDS Forum, New York, New York

ANNE LENHARD REISINGER, Ph.D., Assistant Professor of Public Health and Public Affairs, Columbia University, New York, New York

MARGUERITE RO, M.P.H., Department of Health Policy and Management, Johns Hopkins University School of Hygiene and Public Health, Baltimore, Maryland

DIANE ROWLAND, Sc.D., Senior Vice President, Henry J. Kaiser Family Foundation, and Executive Director, Kaiser Commission on the Future of Medicaid, Washington, D.C.

ALINA SALGANICOFF, Ph.D., Senior policy analyst, Henry J. Kaiser Family Foundation, Washington, D.C.

DANTE S. SPETTER, Ph.D., Research Scientist, Primary Care Outcomes Research Institute, New England Medical Center, Boston, Massachusetts

LISA M. SULLIVAN, Ph.D., Research Scientist, Primary Care Outcomes Research Institute, New England Medical Center, Boston, Massachusetts

CAROL S. WEISMAN, Ph.D., Professor, Department of Health Policy and Management, Johns Hopkins University School of Hygiene and Public Health, Baltimore, Maryland

NANCY FUGATE WOODS, Ph.D., R.N., Director, Center for Women's Health Research, and Professor, School of Nursing, University of Washington, Seattle, Washington

ROBERTA WYN, Ph.D., Associate Director for Research, Center for Health Policy Research, University of California, Los Angeles, California

HONGJIAN YU, M.S., Senior Programmer, Center for Health Policy Research, University of California, Los Angeles, California

Introduction:
Listening to Women's Voices, Learning from Women's Experiences

Marilyn M. Falik, Ph.D.

Health and well-being are complex phenomena. An overly simplistic emphasis on superior longevity as a hallmark of health status all too often masks women's serious health concerns. Mortality statistics, for example, suggest that women are healthier than men. Yet although women tend to live longer, they are far more likely to experience depression, and to have chronic disabilities, and are less likely to have adequate health insurance coverage. Women are more likely than men to use health services—more physician visits and more hospitalizations. It would appear that women are experiencing longer but not necessarily healthier lives.

Certainly a myriad of biomedical and behavioral factors come into play when examining women's health, well-being, and related care-seeking behavior. Women's health is surfacing as a high-visibility topic in the media, but very basic issues remain largely unexamined. Much of the research on women's health continues to emphasize the biomedical model (i.e., a disease orientation) and to focus on reproductive health and related issues of perinatal care. Far less attention has been given to forging a behavioral model that takes into account biopsychosocial factors and to supporting health services research that examines how these factors influence women's health-seeking options, preferences, and behavior.

Until very recently, women's health was viewed principally in terms of maternal and child health, with gynecological services being subordinate to obstetrical care, and both far more prominent than basic primary care and preventive services for women (irrespective of age and procreative status). For too many decades, the biomedical research community excluded women from important clinical trials, thus leaving significant gaps in addressing women's health concerns and redressing disabling conditions. Fears regarding the potential effects of women's participation in clinical trials on their fertility and the health status of their offspring led to the virtual wholesale exclusion of women from most clinical trials.

The National Institutes of Health (NIH) launched a campaign in 1991 to expand the role of women in clinical trials and initiated clinical research on women's midlife health concerns, including osteoporosis, menopause, and hormone replacement therapy. The findings of the NIH women's midlife clinical trial, however, will not be available for some 10 to 15 years. In the interim, women will continue to make health- and care-seeking decisions that reflect their experiences and related psychosocial forces and thus define their health-seeking options, preferences, and behavior.

The health services research community had a similarly myopic focus on women's access to and use of reproductive services—family planning, contraception, perinatal services, and related newborn care issues. Until very recently, women's health services research principally focused on women in their reproductive years, ages eighteen through forty-four. Women's role as birth mother framed both the health issues and the research agenda, with women's health falling within the arena of "maternal and child health" and reproductive specialists, obstetrician-gynecologists, serving as women's principal, if not primary care physicians.

This book, through a series of multidisciplinary analyses of The Commonwealth Fund survey on women's health, seeks to give voice to women by examining their health-related experiences and how these experiences appear to influence health and well-being. The Commonwealth Fund survey is the first nationally representative survey on women's health. It offers a timely opportunity to examine the diversity of women's experiences and their implications for women's health and well-being. Bearing witness to the changing demographics, the survey offers a unique opportunity to begin to explore emergent health-related issues, behaviors, care patterns, and challenges that confront women at various stages of life, including the postreproductive years, which are increasingly likely to comprise over half their lives.

Experts from a variety of disciplines were invited to mine the survey and build on respective disciplines to listen and score the emergent lyrics. The contributors seek to advance our understanding of forces that influence women's health, their choices (or lack of choices), and their behaviors. Listening can be the first constructive step in advancing women's health, mapping changes to improve access to health care, or empowering women to assume a more positive, health-seeking role. Each of the contributing authors highlights implications of the respective findings for public policy and delivery system reforms. The resultant chapters, individually and together, also seek to build research–policy bridges by surfacing care patterns, identifying challenges women face, and, as applicable, highlighting opportunities for enhancing women's health and well-being.

DESIGN AND STRUCTURE OF THE SURVEY

The Commonwealth Fund survey on women's health was designed, with the assistance of expert consultants, by staff members of The Commonwealth Fund and of Louis Harris and Associates, Inc. The questionnaire encompassed a wide range of health and health-related issues, including (1) insurance coverage, access to and use of various health services; (2) sources of health care, satisfaction with care, and patient-physician communication; (3) risk factors and behaviors; (4) measures of health status, psychological well-being, and self-esteem; (5) abuse and domestic violence; (6) employment, familial roles and responsibilities; and (7) socioeconomic characteristics.[1]

Louis Harris and Associates fielded the telephone interviews in 1993. The nationally representative cross-section of adult women and men (age eighteen years or older, residing in the continental United States) included 3,010 completed interviews (2,010 women and 1,000 men). An oversampling of minority women (439 African American women and 405 Hispanic women) permits a more detailed analysis of these two subgroups of minority women. To create projectable results for the U.S. population (95 million women and 87 million men age eighteen or older), the survey data were weighted by age, race, education, insurance status, and Census region, using March 1992 Census Bureau data.

All of the telephone interviews were conducted by female interviewers. Five percent of the women's and 4 percent of the men's cross-section interviews were conducted in Spanish. Seven percent of the women's Hispanic oversample were conducted in Spanish. Women responded to a 25-minute interview and men responded to a 15-minute interview.

The cross-section sample was created in multiple-stage process, using a sampling grid to generate a systematic random selection of respondents, with subquotas set for male and female respondents. Substitutions were not permissible. Excluded from the sampling frame were persons residing in religious, educational, or penal institutions, those associated with the military, homeless persons, those without telephones, and individuals who did not speak English or Spanish. The completion rate was 56 percent. For women, the theoretical margin of sampling error is ±2 percent.

CARE-SEEKING BEHAVIORS

The first section of this book focuses on a variety of factors that can influence health care-seeking behavior. Some aspects of women's care-seeking behavior may well reflect the structure and organization of the health care system itself. Other behaviors may correspond with personal attributes or experiences, such as, women's awareness or knowledge regarding particular health care practices or women's interactions and satisfaction with health care professionals. The authors examine how women view their health-related experiences and how they translate these experiences into behaviors.

That women, even beyond the reproductive years, use more health services than men is a persistent and largely unexplained finding in the health services research literature. Women, for example, are more likely than men to have a usual source of care, to visit a physician, to be hospitalized, and to use prescription drugs.

In chapter 1 Carol Weisman seeks to examine and explain why women have higher rates of health care utilization than men. While recognizing that various predisposing factors (e.g., sociodemographics such as age) and enabling factors (e.g., resources such as insurance) affect utilization, Weisman focuses on the structural attributes of women's health care systems. Via the fragmentation hypothesis, she examines women's utilization patterns in terms of the type of physician (e.g., family practitioner, internist, obstetrician-gynecologist) and the number of physicians a woman regards as her usual source(s) of care. Measures of utilization are the numbers of physician visits over the past year and of preventive services received over the past 2 years. An apparent reliance on both a primary care physician and a reproductive specialist was more evident among women of some means, who were relatively affluent and had private insurance. These women, in turn, were more likely to report higher utilization—making more physician visits and being more likely to receive preventive health services.

Weisman concludes that fragmentation underscores system-driven inefficiencies and inequities. Some women (those of means) are being well served, while others tend to receive less than optimal access, especially as measured by their receiving preventive health services. To ameliorate structural barriers and implications of fragmentation, Weisman presents several recommendations, including a greater emphasis on multidisciplinary medical education, the introduction of cross-cutting guidelines for women's health services, and the application of organizational models that integrate a broader spectrum of women's health services into a single more accessible and efficient entity.

Another analysis of The Commonwealth Fund survey confirms that preventive screening rates are lower than desirable among all women, but especially among low-income and elderly women and some minority women. Roberta Wyn, Richard Brown, and Hongjian Yu in chapter 2 highlight several very disturbing findings in the light of knowledge about the benefits of screening and early detection. Notably, women of lower socioeconomic status are least likely to get timely screenings, women who are uninsured or inadequately insured have comparatively low screening rates, and, somewhat surprisingly, screening rates for mammography decrease with age. Screening rates are also lower among women who do not have a regular source of care, and tend to be lower among women who visit family practitioners or internists rather than obstetrician-gynecologists. The two most frequently cited barriers to obtaining timely screenings were cost (often uncovered service) and time (not surprising for women juggling multiple roles).

Wyn and colleagues conclude by observing that simplistic solutions will not suffice. Effective strategies should redress financial barriers (universal coverage and comprehensive benefits package) as well as deficiencies in the delivery system. To promote timely access to and use of preventive services, Wyn and colleagues recommend efforts directed at enhancing women's knowledge (e.g., targeted education campaigns and outreach) and reinforcing positive care-seeking behavior (e.g., having a regular source of care, physician follow-up with screening information and services).

In chapter 3 Sherrie Kaplan and co-authors Lisa Sullivan, Dante Spetter, Kimberly Dukes, Amina Khan, and Sheldon Greenfield examine aspects of physician-patient communication, seeking to unravel gender-based communication patterns and explore their implications. The recent literature suggests that women and men exhibit different conversational styles and communication preferences—in personal, business, and health care situations. In some settings, men appear to be more dominant. During business meetings, for example, men tend to talk more and interrupt women. In health care settings, women appear to be more assertive than men. Women patients ask more questions, present more complaints, and get more information during their visits. Studies also suggest that women physicians, compared with male physicians, are more attentive and supportive. Women physicians, for example, spend more time with patients, show more positive affect, share concerns and doubts with their patients, and provide more information than their male colleagues. Women patients, in turn, are more likely to value a communication style that encompasses information sharing and rapport.

This analysis of The Commonwealth Fund survey data indicates that women, compared with men, are less satisfied with physician-patient communication and as a consequence, are more likely to change physicians. Women are twice as likely as men to switch physicians. Women are far more likely to indicate that problematic communications with their prior physician led to their switching to another physician. A fair number of women report experiences with a physician who "treated them like a child" or "talked down to them." Female physicians appear to benefit from switchers, as more patients of female physicians had changed physicians.

Less than favorable experiences can lead to dissatisfaction; less than favorable perceptions of physicians' interpersonal and communication skills can lead to doctor shopping. Within the increasingly cost-conscious practice environment, efficiency often translates into more patients per hour and less time per patient. This, in turn, can adversely affect the quality of physician-patient communication, promote switching behavior, and disrupt care. Switching physicians may lead to care-seeking behaviors that result in duplicative services, such as repeat tests and procedures. Kaplan and colleagues conclude by observing that physician-patient communication failures may ultimately raise both cost and quality of care concerns.

CULTURAL AND LIFE SPAN PERSPECTIVES

Various demographic forces shape women's perspectives. Shared norms influence women's expectations and attitudes. Shared expectations shape and give meaning to common experiences. Race, ethnicity, and age-cohorts (e.g., Baby Boomers, midlife women, or seniors) serve as a lens for filtering experiences. This section examines selected aspects of these cultural filters and how they influence women's health and related behavior.

Among African Americans, education and, to a somewhat lesser extent, satisfaction with care correlate with the use of specific preventive health services. Marsha Lillie-Blanton, Janice Bowie, and Marguerite Ro in chapter 4 explore aspects of women's experience and the extent to which social distance shapes the use of health care, especially preventive health services. The two principal measures of social distance are educational attainment and satisfaction with care. Education serves as a proxy for social status, and satisfaction with care serves as an indicator of the perceived value of the physician-patient relationship.

Lillie-Blanton and colleagues found that race was not a significant factor in explaining the differential use of several preventive services. After controlling for sociodemographics that generally influence patterns of use (e.g., socioeconomic variables such as education and income), the least educated women (did not complete high school), irrespective of race, were the least likely to receive preventive health and screening services. As education proved to be a predictor of positive, preventive screening behavior, delivery system recommendations focus principally on improving health promotion information campaigns and elevating women's health-related knowledge. For example, Lillie-Blanton and colleagues suggest developing culturally sensitive consumer health promotion campaigns, culturally competent professional training programs, and more targeted awareness programs to motivate positive, health-seeking behaviors. Education emerges as a means for empowering women and, thus, increasing their seeking timely preventive care.

Understanding cultural differences is essential for listening to women and interpreting their responses to survey questions. Cultural sensitivity begins with the survey questions—how they are stated, how they might be translated, and, most important, how women from different cultures view and present their experiences in the light of these questions.

In chapter 5 Annette Ramírez de Arellano profiles care-seeking behavior of Latinas and highlights the importance of understanding cultural differences when drawing cross-cultural inferences from U.S. survey data. Latinas, for example, reported significantly lower rates of life satisfaction and self-esteem and notably higher rates of depression. Certainly, Latinas' material circumstances, such as lower income and less education, may correlate with and influence such sentiments. Ramírez de Arellano observes, however, that cultural forces must be taken into account when interpreting survey statistics. For example, she observes that there is a tendency among Latinas to downplay self-worth and well-being. Similarly, there is evidence for a religious belief that "suffering cleanses," which may influence Latinas' responses to some survey questions. Culturally derived roles may also influence Latinas' attitudes toward physicians and other medical care professionals and result in greater fear and distrust. For example, within Latinas' culture, silence does not necessarily signal comprehension or acquiescence.

Ramírez de Arellano directs attention to listening to women carefully and recognizing the cultural dimensions of their expressed experiences. It is important to take into account cultural values and norms that affect women's perspectives and, thus, their responses to survey questions. Ramírez de Arellano cautions that while Latinas remain socioeconomically disadvantaged, a culturally sensitive analysis suggests that "lowering financial barriers . . . will increase accessibility . . . [but] will not automatically improve the health status and perceptions of Latino women. More fundamental changes in terms of how care is delivered, and by whom, are required if the health delivery system is to offset the disadvantages intrinsic to poverty and marginalization."

Age can be viewed as a dynamic force in shaping women's perspectives, priorities, and care-seeking behavior. Convergent environmental, medical, lifestyle, and economic advances have increased the number of women who live longer today. For most women, childbirth and reproductive risks have been substantially eliminated. Midlife is difficult to demarcate. Women continue their reproductive experiences well beyond age forty, and women's perimenopausal phase has a 10- to 15-year window of opportunity. Age sixty-five continues to be viewed as retirement age, a transition phase in women's life cycle. Among aging women, new, unchartered health concerns exist. Midlife and elderly women in the 1990s might be viewed as pioneers whose experiences will pave the way for understanding the aging process and its challenges.

In chapter 6 Nancy Fugate Woods profiles midlife women—women ages forty to sixty-five. The Commonwealth Fund survey provides a unique opportunity to examine midlife women's health and to explore their health promotion and care patterns. Woods examines women's knowledge and behavior with respect to health-promoting practices— screening for breast and cervical cancers, positive health behaviors such as exercise, diet (cholesterol), and calcium supplements (osteoporosis), and hormone therapy for perimenopausal women. Certainly, the use of hormone therapy remains somewhat controversial, as we await the results of large-scale clinical trials. In the interim, perimenopausal women must make decisions based on insufficient information.

Woods's analysis indicates that access correlates appear to apply to women who receive hormone therapy. Taking into account a variety of factors, hormone therapy is more likely among women who are educated, have higher incomes and health insurance, are knowledgeable about midlife health risks (e.g., cholesterol, osteoporosis), and engage in health-promoting practices (e.g., calcium supplementation, exercise). Woods concludes with a thoughtful agenda for advancing the health and well-being of midlife women, including better access to timely, scientific information to assist them in making responsible health care decisions and adopting positive, health-promoting behaviors.

Linda Fried in chapter 7 profiles the nation's older women—women in their senior and retirement years. Importantly, she begins by acknowledging that chronic diseases associated with aging are not inevitable and emphasizing the value of preventive health practices for elderly women. Fried sets forth a positive, health-promoting framework for exploring elderly women's health behaviors. Her profile gives voice to elderly women by examining the full spectrum of health status measures, including a variety of physical, psychological (depression, self-esteem), and behavioral indicators.

Fried's analysis indicates that for a minority (albeit a sizable minority) a negative portrait emerges, with convergent shades of disability, depression, low self-esteem, low self-efficacy, and, not surprisingly, overall inferior health status. Some populations are more vulnerable, with low-income and minority elderly women most likely to suffer an array of physical, socioeconomic, and psychological burdens. On the positive side, the better-informed, more knowledgeable elderly women are more likely to practice positive health behaviors such as taking calcium supplements and receiving hormone therapy. Other correlates for obtaining preventive health care are having a chronic condition, having a usual source of care, and thinking that insurance paid for specific preventive services.

Fried observes the importance of knowledge and resources as key motivators and enablers. In this context, she examines the role of work (ability or preference) and extrapolates several recommendations for promoting health-seeking behaviors among seniors. She suggests combining targeted educational campaigns and enhanced health care coverage to promote positive behaviors and access to critical, preventive services. Furthermore, she advocates public policies that would promote work opportunities for older women. Her analysis suggests that work might serve as a health-promotion strategy by redressing some women's feelings of uselessness, low self-efficacy, and depression (see chaps. 8 and 11).

BEHAVIORAL WELL-BEING

The third section of this book examines two aspects of behavioral well-being: psychological distress and violence/victimization. Psychological distress, especially depression, has come to be viewed as a "woman's malady." There are ample data and research to document women's substantially higher rates of psychological distress and depressive disorders, as compared with men's. Mary Clare Lennon examines two aspects of psychological well-being: depressive symptoms and self-esteem. She seeks to identify correlates and thereby begin to unravel the subtext for some women's expressed psychological distress.

In a violent society, the victimization of women is all too frequent and takes many forms, commencing early (child abuse, molestation), within families (domestic battering), and within communities (rape, assault). As any other serious trauma, childhood abuse and domestic violence can have striking, if not lifelong, biopsychosocial consequences. Stacey Plichta examines the implications of violence for health and psychological status and the use of health services.

Lennon's analysis in chapter 8 reaffirms that, even after we control for various demographic factors (age, marital status, income, education, race), women report higher rates of depressive symptoms than men. Among women, education, income, and race are critical variables. Education and income may not "buy" happiness but certainly appear to improve some women's chances for expressing positive feelings about themselves and their overall emotional status. Broad, bivariate comparisons of women by marital, employment, and parenting status, however, do not reveal striking differences in depressive symptoms or self-esteem. Lennon extends her analysis to examine women in terms of their more complex, multiple roles, such as working, single mothers or married, nonworking mothers, available supports, or parenting assistance. She explores the implications of social role for women's expressions of psychological well-being.

Lennon's analysis reveals a treasure trove of findings regarding women's roles, circumstances, and preferences. For example, unemployed women who would prefer to work experience more depressive symptoms and reveal lower self-esteem than other women. Voluntarily "unemployed" women, however, report higher self-esteem than women who prefer to be working. Role satisfaction rather than employment status appears to be determinant. Among respondent women, Lennon confirms the anticipated nexus of mind–body well-being—depressive symptoms, self-esteem, and overall health status. Underscoring women's depression and low self-esteem are several social circumstances, notably, poverty, victimization, poor health, and absence of social supports. Women's well-being may well resonate from positive experiences with social role(s), an ability to achieve role, lifestyle, and work preferences (see chaps. 7, 9, 10, and 11).

A broad behavioral definition of women's health and well-being must consider the extent, role, and implications of violence. Stacey Plichta begins chapter 9 by observing that The Commonwealth Fund survey is the first nationally representative survey to permit an examination of violence as experienced by women and how that violence relates to various measures of health status (physical and psychological), use of health care, and patient-physician communication. Plichta's analysis gives voice to women as victims of violence. She unfolds horrific rates for various forms of violence that may be viewed as conservative estimates: 11.5 percent of women experienced child sexual abuse, 8 percent reported some form of spousal abuse, and nearly 3 percent were sexually assaulted or raped. Moreover, violence has a compounding effect on women's lives. For example, women who have experienced childhood or spousal abuse are twice as likely to report compromised health status and are far more likely to experience disabilities, depression and depressive symptoms, and low self-esteem. And, experiencing familial violence, especially child abuse, is a risk factor for future adult victimization.

Plichta finds that abused women often remain outside the health care system. Abused women, especially abused spouses, report difficulties getting necessary care, identify emergency rooms as their primary source of care, and express greater problems in their communication with physicians. The challenge is to reach women and remove them from harm's way. As Plichta recommends, health care professionals have a prominent role to play—getting beyond mending wounds to develop the skills and resources to achieve primary prevention.

SOCIOECONOMIC CIRCUMSTANCES

Several socioeconomic circumstances are particularly revealing in analyzing women's health—experiences, options, and constraints. In the fourth section of this book, contributors focus on three life circumstances that affect women's differential ability to gain access to and benefits from the U.S. health care system: poverty, employment, and health insurance.

The seeming vortex of poverty disproportionately affects far too many women. Women comprise one-third of the U.S. population under age sixty-five living in poverty; their children account for 45 percent. In chapter 10 Barbara Lyons, Alina Salganicoff, and Diane Rowland profile low-income women (poor and near-poor), documenting a host of interrelated economic, social, and health vulnerabilities. Low-income women are likely to be young, to be minority, and to lack formal education and marketable employment skills. Compared with higher-income women, poor and near-poor women are twice as likely to rate their health status as fair/poor, to express feelings of low self-esteem, and to be dissatisfied with their lives.

Lyons and colleagues document the extent to which Medicaid has had a significant impact on some women's ability to gain access to health services. For example, the utilization rates of Medicaid women are similar to those of privately insured women and notably higher than those of uninsured, low-income women. Lyons and colleagues seek to build on Medicaid successes and to advance policies to guide reforms and managed care policies for reducing, if not eliminating, the remaining financial, societal, and behavioral barriers to care.

For many women, employment appears to empower, to convey a variety of benefits, including monetary, social, psychological, and physical well-being. In chapter 11 Heidi Hartmann, Joan Kuriansky, and Christine Owens seek to unravel the relationship between women's employment status and various measures of biopsychological well-being. Since the mid-1960s various studies have found that employed, salaried women report being healthier than nonemployed women. Hartmann and colleagues similarly found that working women were healthier. Among employed women, insured women were less likely to report medical conditions or other disabilities and more likely to report their overall health status as being excellent or good.

Hartmann and colleagues seek to examine the extent to which women's work preferences play a role. They examine nonemployed women and compare those who reported a preference for employment with those who reported being voluntarily out of the job market. Several disturbing findings surface. Notably, women who were more likely to need health services were less likely to be insured; the least healthy were nonemployed women who reported a preference to be working (i.e., involuntarily unemployed). These "work preferrers" were the least likely to have health insurance and were the most disadvantaged (least educated and in the lowest income strata). Three-quarters of all nonworking women of color would prefer to work (compared with fewer than half of the nonworking white women). Hartmann and colleagues reveal that the involuntarily unemployed women can be viewed as a new voice that warrants special attention. They recommend that public policies assist women seeking employment, to exploit more fully the potential of and positive relationship between employment and women's well-being.

Health insurance is often the foremost vehicle for promoting (though perhaps not necessarily achieving) real access to health services. In chapter 12 Anne Lenhard Reisinger examines socioeconomic factors such as income, education, marital status, and race/ethnicity as they may influence women's insurance status and, in turn, access to health services. Controlling for health status, age, and insurance, her analysis indicates that income remains a relatively powerful predictor of women's access and care-seeking behavior. Interestingly, women enrolled in HMOs were more likely to report difficulties obtaining necessary care than other insured women. Nonfinancial forces (e.g., knowledge about care-seeking behaviors and motivation to adopt health-seeking behaviors) remain powerful enablers and, thus, correlates of access and utilization. Consequently, Reisinger concludes, health insurance reforms that principally finance care by extending insurance coverage to more women are important but would not automatically eliminate behavioral barriers to care.

A WOMEN'S HEALTH AGENDA

Women's Health offers a new and solid foundation for advancing women's health and well-being through enlightened public policies and health care practices. In their concluding chapter, Karen Scott Collins and Joan Leiman set forth five strategic areas for promoting women's health: (1) expanding economic and education opportunities, (2) assuring adequate financial coverage and access to health care, (3) training of health care professionals, (4) enhancing women's awareness of their health needs and constructive health behaviors, and (5) further biomedical and behavioral health services research. Reflecting the *Women's Health* findings, their agenda underscores the saliency of social, economic, and behavioral forces such as education and employment for understanding women's health and well-being. Collins and Leiman also reaffirm the overriding importance of financial access to women's health services and the necessity of monitoring changes in the health care market, the structure of publicly financed health programs, and the impact of managed care on access and quality.

The Commonwealth Fund and its Commission on Women's Health are pursuing aspects of this evolving agenda. These knowledge-building and dissemination activities support national surveys (e.g., minority women, managed care), a variety of best-practice studies, development (design and testing) of interventions (e.g., domestic violence curricula, interactive videos), and various media and "knowledge dissemination" forums. In moving forward, Collins and Leiman acknowledge that *Women's Health* and related Commonwealth Fund research activities are beginnings, with much more being both necessary and valuable for establishing "a platform on which to build future advances in women's health." We hope and anticipate that we and you, our readers, will continue to be interested in and committed to enhancing our knowledge of and thus our ability to improve women's health and well-being.

NOTE

1. Humphrey Taylor, Ron Bass, and Lois Hoeffler, *The Health of American Women* (Louis Harris and Associates, Inc., 1993). The Commonwealth Fund survey permits analysis of a variety of timely topics in women's health, but not necessarily all areas of potential interest. For example, we were unable to examine substance abuse behaviors such as smoking, alcoholism, or use of illicit drugs. Not surprisingly, very few women indicated their use of specific illicit drugs, such as cocaine, or high levels of drinking, and the respondent sample was viewed as too small for analysis.

I

Care-Seeking Behaviors

1

Women's Use of Health Care

Carol S. Weisman, Ph.D.

Growing interest in women's health and the debate over health care reform have raised a number of questions about how women use health care and how the U.S. health care system serves women. One issue has to do with women's access to adequate health insurance coverage, either public or private, which enables them to obtain needed services in a timely fashion. Another concern is women's access to appropriate primary care services throughout the life span. As efforts to redesign the health care system continue, key responsibilities for policy makers and providers will be to define appropriate primary care for women and to ensure that women in all age groups and socio-economic circumstances can obtain primary care services.

Generally accepted components of primary care include comprehensive services (preventive, curative, and rehabilitative services) coordinated over time by a first-contact provider who is familiar with the patient (Starfield 1992). There is considerable evidence that women are more likely than men to have a usual source of health care and that women consume more services than men. However, it is not known whether the higher overall utilization reflects appropriate care, and surprisingly little research has addressed the organization of primary care services for women. This chapter considers possible explanations for the gender difference in utilization and then examines the types of physicians women see for regular health care and how these physicians influence the use of services.

WHY DO WOMEN USE MORE HEALTH CARE?

A ubiquitous finding in health services research is that adult women use more health services than men and that this difference persists beyond the reproductive years and thus cannot be fully explained by use of obstetrical care (Wilensky and Cafferata 1983; Horton 1992; Aday 1993). National data on these issues come largely from the National Health Interview Survey, based on household interviews, and the National Ambulatory Medical Care Survey, based on records of visits to physicians' offices; both surveys are conducted periodically by the National Center for Health Statistics. These and other sources show that women are more likely than men to have a usual source of health care; women make more medical visits per year; women are more likely to be hospitalized (even after excluding admissions for obstetrical reasons); and women receive more drug prescriptions.

Three possible explanations for the gender difference in utilization have been posed and debated. First, despite their lower overall mortality rates, women may have poorer health status than men and hence have greater need for health care. Poorer health status may be caused by biological or acquired risks, the latter including environmental exposures, poor health habits, and stresses associated with women's social roles (Nathanson 1975; Verbrugge 1989; Bird and Fremont 1991). Second, women may engage in more health-seeking behavior, including the use of health services, because they are socialized to acknowledge symptoms or to perceive a need for health care more readily than men (Mechanic 1976). Third, the structure of the health care system might produce more utilization by women. Although this has not been well investigated, aspects of the health care system that might contribute to women's higher rates of utilization include aggressive marketing of health services to women, medicalization of such biological life events as pregnancy and menopause (Ruzek 1978; Riessman 1983), inadequacies of standard treatments for women (e.g., as the result of the exclusion or underrepresentation of women in clinical trials), physicians' biases about women's health care needs, or the fragmentation of basic health services for women.

Fragmentation refers to the tendency in U.S. health care to separate reproductive health care (pregnancy-related services, medical and surgical care related to the female reproductive system, and gender-specific preventive services including family planning and cancer screening tests) from other components of primary care (Clancy and Massion 1992). The result is that adult women may obtain basic health care services from a variety of physicians, including general internists, family or general practitioners, and obstetrician-gynecologists. There is considerable controversy over which specialists should qualify as primary care providers for women. Fragmentation would tend to increase utilization if women see more than one physician (i.e., both a reproductive health care specialist and another physician) to obtain comprehensive services. Yet to date there have been no studies of women's use of multiple physicians for basic health care. This chapter addresses this issue through analysis of The Commonwealth Fund survey data.

THE CAUSES AND IMPLICATIONS OF FRAGMENTATION

Fragmentation is encouraged by two phenomena. The first is medical specialization, which largely determines physicians' roles and practice patterns. Obstetrician-gynecologists are trained as specialists in reproductive health care for women and are major providers of such gender-specific preventive screening services as Pap smears, clinical breast examinations, and mammography. Some women rely on obstetrician-gynecologists as their primary physicians, although the proportion who do so is unknown (Aiken et al. 1979; Marieskind 1980).[1] Studies of practice patterns, however, have shown that many obstetrician-gynecologists do not provide such preventive services as blood cholesterol screening and adult immunizations (Horton, Cruess, and Pearse 1993). Conversely, the major adult primary care providers (general internists, family practitioners, and general practitioners) are less likely than obstetrician-gynecologists to provide reproductive health care, including family planning and preventive services such as pelvic examinations, Pap smears, and clinical breast examinations that are required by women both during and after the reproductive years (Weisman et al. 1989; Bartman and Weiss 1993; Lurie et al. 1993).

The second factor that encourages fragmentation is the tendency to segregate organizationally reproductive health services from other aspects of care (e.g., in family planning or prenatal care clinics). This occurs in part because of the ways in which reproductive services are financed for low-income women through the Medicaid program, Title X of the Public Health Service Act, or Maternal and Child Block Grants (Muller 1990). In addition, the politicization of certain aspects of women's reproductive health care (e.g., family planning services for adolescents, abortion services) tends to promote organizational segregation when traditional providers are unwilling to offer such controversial services.

As a consequence of fragmentation, some women might receive only a component of what would be considered appropriate primary

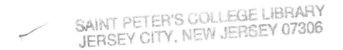

care, while others who seek comprehensive care might have to see a number of physicians and make more visits. Although receiving care from multiple physicians could result in more comprehensive services to the woman, especially if she is seen in a health maintenance organization (HMO), it also introduces the potential problem of lack of coordination among providers and resultant gaps or duplications in services received. The implications of fragmentation for women's receipt of comprehensive, coordinated primary care services at all stages of life, for women's health status, and for women's satisfaction with the health care received are just beginning to be investigated.

Furthermore, the recent debate over national health care reform and the growth of managed care have focused attention on appropriate organizational mechanisms for providing primary health care in an efficient manner. It is of interest, therefore, whether fragmentation of women's health services results in use of more health care services and higher costs to a woman and her insurer than might be indicated by her health care needs. To date, women's patterns of using health care have not been examined from this perspective.

METHODOLOGY

Data from The Commonwealth Fund survey are used here to present a population-based analysis of women's patterns of using health care that focuses on the types of physicians used for regular care and the effects on services used. This is a unique data set because it provides information on women's use of multiple physicians. Measures include: (1) whether or not the woman has a regular source of care; (2) the specialty of the regular physician; (3) whether or not an obstetrician-gynecologist is seen in addition to the regular physician (if the regular physician is not an obstetrician-gynecologist); and (4) which types and combinations of physicians are seen for regular care.

Measures of the use of services include the number of physician visits made during the past year and the number of key preventive services received during the past 2 years. Each of these variables is described in more detail as the results are presented.

Women's use of health services is examined in the context of a behavioral model of health services utilization proposed by Andersen and colleagues (Andersen 1968; Aday, Andersen, and Fleming 1980). This model specifies three categories of variables that affect individuals' use of health services: predisposing, enabling, and need variables. Predisposing variables include sociodemographics (such as gender, age, and educational level), social role obligations, and attitudes and beliefs about health care (such as the efficacy of treatment). Enabling variables enhance access to the health care system and include resources available to the individual, such as health insurance and income, as well as geographic proximity to services. Need variables include health status indicators as well as perceived need for care. Research based on this model of utilization consistently finds that need variables are the strongest predictors of utilization, which usually is measured as having a regular source of care or the frequency of visits to a physician.

This analysis uses several predisposing, enabling, and need variables.[2] Predisposing variables include the woman's age, education, race/ethnicity, marital status, and the presence or absence of children under age eighteen in her household. (No attitudes or beliefs about one's need for health care or the efficacy of health care are available in this data set.) Enabling variables include the woman's employment status, household income, health insurance status, receipt of any welfare benefits (food stamps, Aid for Families with Dependent Children [AFDC], Supplemental Security Income [SSI], or state or local public assistance), urban or rural location, and region of the country.

Need variables include indicators of the woman's physical and mental health status: (1) perceived health status; (2) number of chronic conditions reported by the woman as having been confirmed by a physician within the past 5 years; (3) presence of any disability that interferes with regular social roles or causes the woman to need help with activities of daily living; (4) reporting that anxiety or depression was confirmed by a physician within the past 5 years; and (5) a health risk index constructed from four behaviors (smoking, drinking three or more alcoholic beverages a day during the past 2 weeks, using illicit drugs during the past month, and never engaging in strenuous exercise). No measures of pregnancy-related needs are available in this data set.

RESULTS OF SURVEY ANALYSIS

Gender Comparisons

Consistent with previous research, the survey revealed that women are significantly more likely than men to report that they have a regular source of health care. Eighty percent of women, compared with 72 percent of men, reported having a regular source of care. (These figures compare with 84% of women and 78% of men in the 1987 National Medical Expenditures Survey [Cornelius, Beauregard, and Cohen 1991].) Among the women who reported having a regular source of care, 75 percent reported that they go to a physician's office, 16 percent go to a clinic, 5 percent go to a hospital emergency room, and 3 percent go to other places. Fewer than 0.5 percent reported using a nurse practitioner or nurse midwife as the usual source of care. Men were not asked about the type of regular source of care they used.

Ten percent of women, compared with 15 percent of men, reported having no regular physician, but among those who had a regular physician, men and women used different types. Sixty-three percent of men used a family or general practitioner, compared with 54 percent of women, and 12 percent of men and 16 percent of women used an internist. Thirteen percent of women reported that their regular doctor is an obstetrician-gynecologist.[3]

Women made significantly more visits to a physician than men during the past year. Women reported an average of 5.20 "doctor visits," compared with 4.14 made by men (the median number of visits was 3 for women and 2 for men). (These figures compare with a mean of 5.9 physician visits in the past year by women, and 4.8 by men, in 1989 data from the National Center for Health Statistics [Aday 1993].) The average gender difference of one visit a year is accounted for by the fact that men were twice as likely as women to have made *no* visits in the past year (18% of men compared with 9% of women), and women are more likely than men to have made 5 or more visits (34% of women compared with 24% of men).

The largest gender difference occurs during the reproductive years: women ages eighteen to forty-four made an average of 1.84 more visits than men of comparable age.[4] In the middle years (ages forty-five to sixty-four), women made an average of 0.48 more visits than men. Among those ages sixty-five or older, the gender difference is reversed, with men making an average of 0.81 more visits than women. For men the average number of annual physician visits increases with age, but for women the highest number of annual visits occurs during the reproductive years and the lowest during the middle years. This pattern is consistent with women making more visits for pregnancy-related or family planning services during the reproductive years.

Women saw significantly more physicians than men did during the past year. Women reported seeing 2.08 "different doctors" during the past year, compared with 1.86 by men (the median number of physicians was 2 for women and one for men). The average difference in number of physicians seen is accounted for by the fact that men are twice as likely as women not to have seen any physicians in the past year (18% of men compared with 9% of women), and women are more likely than men to see 2 different physicians (33% of women compared with 25% of men). Men and women do not differ in the rate at which they saw more than two physicians.

Women in the reproductive years see an average of 2.07 physicians, compared with 1.58 by men of comparable age. In the middle years, women see an average of 2.09 physicians, compared with 2.01 by men. Among those ages sixty-five or older, the gender difference is reversed: men see an average of 2.68 physicians, compared with 2.09 for women. For men the average number of physicians seen increases with age, whereas for women the average number of physicians seen holds steady, at just over 2 physicians, across age groups.

Women's Patterns of Using a Physician

The predominant patterns of women's physician use are identified by combining information about the specialty of the regular physician with information in response to the question, "In addition to your regular doctor, do you see a separate doctor for female-related problems, or not?" If the woman reported that she did, the specialty of this physician was requested; these doctors are obstetrician-gynecologists in nearly all cases. Three percent of women were excluded because they could not identify the specialties of their physicians.

Women's patterns of physician use for regular care vary (fig. 1.1).Thirty-nine percent of women reported that their regular doctor was a family practitioner or internist and that they do *not* also see an obstetrician-gynecologist. Thirty-three percent reported that their regular physician is a family practitioner or internist and that they also see an obstetrician-gynecologist. Sixteen percent reported that their regular physician is an obstetrician-gynecologist, or that the regular physician is another specialist but that an obstetrician-gynecologist was also seen.[5] (Eighty-four percent of this group identified the obstetrician-gynecologist as their regular provider.) Three percent reported that their regular doctor is another type of specialist (e.g., cardiologist, rheumatologist, oncologist) and that they do *not* also see an obstetrician-gynecologist. Ten percent of women reported having no regular physician of any kind.

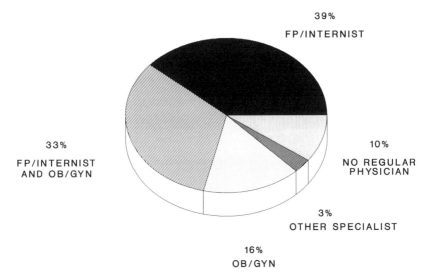

Fig. 1.1. Women's Regular Physicians
Source: Analysis of The Commonwealth Fund survey on women's health, 1993.

The pattern of physician use varies with the predisposing, enabling, and need variables (tabs. 1.1–1.3). Because of the large sample size, all of the associations are highly statistically significant ($p < 0.02$) by the chi-square test. This discussion therefore highlights only the most important differences.

A noteworthy finding among the predisposing variables (tab. 1.1) is that the women most likely to use both a family practitioner or internist and an obstetrician-gynecologist are between the ages of eighteen and sixty-four; women in the middle years (ages forty-five to sixty-four) are no less likely than women in the reproductive years to use both types of physicians. This suggests that the use of two physicians is not associated with pregnancy or family planning needs alone, but may reflect patterns of utilization established earlier in life or specific health care needs of perimenopausal women. In addition, increasing age is associated with a greater likelihood of seeing only a family practitioner or internist and with a lower likelihood of seeing an obstetrician-gynecologist (with or without another physician). Women in the reproductive years (ages eighteen to forty-four) are more likely than older women to have an obstetrician-gynecologist as their regular physician.

Table 1.1. Patterns of Physician Use, by Predisposing Variables

Variable	All Women	Family Practitioner/ Internist	Family Practitioner/ Internist + Ob/Gyn	Ob/Gyn	Other	No Regular Physician
Age (N = 2,435)						
18–44 years	53	28	37	22	2	11
45–64 years	30	43	36	11	2	8
65+ years	17	65	16	4	6	9
Education (N = 2,443)						
Not high school graduate	12	53	18	8	4	17
High school graduate	34	43	33	13	2	8
Some post–high school	28	35	35	18	4	9
College graduate	26	30	37	21	2	10
Race/Ethnicity (N = 2,447)						
White	67	41	34	14	3	8
African American	16	36	27	24	3	11
Hispanic/Latina	16	32	34	16	3	15
Other[a]	1	39	18	15	0	27
Marital status (N = 2,447)						
Married/living together	61	36	37	18	2	8
Not married	39	44	25	13	4	13
Children in household (N = 2,447)						
Yes	39	29	39	21	2	9
No	61	45	29	12	3	10

Source: Data from The Commonwealth Fund survey on women's health, 1993.

Note: Base N for each cross-tabulation is given in parentheses after the variable name. Numbers cited are percentages.

[a] "Other" (N = 33) includes Asian or Pacific Islanders and "not sure."

Table 1.2. Patterns of Physician Use, by Enabling Variables

Variable	All Women	Family Practitioner/ Internist	Family Practitioner/ Internist + Ob/Gyn	Ob/Gyn	Other	No Regular Physician
Employment status ($N = 2,447$)						
Not employed	40	47	25	13	4	12
Employed part-time	15	37	34	17	2	10
Employed full-time	45	33	39	18	2	8
1992 household income ($N = 2,183$)						
$0–$15,000	27	50	19	12	4	14
$15,001–$25,000	36	42	31	15	3	10
$25,001+	38	29	45	19	2	6
Health insurance[a] ($N = 2,447$)						
Private	49	32	38	20	2	8
HMO	17	34	43	15	1	6
Medicare	20	62	17	7	6	8
Medicaid	5	38	23	20	4	14
None	9	31	22	15	4	29

Welfare status[b] (N = 2,447)						
Receives	12	46	18	15	5	15
Does not receive	88	38	35	16	2	9
Location[c] (N = 2,447)						
Urban	78	35	35	18	2	10
Rural	22	53	26	10	4	8
Region (N = 2,447)						
Northeast	21	31	41	16	2	10
North central	22	45	32	11	4	8
South	37	37	32	18	3	10
West	20	44	26	16	2	12

Source: Data from The Commonwealth Fund survey on women's health, 1993.

Note: Base N for each cross-tabulation is given in parentheses after the variable name. Numbers cited are percentages.

[a] Health insurance categories were created in hierarchical fashion, because 34 percent of women had more than one type of insurance. When multiple types were reported, the order of priority for coding was: Medicare, Medicaid, HMO, private insurance (through either the woman's or her spouse's employer or purchased directly).

[b] Whether the woman receives any of the following: food stamps, AFDC, SSI, state or local public assistance.

[c] "Urban" includes inner cities or their suburbs.

Table 1.3. Patterns of Physician Use, by Need Variables

Variable	All Women	Family Practitioner/ Internist	Family Practitioner/ Internist + Ob/Gyn	Ob/Gyn	Other	No Regular Physician
Perceived health status[a] ($N = 2,447$)						
Excellent	22	36	30	19	3	11
Very good	35	36	36	17	2	9
Good	28	41	33	13	3	10
Fair to poor	14	46	27	13	4	10
Chronic conditions[b] ($N = 2,447$)						
None	47	33	33	20	2	12
One	28	42	34	14	2	8
Two	14	46	31	12	4	7
Three or more	10	49	31	6	6	8
Disability[c] ($N = 2,447$)						
No	82	37	34	17	2	10
Yes	18	47	28	10	5	10

Depression/anxiety[a] (N = 2,447)						
No	86	39	33	17	2	10
Yes	14	40	33	10	5	11
Risk index[e] (N = 2,447)						
No risks	54	36	35	18	3	9
One risk	38	42	32	14	2	11
Two or more risks	8	46	26	12	4	12

Source: Data from The Commonwealth Fund survey on women's health, 1993.

Note: Base N for each cross-tabulation is given in parentheses after the variable name. Numbers cited are percentages.

[a] Response to: "Would you say your health in general is excellent, very good, good, fair, or poor?"

[b] Number of the following chronic conditions respondents had been told by a doctor that they had within the past 5 years: hypertension, cardiovascular disease, cancer, arthritis, diabetes, lung disease, osteoporosis, severe menstrual problems, endometriosis. Responses ranged from zero to seven chronic conditions.

[c] The respondent was coded as having a disability if she reported any one of the following: a "disability, handicap, or chronic disease" that interferes with participation in regular social roles; needing help in activities of daily living "because of any impairment or health problem"; or needing help in instrumental activities of daily living "because of any impairment or health problem."

[d] Reporting having been told by a doctor within the past 5 years that she had "anxiety or depression."

[e] Number of the following risk behaviors reported by the respondent: being a current smoker; drinking three or more alcoholic beverages per day, on average, during the past 2 weeks; using marijuana or other illicit drugs during the past month; never exercising strenuously. Responses ranged from zero to three risk behaviors.

With regard to education, increasing levels of education are associated with a declining likelihood of seeing only a family practitioner or internist and with an increasing likelihood of seeing an obstetrician-gynecologist, with or without another physician. Women who have not graduated from high school are least likely to see two physicians.

With regard to race/ethnicity, African American women are more likely than non-Hispanic white women to see only an obstetrician-gynecologist. Although the numbers are small (only thirty-three women are classified as "other"), women in the "other" race/ethnicity category are least likely to see two physicians and more likely to have no regular physician.

Married women and women who are living with a partner are more likely than unmarried women to see two physicians. Women with children under age eighteen living in the household (who tend to be younger women) are less likely than other women to see only a family practitioner or internist and more likely than other women to see an obstetrician-gynecologist.

The enabling variables (tab. 1.2) are strongly associated with seeing two physicians. Women who are not employed are more likely than employed women to see only a family practitioner or internist and less likely than employed women to see two physicians. Household income data (for which there was a relatively large amount of missing data due to refusals or "not sure" responses) suggest that increasing levels of household income are associated with a declining likelihood of seeing only a family practitioner or internist and of having no regular physician. Increasing income is associated with an increasing likelihood of seeing an obstetrician-gynecologist, especially in combination with a family practitioner or internist.

Women who have private health insurance or who are enrolled in private HMOs are more likely than other women to see two physicians. Women on Medicare are more likely than other women to see only a family practitioner or internist or only a specialist, and they are less likely than other women to see an obstetrician-gynecologist. Women with no health insurance of any kind are more likely than insured women to have no regular physician. Women receiving some form of welfare are less likely than other women to see two physicians.

Women in urban areas (inner cities or suburbs) are less likely than rural women to use only a family practitioner or internist and more likely than rural women to see an obstetrician-gynecologist (with or without another physician). This reflects the fact that specialists, including obstetrician-gynecologists, tend to be concentrated in urban areas. Residing in the North Central or Western regions of the country is associated with seeing a family practitioner or internist; residing in the Northeast is associated with seeing both a family practitioner or internist and an obstetrician-gynecologist.

The need variables (tab. 1.3) have no clear pattern of association with types of physicians seen. An increasing number of chronic conditions appears to be associated with an increasing likelihood of seeing only a family practitioner or internist and with a decreasing likelihood of using an obstetrician-gynecologist as the regular physician. Women reporting a disability are more likely to see only a family practitioner or internist and less likely to see an obstetrician-gynecologist. An increasing number of health risk behaviors appears to be associated with an increasing likelihood of seeing only a family practitioner or internist and with a decreasing likelihood of seeing an obstetrician-gynecologist.

Who Sees Multiple Physicians?

Because one-third of women use two types of physicians for regular care, the relative importance of all of the predisposing, enabling, and need variables in determining this pattern of utilization has been examined by multiple logistic regression analysis. This analysis shows that the variables differentiating women who see both a family practitioner or internist and an obstetrician-gynecologist from all other women are, in declining order of importance, region of the country (women in the Northeast were more likely to see both types of physicians), type of health insurance (women with private health insurance or enrolled in an HMO were more likely to see both types of physicians), having a chronic condition, race/ethnicity (African American women were less likely to see both types of physicians), residence in an urban area, being married or living with a partner, and being at least a high school graduate. Thus women seeing both types of physicians are relatively affluent.

Age, which is strongly associated with the use of obstetrician-gynecologists in general, is not a significant predictor of seeing both types of physicians when all other variables are controlled. This again suggests that health care needs unique to the reproductive years (i.e., pregnancy and family planning needs) do not account for women's use of two physicians.

Health Services Used

To examine how the types of physicians seen affects the use of health services, two indicators of services consumed are considered: the number of physician visits during the past year, and the number of preventive services received during the past 2 years. The latter measure is a sum based on seven services: complete physical examination (74% of women received this service in the past 2 years), blood pressure screening (95%), blood cholesterol screening (66%), clinical breast examination (79%), mammogram (47%), pelvic exam (75%), and Pap smear (76%). With the exception of mammograms, these services are recommended periodically for all adult women. The average number of services received during the past 2 years was 5.11.

The average number of physician visits made in the past year varies significantly by the pattern of physician use (tab. 1.4). Women who did not have a regular physician have the lowest number of visits (3.02), while women seeing only specialists have the highest number (7.28

Table 1.4. Use of Services, by Physician Pattern

	Number of Physician Visits in Past Year[a]		Number of Preventive Services in Past 2 Years[b]	
	Mean	SD	Mean	SD
Family practitioner/internist	5.02	(7.04)	4.86	(2.09)
Family practitioner/internist + obstetrician-gynecologist	5.84	(6.92)	5.64	(1.54)
Obstetrician-gynecologist	5.36	(6.88)	5.50	(1.44)
Other	7.28	(8.41)	4.97	(2.10)
No regular physician	3.02	(4.16)	3.79	(2.30)
Total	5.21	(6.84)	5.11	(1.94)

Source: Analysis of The Commonwealth Fund survey on women's health, 1993.

[a] Kruskal-Wallis analysis of variance is significant ($H = 91.2$, $p < 0.001$, $N = 2{,}372$). In tests for multiple comparisons, the mean number of visits for women with no regular physician is significantly different ($p < 0.05$) from all others.

[b] Kruskal-Wallis analysis of variance is significant ($H = 167.7$, $p < 0.001$, $N = 2{,}447$). In tests for multiple comparisons, the mean number of services for women with no regular physician is significantly different ($p < 0.05$) from all others, and the mean number for women seeing a family practitioner/internist is different from the mean number for women seeing a family practitioner/internist and an obstetrician-gynecologist and for women seeing an obstetrician-gynecologist.

during the past year). Women seeing both a family practitioner or internist and an obstetrician-gynecologist have the second highest number of visits (5.84). The average number of visits made by women seeing a family practitioner or internist without an obstetrician-gyne- cologist (5.02) is closest to the overall average for men (4.14 visits).[6]

The number of preventive services received during the past 2 years also varies significantly by the pattern of physician use (tab. 1.4). Wom- en with no regular physician received the lowest number of services (3.79). On the other hand, women who (1) not only have a regular physician (family practitioner or internist) but also saw an obstetrician- gynecologist or (2) see only an obstetrician-gynecologist received the highest average number of preventive services (5.64 and 5.50, respec- tively). Women seeing a family practitioner or internist alone received significantly fewer services (4.86).[7]

Each of these indicators of the services used was analyzed using multiple linear regression. Regression models include the pattern of physician use and predisposing, enabling, and need variables as pre- dictors. They show the relative importance of the types of physicians used in determining the quantity of services consumed while control- ling need, access, and sociodemographics (tab. 1.5).

The key result is that in both models the pattern of physician use contributes significantly to variance explained after financial access (health insurance) and need have been controlled. With regard to vis- its, having any type of regular physician, compared with having no regular physician, increases the number of visits. However, using both

Table 1.5. Predictors of the Number of Physician Visits in the Past Year and the Number of Preventive Services in the Past 2 Years

	Number of Visits[a]	Preventive Services[b]
Pattern of physician use		
No regular physician	(reference)	(reference)
Family practitioner/internist	0.17[c]	0.18[c]
Family practitioner/internist + obstetrician-gynecologist	0.25[c]	0.35[c]
Obstetrician-gynecologist	0.18[c]	0.27[c]
Other	0.08[c]	0.07[c]

(*continued*)

Table 1.5. (*Continued*)

	Number of Visits[a]	Preventive Services[b]
Predisposing variables[d]		
Age		
18–44 years	(reference)	(reference)
45–64 years	−0.09[c]	0.13[c]
65+ years	−0.12[c]	0.01
Education		
Not high school graduate	(reference)	(reference)
High school graduate	−0.04	0.05
Post–high school education	0.02	0.13[c]
Race/ethnicity		
White	(reference)	(reference)
African American	−0.01	0.04[c]
Hispanic/Latina	−0.02	−0.03
Other	−0.04[c]	−0.02
Married/living with partner	0.01	0.06[c]
Enabling variables[d]		
Health insurance		
None	(reference)	(reference)
Private	0.14[c]	0.16[c]
HMO	0.16[c]	0.18[c]
Medicare	0.16[c]	0.20[c]
Medicaid	0.11[c]	0.13[c]
Need variables		
Perceived health status (fair/poor)	0.07[c]	−0.02
Chronic illness (any)	0.21[c]	0.10[c]
Disability	0.13[c]	0.00
Depression/anxiety	0.10[c]	0.04[c]
Risk index	−0.03	−0.09[c]

Source: Analysis of The Commonwealth Fund survey on women's health, 1993.

Note: Numbers are standardized partial regression coefficients.

[a] The dependent variable is the square root transformation of the number of physician visits in the past year. R^2 for the full model = 0.18, F = 17.18, $p < 0.0001$, $N = 2,357$.

[b] The dependent variable is the number of preventive services received in the past 2 years. R^2 for the full model = 0.16, F = 15.55, $p < 0.0001$, $N = 2,431$.

[c] Univariate F-test significant ($p < 0.05$).

[d] Number of children, employment status, welfare status, region, and urban/rural location are not shown because they were not statistically significant in either model. Household income was not included due to missing data.

an internist or family practitioner and an obstetrician-gynecologist results in the greatest increase in the number of visits.

Having any type of health insurance coverage also predicts a higher number of visits. All of the indicators of need, except for the risk index, are significant, positive predictors as well. Among the predisposing variables, the effect of age is noteworthy: being beyond reproductive age predicts fewer visits. This is consistent with the expectation that pregnancy-related or family planning needs would increase the number of visits.

The possible interaction of age and the pattern of physician use was examined by generating this regression model separately for women in the three age groups (ages eighteen to forty-four, forty-five to sixty-four, and sixty-five or older). Patterns of physician use are statistically significant predictors of the number of visits for all age groups, with the combination of a primary care physician and an obstetrician-gynecologist having a particularly strong effect on the number of visits made by women in the middle years (ages forty-five to sixty-four).

For preventive services, the pattern of physician use again exerts an independent effect on preventive services received after controlling for financial access (health insurance). Women who have any type of regular physician receive more preventive services than women who have no regular physician. However, seeing both an internist or family practitioner and an obstetrician-gynecologist has the greatest impact on the number of preventive services, followed by seeing an obstetrician-gynecologist as the regular physician or in combination with other specialists. Thus, seeing an obstetrician-gynecologist has a strong effect on receiving the set of preventive services measured in this study.

Having any type of health insurance also increases the number of preventive services received. Three need variables have significant but weaker effects on the preventive services received: having a chronic illness and being depressed or anxious predict more preventive services; and having more risk behaviors predicts fewer preventive services. The latter finding suggests that not obtaining preventive services might be interpreted as another health risk behavior.

Women ages forty-five to sixty-four receive more preventive services than women of reproductive age (possibly because this is the age group for which mammography is first recommended on a regular basis). Women with post–high school education receive more preventive services than women who were not high school graduates. African American women receive more preventive services than non-Hispanic white women. And women who were married or living with a partner receive more preventive services.

The possible interaction of age and the pattern of physician use was examined by generating this regression model separately for women in the three age groups. For women in their reproductive years, seeing an obstetrician-gynecologist, with or without another physician, is predictive of receiving more preventive services. No other patterns of physician use are associated with the number of preventive services in this age group. For older women, all patterns of regular physician use increase the number of preventive services, compared with not having a regular physician, but the combination of a family practitioner or internist and an obstetrician-gynecologist has the strongest effect on the number of preventive services received.

Summary of Key Findings

This chapter has explored how fragmentation in women's health services affects women's patterns of using health care; it is the first study to attempt to document women's use of multiple types of physicians for regular care. Analyses confirm that nonelderly women make more physician visits than men; that women use about two physicians, on average, throughout the life span; and that there is considerable variation among women in the types of physicians used for regular care. Variables other than need—particularly socioeconomic circumstances—affect the types of physicians women use for regular care. The types of physicians seen, furthermore, are related to services used, independent of other variables, including the type of health insurance and health care needs.

The findings show that many women divide their regular health care between an obstetrician-gynecologist and either a family practitioner or an internist. One-third of the women surveyed reported that they use both types of physicians for regular care. These women are characterized by relative affluence and financial access to health care through private health insurance or enrollment in an HMO. The use of two physicians does not appear to be a function primarily of pregnancy or family planning needs, because it is not a pattern of utilization confined to women in the reproductive years. Using two physicians, in turn, is associated with making more annual physician visits (independent of age and the need for health care) and with receiving more preventive services.

Thus, this analysis shows that some women cannot gain access to a regular source of health care; others are at risk for receiving only a component of basic care; still others, who are relatively affluent, see both a reproductive health specialist and another primary care physician for regular care. The use of two providers introduces the possibility of more visits (independent of need), with associated costs to the woman and her insurer, and of duplication of services, including preventive services. On the other hand, such use also increases the woman's chances of receiving key preventive services.

IMPLICATIONS FOR POLICY

One implication of this study is that the current health care system for women is inefficient because it impedes women's access to appropriate primary care services and encourages some women to make more visits than they may need to obtain comprehensive care. The observed variations in patterns of physician use also suggest that subgroups of women may have quite different perceptions of their primary health care needs, the appropriateness of different types of physicians as primary care providers, and the balance of costs and benefits associated with a greater quantity of services consumed.

The most compelling policy implication of this study is the need within the U.S. health care system to integrate routine reproductive health services with other components of women's primary care and to make such services available to all women. Part of the challenge lies in conceptualizing what services should be part of the routine health care of adult women and what services are more appropriately defined as specialty services for women who are ill or have special needs. A basic fallacy in contemporary health care of the well woman is that routine preventive services that should be part of each adult woman's regular care (such as family planning services, pelvic examinations, and Pap smears) are often defined as specialty services and are not provided by many primary care physicians. In HMOs, for example, these services often require a referral to a physician other than the primary care provider and an additional visit.

There are a number of approaches, including public and private initiatives, for addressing these issues. These include health care financing initiatives that expand access to health insurance and define a basic benefits package; establishing guidelines for women's health services and disseminating them to providers and consumers; changing medical education and certification; and developing new organizational models for women's health care.

Health Care Financing

A number of opportunities exist to integrate components of women's basic health care and to improve access within the context of health care financing. State or national adoption of universal health insurance coverage would improve access to health care for women who are currently uninsured or underinsured. The development of a comprehensive benefits package that includes reproductive health care, as well as other aspects of primary care, would improve women's access to basic services, assuming co-payments are minimal.[8]

A recent study by the Women's Research and Education Institute (1994) underscores the importance of including reproductive health services in a basic benefits package for women. The study found that expenditures for reproductive services (broadly defined to include pregnancy-related services, contraception and abortion services, and preventive and curative services related to the female reproductive system) accounted for one-third of all health expenditures by women ages fifteen to forty-four in 1987. A further finding was that women in this age group have higher out-of-pocket expenditures than men of comparable age because they frequently have inadequate or no health insurance coverage for reproductive health services. These higher costs, in turn, are thought to discourage many women from obtaining needed reproductive and preventive services.

Health care financing initiatives that expand access to health insurance and provide a basic benefits package for women, including reproductive health services with minimal or no cost sharing, would go far toward improving women's access to integrated primary care services.

Guidelines for Women's Health Services

A critical need exists to develop and disseminate guidelines for the content and frequency of services that make up women's primary care. These guidelines should incorporate reproductive and other components of women's primary care and should specify a schedule for preventive services by age group. The guidelines could be developed by a multidisciplinary panel of experts and adopted as institutional policy by health care organizations providing primary care to women.

Current guidelines generally are not gender-specific and do not address a comprehensive set of conditions and services relevant to women. For example, the U.S. Preventive Services Task Force's *Guide to Clinical Preventive Services* (1989) is not based on a review of an exhaustive set of preventive services and notes that the task force did not examine endometrial disease, among other conditions. In addition, current recommendations and controversies pertaining to specific preventive services have generated considerable confusion among women and their providers. A case in point is the controversy surrounding the efficacy of routine mammography for women under age fifty.

The guidelines should be disseminated to consumers as well as to health care providers. Although women's knowledge, attitudes, and beliefs about health care were not measured in this study, they might account for some of the unexplained variance in patterns of physician use and the receipt of preventive services. For example, women's awareness of the current recommended intervals for obtaining key preventive services, their perceived risks for key conditions, and their beliefs about the efficacy of health care may be important determinants of their utilization patterns.

Women also may be unaware that certain types of physicians are less likely than others to offer specific preventive services. Informing women about the care that is recommended for their age group would provide an incentive to physicians in various specialty areas to offer the recommended services directly or to coordinate their provision through referrals.

Changing Medical Education

Another strategy aimed at integrating the components of women's primary health care without contributing to an overutilization of services is to train and certify physicians as primary care providers to women. The cross-training of physicians in several specialty areas is one option. For example, internists and family practitioners could be trained in the provision of routine reproductive health care, including pelvic exams and gender-specific preventive services now provided largely by obstetrician-gynecologists, with the expectation that referrals would be made to an obstetrician-gynecologist for obstetrical services or for gynecologic problems that cannot be diagnosed or treated by the primary care provider. In addition, obstetrician-gynecologists could be trained in the provision of nonreproductive aspects of primary care (including adult immunizations, blood cholesterol screening, etc.) for women during and beyond the reproductive years.

There is much debate over which types of physicians are or should be primary care providers for women, and, based on the utilization patterns observed here, there is likely to be much disagreement among women. Concerned that women might not be able to access obstetrician-gynecologists directly in managed care systems, the American College of Obstetricians and Gynecologists (1993) argued that obstetrician-gynecologists function as primary care providers for women and should be formally designated as such. This position is difficult to reconcile with data from the National Ambulatory Medical Care Survey showing that the most common reason for visits to office-based obstetrician-gynecologists in 1989–90 was routine prenatal examinations (accounting for 32.8% of visits) and that 86.3 percent of visits were made by women under the age of forty-five (Schappert 1993). The potential exists, however, to improve the ability of, and incentives to, obstetrician-gynecologists to provide a broader array of primary care services to women in the reproductive years and beyond, who may rely on these physicians as their regular providers.

Physicians in the traditional specialties seeking to be designated as primary care providers could be certified in these areas and be required to provide comprehensive primary care services to women according to recommended guidelines. For example, the protocol for a regular physical examination for a woman might include a pelvic examination, gender-specific preventive tests appropriate to the woman's age group, and other age-appropriate components of routine care.

Another strategy to reduce fragmentation is to create a new type of women's health care provider, either a new medical specialist in women's health or an advanced practice nurse. Of these options, a new medical specialist has received the most attention. The rationale for this proposal is that men can now obtain comprehensive primary care services from one provider—an internist or family practitioner—and that women should have the same option, but there is no medical specialist currently trained to provide comprehensive primary care to women (Johnson 1992). The main arguments against this proposal are that the creation of a new specialty might further isolate women's health care and that reforms in medical education and specialty training can remedy existing deficiencies in practice (Harrison 1992). Another argument against a new specialty is the considerable time lag that would occur between training the new specialists and their availability to women.

New Organizational Models

Another strategy is the creation of organizational entities designed to integrate components of women's primary health care and provide care to women in a more coordinated and efficient manner (i.e., requiring fewer visits and reducing financial and time costs). Increased emphasis on primary and preventive care and the growth of managed care provide an incentive for physicians and health plans to reassess how efficiently they provide primary care to women and how well they satisfy women as customers.

Staff- or group-model HMOs would be expected to increase the likelihood of coordination between the primary care physician and the obstetrician-gynecologist and to reduce redundancies and gaps in services, compared with other models of care. No data exist to test this hypothesis. However, the primary care physician in HMOs usually is a family practitioner or internist, and referrals to an obstetrician-gynecologist require additional visits by the patient. Our data revealed that women enrolled in HMOs were slightly more likely than women with other private health insurance to use multiple physicians, and women enrolled in HMOs also made an average of 2.5 more visits per year than men enrolled in HMOs. Thus, we do not yet have evidence that HMOs provide primary care to women in a more efficient manner than other service options.

Another model for the provision of comprehensive health services to women is the multidisciplinary women's health center designed to provide comprehensive care in a "one-stop shopping" format. These organizations, which include hospital-affiliated and independent centers, are thought to be increasing in number (Looker 1993). The American Hospital Association (1993) reported that in 1992, 1,394 U.S. hospitals (24% of those reporting) had women's health centers providing a range of services that may or not include obstetrics; this was an increase of 19 percent over 1991. However, the services provided in these centers were not studied.

A 1994 survey estimated that there were 3,600 women's health centers nationwide, of which only 12 percent provide primary care services (Weisman, Curbow, and Khoury 1995). These centers come closest to implementing the core values for women-centered care proposed by

The Jacobs Institute of Women's Health (Schaps et al. 1993). Neither women's attitudes toward these centers nor the quality of care provided has been assessed, however.

IMPLICATIONS FOR RESEARCH

This study suggests a number of avenues for future research. One obvious need is for population-based descriptive studies that measure women's use of health care with a set of indicators based on the recognition that women may use multiple providers for regular care and various types of health care settings other than a private physician's office (e.g., family planning clinics, women's health centers). Typical measures of whether a woman has a usual source of care or of the number of annual physician visits are not adequate because they do not capture the variation among women in types of providers used and services received.

In measuring the services received, furthermore, it is important to assess the source of these services by physician type and setting. For example, to test hypotheses about how the types of providers affect the number of preventive services women receive, it would be necessary to measure which preventive services were received from each provider seen during a specified time period. An inventory of the services received by the type of provider also would permit an assessment of the appropriateness of care received—whether care is comprehensive (no major gaps in basic services), consistent with accepted guidelines (with regard to preventive services appropriate for the woman's age group), coordinated across providers (no major redundancies in care, physicians communicate with each other), or associated with better health outcomes. Currently, it is not known what type or combination of providers is optimal with regard to women's primary care.

Given the variation in women's patterns of using health care, research is badly needed that compares the services received and the health outcomes of women who obtain health care from different types of physicians or in different types of delivery settings. Comparison of care patterns in multidisciplinary women's health centers with those in other settings is one research need. Another key question for research is whether managed care plans produce more integrated primary care services for women in different age groups than would be obtained, for instance, from private physicians. In theory, HMOs should not only balance the woman's needs for primary and specialty care (through the gatekeeping function) but also enhance coordination among the various providers of services to the woman, thereby reducing redundancies and gaps in preventive services. As has been suggested, it is not clear from the utilization patterns observed here that HMOs provide women with efficient primary care. At present, there are no national data on how managed care plans define basic benefits for women or on the types of physicians women use as primary care providers within these plans. Because managed care plans are increasingly prevalent and diverse, these issues need attention.

ACKNOWLEDGMENTS

I gratefully acknowledge the assistance of Stacey B. Plichta, Sc.D., and Sandra D. Cassard, Sc.D., with data analysis.

NOTES

1. A 1993 national survey sponsored by the American College of Obstetricians and Gynecologists (Gallup Organization 1993) found that of 1,005 women (ages eighteen to sixty-five) 72 percent reported having a physical examination by an obstetrician-gynecologist within the past 2 years and, of these, 54 percent considered their obstetrician-gynecologist to be their "primary physician." Thus, about 39 percent of women surveyed might rely on an obstetrician-gynecologist as their primary physician.

2. The assignment of variables to these three categories follows conventions in the literature in cases where variables might indicate more than one component. For example, age is typically regarded as a predisposing variable, although it also may be a proxy for the need for health care. Similarly, employment status may be regarded as a predisposing variable if it is considered as a social role indicator, or as an enabling variable if it is regarded as an indicator of access to health insurance.

3. Throughout this chapter, the term *family practitioner* refers to a family or general practitioner; *obstetrician-gynecologist* refers to a physician identified as only an obstetrician, only a gynecologist, or both.

4. The terms *reproductive years* and *childbearing years* refer to that portion of the life span when women are capable of reproduction (between menarche and menopause). The age group of fifteen years to forty-four years conventionally is used to reflect this period. In this study, women in the reproductive years are defined as those between ages eighteen and forty-four, because women younger than eighteen were not included in the survey.

Although the use of this age category permits comparisons with other studies, it should be noted that the term *reproductive years* is something of a misnomer. According to 1988 U.S. data, only 4 years typically elapse between the births of a woman's first and last children, and 75 percent of women have completed their desired family size by age thirty-five (Forrest 1993). Also, the transition to menopause typically occurs around age fifty.

5. Because of the way the questions were structured, 325 women who reported that their regular physician was an obstetrician-gynecologist were not asked about additional physicians seen. Some of these women might also see an internist or family practitioner but might not regard that physician as the regular doctor. Thus, the total number of women seeing both an obstetrician-gynecologist and an internist or family practitioner could be underestimated.

6. Women were also asked, "In the past 12 months, was there a time when you needed medical care but did not get it, or not?" Reporting an unmet need for care did not differ substantially by the pattern of physician use, except that women who had *no* regular physician were more likely than other women to report an unmet need (26% compared to 10%).

7. This list of preventive services is skewed toward reproductive health care (four out of the seven services involve breast or pelvic examinations or tests). A more comprehensive list of recommended preventive services for adult women might include immunizations and other procedures recommended by the U.S. Preventive Services Task Force (1989).

8. Research has shown that cost sharing reduces the use of preventive services, which could be a major problem for women who receive recommended services less often than normally recommended. See, for example, Newhouse and the Insurance Experiment Group (1993).

REFERENCES

Aday, L. A. 1993. Indicators and predictors of health services utilization. In S. J. Williams and P. R. Torrens, eds., *Introduction to Health Services*. Albany, N.Y.: Delmar.

Aday, L. A., Andersen, R., and Fleming, G. V. 1980. *Health Care in the U.S.: Equitable for Whom?* Beverly Hills, Calif.: Sage Publications.

Aiken, L. H., et al. 1979. The contribution of specialists to the delivery of primary care: a new perspective. *New England Journal of Medicine* 300:1363–70.

American College of Obstetricians and Gynecologists. 1993. *Obstetrics and Gynecology: Primary Care—A Guide to Communicating with Lawmakers, the Public, and Patients*. Washington, D.C.: American College of Obstetricians and Gynecologists.

American Hospital Association. 1993. *AHA Hospital Statistics, 1993–94 Edition*. Chicago: American Hospital Association.

Andersen, R. 1968. *A Behavioral Model of Families' Use of Health Services*. Research

Series no. 25. Chicago: Center for Health Administration Studies, University of Chicago.

Bartman, B. A., and Weiss, K. B. 1993. Women's primary care in the United States: a study of practice variation among physician specialties. *Journal of Women's Health* 2:261–68.

Bird, C. E., and Fremont, A. M. 1991. Gender, time use, and health. *Journal of Health and Social Behavior* June:114–29.

Clancy, C. M., and Massion, C. T. 1992. American women's health care: a patchwork quilt with gaps. *Journal of the American Medical Association* 268:1918–20.

Cornelius, L., Beauregard, K., and Cohen, J. 1991. Usual sources of medical care and their characteristics. *National Medical Expenditure Survey Research Findings 11*. Rockville, Md.: Agency for Health Care Policy and Research.

Forrest, J. D. 1993. Timing of reproductive life stages. *Obstetrics and Gynecology* 82:105–11.

Gallup Organization. 1993. A Gallup Study of Women's Attitudes toward the Use of OB/GYN for Primary Care. Princeton, N.J.

Harrison, M. 1992. Women's health as a specialty: a deceptive solution. *Journal of Women's Health* 1:101–6.

Horton, J. A., ed. 1992. *The Women's Health Data Book*. Washington, D.C.: Jacobs Institute of Women's Health.

Horton, J. A., Cruess, D. F., and Pearse, W. H. 1993. Primary and preventive care services provided by obstetrician-gynecologists. *Obstetrics and Gynecology* 82:723–26.

Johnson, K. 1992. Women's health: developing a new interdisciplinary specialty. *Journal of Women's Health* 1:95–99.

Looker, P. 1993. Women's health centers: history and evolution. *Women's Health Issues* 3:95–100.

Lurie, N., et al. 1993. Preventive care for women: does sex of the physician matter? *New England Journal of Medicine* 329:478–82.

Marieskind, H. I. 1980. *Women in the Health System: Patients, Providers, and Programs*. St. Louis: Mosby.

Mechanic, D. 1976. Sex, illness, illness behavior, and the use of health services. *Journal of Human Stress* 2:29–40.

Muller, C. F. 1990. *Health Care and Gender*. New York: Russell Sage Foundation.

Nathanson, C. A. 1975. Illness and the feminine role: a theoretical review. *Social Science and Medicine* 9:57–62.

Newhouse, J. P., and the Insurance Experiment Group. 1993. *Free for All?: Lessons from the RAND Health Insurance Experiment*. Cambridge, Mass.: Harvard University Press.

Riessman, C. K. 1983. Women and medicalization: a new perspective. *Social Policy* 14:3–18.

Ruzek, S. B. 1978. *The Women's Health Movement: Feminist Alternatives to Medical Control*. New York: Praeger.

Schappert, S. M. 1993. National Ambulatory Medical Survey: 1991 summary. *Advance Data* 230. Hyattsville, Md.: National Center for Health Statistics.

Schaps, M. J., et al. 1993. Women-centered care: implementing a philosophy. *Women's Health Issues* 3:52–54.

Starfield, B. 1992. *Primary Care: Concept, Evaluation, and Policy.* New York: Oxford University Press.

U.S. Preventive Services Task Force. 1989. *Guide to Clinical Preventive Services: An Assessment of the Effectiveness of 169 Interventions.* Baltimore: Williams and Wilkins.

Verbrugge, L. M. 1989. The twain meet: empirical explanations of sex differences in health and mortality. *Journal of Health and Social Behavior* September:282–304.

Weisman, C. S., et al. 1989. Cancer screening services for the elderly. *Public Health Reports* May–June:209–14.

Weisman, C. S., Curbow, B., and Khoury, A. J. 1995. The national survey of women's health centers: current models of women-centered care. *Women's Health Issues* 5:103–17.

Wilensky, G. R., and Cafferata, G. L. 1983. Women and the use of health services. *American Economic Review* May:128–33.

Women's Research and Education Institute. 1994. *Women's Health Care Costs and Experiences.* Washington, D.C.: Women's Research and Education Institute.

2

Women's Use of Preventive Health Services

Roberta Wyn, Ph.D.
E. Richard Brown, Ph.D.
Hongjian Yu, M.S.

A key issue in health care reform, which often is overshadowed by cost and financing concerns, is how best to structure a health care system to promote and maintain the health of the population. One of the many criticisms leveled against the current health care system is that it does not emphasize or promote a cohesive preventive orientation. Historically, the delivery of care and its financing have been structured around acute curative care, with a bias toward better financing for inpatient care and procedures. Although a reduction of risk factors and early detection of disease have been public health goals for several decades, the integration of these goals into the health care system through financial incentives and practice patterns has been slow. One of the main opportunities for this integration is in providing and paying for clinical preventive services.

Health care reform focuses primarily on extending insurance coverage and controlling the costs of health care, changes that would benefit many women and men. But women have gender-specific health needs—conditions that are specific to women, that occur more frequently in women, that affect women differently than men, or that, combined with women's multiple roles and socioeconomic status, have different consequences for women—that must be considered in health care reform. This chapter focuses on women's use of clinical preventive health services by examining: (1) which women are under-screened for clinical preventive health services; (2) how health insurance and other noninsurance health care system factors affect use; (3) what barriers to screening women report; (4) what is needed in a reformed health care system to promote the use of preventive services consistent with recommendations; and (5) what areas require additional research to improve our understanding of women's use of clinical preventive services.

WOMEN AND ACCESS TO HEALTH CARE

Women have serious problems of access to health care. Although it is often assumed that women have better access to the health care system than men (based on women's higher rates of utilization) part of the difference in the use of health care between the genders is attributable to women's use of obstetrical and reproductive services. Women of all ages are more likely than men to have had at least one physician visit in the past year, but the differences are greatest among women of reproductive age (Collins et al. 1994). Rates of hospital discharge are also higher for women than for men ages eighteen to forty-four, but when hospital stays for childbirth are excluded, the difference narrows. Hospital discharge rates are similar for women and men after age forty-five (Collins et al. 1994). Furthermore, among women, access to the health care system varies by such nonhealth status factors as income, ethnicity, and education. Factors unrelated to the need for health care too often determine use.

One important indicator of the adequacy of women's access to health care is their use of clinical preventive services. This utilization measure is useful for several reasons. It provides information about whether a woman has received a screening. It also is a very robust population-based measure of differences among subgroups of women in access to services because there is considerable agreement about the efficacy of these screenings and, in most cases, the frequency at which such services should be received. This consensus provides an independent criterion of use that is applicable across different groups of women. Finally, whether women receive clinical preventive services at recommended intervals and the determinants of their use provide evidence about the organization and delivery of care and its quality.

This chapter examines women's use of five clinical preventive services: Pap smear, clinical breast examination, mammography, blood pressure screening, and blood cholesterol screening. These five screenings provide a contrast along several dimensions. First, these tests differ in their gender specificity. The Pap smear, clinical breast examination, and mammography are gender-specific, whereas blood pressure screening and blood cholesterol screening are gender-neutral. Second, the technology involved in these screenings and the skill level required to perform them vary. For example, mammography is more technologically intensive than clinical breast examination and the other screenings and typically requires a referral. Third, insurance coverage for these services differs. The Pap smear, mammography, and blood cholesterol screening are typically covered as procedures, whereas the blood pressure screening and the clinical breast examination are viewed as part of a physical examination.

Several national and subnational studies have been conducted during the past 10 years on women's use of clinical preventive services. Many of these studies have focused on screening for cancer and examined women's access to the Pap smear, clinical breast examination, and mammography. Although there is some variation across the studies in screening rates and predictors of screening, several trends emerge. One of the most consistent findings across the studies is the inverse relationship between age and rates of screening: rates of cancer screening decrease with age for the Pap smear (Hayward et al. 1988; Calle et al. 1993), for a mammogram (Hayward et al. 1988; Burg, Lane, and Polednak 1990; Marchant and Sutton 1990; Calle et al. 1993), and for clinical breast examination (Hayward et al. 1988; Burg, Lane, and Polednak 1990), even though higher rates of breast cancer and invasive cervical cancer are found among older women.

Although all groups of women remained underscreened, studies have shown that Latinas in particular have low rates of use of clinical preventive services. They have much lower Pap smear rates than either Anglo or African American women (Hayward et al. 1988) and are less likely to be screened for breast cancer (Hayward et al. 1988; Calle et al. 1993). African American women's access to clinical breast examination has improved, and in some studies the rates of clinical breast examination are equivalent to or higher than those for Anglo women (Makuc, Freid, and Kleiman 1989), but the rates of mammography still lag behind (Marchant and Sutton 1990); moreover, lower-income African American women experience serious problems of access (Mandelblatt et al. 1993).

Another consistent finding is the lower rates of use of these clinical preventive services among socially disadvantaged women. Women with lower income or less education have poorer access to clinical preventive services, contributing to their already compromised health condition and increasing the risk of preventable morbidity and mortality. Education and income were independent predictors of having had a Pap smear within the preceding year, after controlling for several other factors (Hayward et al. 1988; Calle et al. 1993), and income was found to be independently associated with clinical breast examination and education with mammography (Hayward et al. 1988), after accounting for the effects of health insurance coverage. It is clear from these and other studies that women with lower incomes and less education have, for a combination of complex factors, reduced access to these services. These women are also diagnosed with cancer at a later stage (Farley and Flannery 1989), increasing the risk of morbidity and mortality.

Among the health care system factors associated with the use of clinical preventive services, health insurance coverage is one of the strongest and most consistent predictors. The risk of being under-screened for breast and cervical cancer was much higher for women without coverage (Hayward et al. 1988; Woolhandler and Himmelstein 1988)—a relationship that remains after controlling for other demographic and health service variables. One limitation of these studies, however, is the global designation of coverage as insured versus uninsured: specific information about whether a procedure or screening is covered is lacking. A city-level study of Latinas found that the likelihood of a mammogram was positively related not only to coverage but also to the amount of coverage for the procedure (Longman, Saint-Germain, and Modiano 1992).

Factors related to the delivery and organization of health care are also associated with use of these cancer screenings. Women who do not have a regular place where they receive medical care or a regular provider are less likely to receive breast cancer screening (Hayward et al. 1988; Longman, Saint-Germain, and Modiano 1992) or cervical cancer screening (Harlan, Bernstein, and Kessler 1991). Once in the system, provider-related factors such as the specialty of the physician and, as recent studies have shown, the physician's gender may also be associated with the receipt of gender-specific screenings (Franks and Clancy 1993; Lurie et al. 1993). The practice and referral patterns of physicians are important determinants of use for women; nearly three-quarters of women who had a mammogram reported a physician's recommendation as the reason for the screening (Romans et al. 1991).

The factors associated with blood pressure and blood cholesterol screening in women have been less extensively examined than those associated with reproductive system–related cancer screenings. Most women have had their blood pressure checked in the past year, and only small differences in rates are observed among women by income and education. There are greater differences among subgroups of women for blood cholesterol screening than were seen for blood pressure, with poorer, less-educated, and minority women less likely to have ever been screened (Piani and Schoenborn 1993).

Several recent changes have occurred in women's health since the time many of these studies, especially those on cancer screening, were conducted. During the past few years, there has been increasing awareness of women's health needs in the scientific and legislative arenas. Examples of this include the creation of the Women's Office of Health, the implementation of the Women's Health Initiative, and the passage of the Women's Health Equity Act. Also, Medicare recently passed legislation that includes the Pap smear and mammography screening as covered benefits (Schauffler 1993), and several states have passed legislation requiring the coverage of these two preventive services (American College of Obstetricians and Gynecologists 1992).

This chapter provides the most recent information available on women's use of clinical preventive services. This study contains information on several clinical preventive services, allowing for comparisons across different services, and on several critical health care system factors, enabling analysis of the implications of these factors for health care reform.

THE IMPORTANCE OF SCREENING

The use of screening tests for early detection of disease has been credited with major reductions in morbidity and mortality. The goal of the five clinical preventive services examined in this chapter—Pap smear, clinical breast examination, mammography, blood pressure screening, and blood cholesterol screening—is either early identification of disease or the reduction of risk factors (U.S. Preventive Services Task Force 1989) for the three major causes of women's mortality: cancer, cardiovascular disease, and cerebrovascular disease.

Early detection of cervical cancer through the Pap smear has been credited with the overall reduction during the past 40 years in the incidence of and mortality from invasive cervical cancer (Fink 1991). Cervical cancer is one of the most commonly occurring cancers in women; approximately 50,000 new cases in situ occur annually, and in 1990 approximately 13,500 cases of invasive cancer were diagnosed (Fink 1991). The benefit of the Pap smear is its ability to identify precancerous lesions still confined to the epithelium of the cervix (carcinoma in situ) before invasion of the uterine cervix. For women diagnosed with cancer in situ, the 5-year survival rate is 88 percent; for women who have an initial diagnosis of invasive cancer, the 5-year survival rate is 13 percent (National Cancer Institute 1993a).

The consensus among several major organizations, including the American Cancer Society, the National Cancer Institute, the American Medical Association, and the American College of Obstetricians and Gynecologists, is that all women who have been sexually active or who have reached the age of eighteen should receive a Pap smear each year. After three or more consecutive negative tests, the screening may be performed less frequently at the discretion of the physician (Fink 1988). There is no upper age limit on testing. In contrast, the U.S. Preventive Services Task Force recommends that all women who are sexually active be screened every one to three years at their physician's discretion; screening may be discontinued at age sixty-five if previous tests were normal (U.S. Preventive Services Task Force 1989).

There are also differences among organizations regarding the appropriate frequency and age intervals for breast cancer screening, especially mammography. Breast cancer is the most frequently occurring cancer among women in the United States, with an estimated 182,000 new cases in 1993 (Boring, Squires, and Tong 1993). The lifetime odds of a woman developing breast cancer is one in eight (National Cancer Institute 1993b). Breast cancer is the second leading cause of death due to cancer among women, exceeded only by lung cancer. The stage at which breast cancer is diagnosed is a major predictor of survival; therefore, secondary prevention efforts have focused on the early identification of tumors through clinical breast examination and mammography.

There is general agreement among experts about the benefits of clinical breast examination and mammography for women fifty to sixty-nine years of age; this is supported by analytic studies and clinical experience. There is surprisingly little information, however, about the efficacy of screening in women over seventy, even though the risk of breast cancer increases with age. The rate of breast cancer increases with age from 187.4 per 100,000 women ages forty-five to forty-nine, to 267.7 among women ages fifty-five to fifty-nine, and to 451.3 among women ages eighty to eighty-four (National Cancer Institute 1991).

Approximately 78 percent of all breast cancers occur in women over the age of fifty (National Cancer Institute 1993b).

Most of the controversy over mammography screening surrounds women younger than fifty. The American Cancer Society, the American College of Radiology, the American College of Obstetricians and Gynecologists, and several other organizations recommend that women ages forty to forty-nine have mammography screening every one to two years and then yearly beginning at age fifty (Dodd 1992; American College of Obstetricians and Gynecologists 1993). In the past, the National Cancer Institute recommended mammography screening for women under and over forty years of age. In a recent change of policy, however, the institute now discourages women under fifty from being screened, citing a lack of clinical evidence that regular screening reduces mortality in women in that age group (Volkers 1993).

The guidelines for clinical breast examination are less controversial, but still differ among organizations. The American Cancer Society recommends clinical breast examination every 3 years for women twenty to thirty-nine years of age and an annual examination for women over forty years of age (Dodd 1992). Organizations disagree over the screening intervals for women under forty. For example, the National Cancer Institute (1993b) recommends annual clinical breast examination for women over forty, but makes no recommendation for younger women.

The guidelines for blood pressure and blood cholesterol screening are relatively straightforward. Organizations recommend either annual or biennial (for nonhypertensive patients) screening for blood pressure. For blood cholesterol, measurement within the preceding 5 years is recommended (U.S. Preventive Services Task Force 1989).

The Commonwealth Fund survey provides updated information on women's access to clinical preventive services. This survey, which provides the data for the remainder of this chapter, shows that a high percentage of women are still not receiving clinical preventive services at recommended intervals.

Older, Minority, and Socially Disadvantaged Women

The Pap smear has been identified as one of the most efficacious screening tests for cancer, yet a significant portion of women are not adequately screened. Two-thirds of women (65%) had a Pap smear in the previous year (tab. 2.1), but one out of every five women (19%) does

Table 2.1. Percentage of Women Ages Eighteen Years and Older Who Received Clinical Preventive Service, by Demographic Factors, 1993

	Pap Smear[a]	Clinical Breast Examination[a]	Mammography (50+ only)[a]	Blood Pressure Screening[a]	Blood Cholesterol Screening[b]
Age group					
18–39	73	68	—	88	75
40–64	65	69	—	90	88
65+	44	59	—	90	92
Age group (mammography only)					
50–59	—	—	63	—	—
60–69	—	—	54	—	—
70+	—	—	49	—	—
Ethnic group					
Anglo	64	68	c	89	83
Latina	60	56	c	82	77
African American	73	67	c	91	85
Income					
<$25,000	57	58	49	88	80
$25,000+	73	75	67	91	85
Education					
Not a high school graduate	54	55	43	86	78
High school graduate	61	64	58	88	82
College	73	75	64	91	86
Total	65	67	—	89	83

Source: Data from The Commonwealth Fund survey on women's health, 1993.

[a] Criterion used: screening within the past year.

[b] Criterion used: ever received a screening.

[c] Sample size too small to produce reliable estimates.

not meet even the minimum interval of a screening test within the past 3 years.[1]

Rates of Pap smear screening decrease dramatically with increasing age. Older women have lower annual screening rates than younger women and go longer intervals without screening. Three out of four women eighteen to thirty-nine years of age (73%) had a recent Pap smear, compared to fewer than one-half of women over sixty-five (44%) (tab. 2.1). Furthermore, two out of five older women (39%) had not had a Pap smear in the past 3 years, including 6 percent who reported that they have never been tested. These low screening rates are in contrast to the epidemiology of the disease in older women: the incidence of invasive cancer increases with age. Compared with younger women, older women are less likely to have cancer in situ and more likely to have advanced invasive cancer when diagnosed (Muller et al. 1990). It is uncertain whether the pattern of disease observed in older women is the result of lower screening rates in elderly persons or a different progression of disease.

Differences in rates emerge for other subgroups as well. Anglo women and Latinas have lower screening rates for the Pap smear than African American women. Sixty-four percent of Anglo women and 60 percent of Latinas were screened during the past year, compared with 73 percent of African American women (tab. 2.1). Other studies have also shown higher screening rates among African American women (Hayward et al. 1988; Woolhandler and Himmelstein 1988; Makuc, Freid, and Kleinman 1989). Even when screening rates are examined over a 3-year period, a sizable portion of Anglo women and Latinas remain underscreened. Nearly one out of every four Latinas (24%) and one out of every five Anglo women (19%) have not had a Pap smear in the past 3 years.

But screening is by itself insufficient to reduce mortality. Even with the advantage of higher reported rates of screening, African American women have higher mortality rates from cervical cancer than Anglo women (Boring, Squires, and Tong 1992). A combination of several factors could account for African American women's higher cervical cancer death rates: diagnosis at a later stage, poorer survival experience, access barriers to treatment, poorer quality of care, and, perhaps related to all the above, social and cultural disadvantage (Bal 1992; Boring, Squires, and Heath 1992).

Screening rates are lower for poorer women and for those with less education, further compromising women already at risk for poor health status. Fifty-seven percent of women with household incomes below $25,000 had a Pap smear in the past year, compared with 73 percent of women with income over $25,000 (tab. 2.1). This disparity by income persisted when rates are examined separately for non-elderly and elderly women: 63 percent of low-income women ages eighteen to sixty-four had a Pap smear in the past year, compared with 74 percent of women with incomes over $25,000, and 42 percent of low-income elderly women were screened, compared with 50 percent of women with higher incomes. Not only do low-income women have less access to a Pap smear but they are also more likely than affluent women to have a screening interval greater than 3 years (25% and 12%, respectively). Like those with lower income, women with less education are less likely to have received a Pap smear in the past year (tab. 2.1)—a pattern seen for nonelderly and elderly women.

Breast Cancer Screening

Overall, two-thirds of women surveyed (67%) had had a clinical breast examination in the past year (tab. 2.1). Rates of annual breast examination are similar for women under forty years of age and those forty to sixty-four (68 and 69%, respectively), but drop to 59 percent for women over sixty-five, despite their greater risk for developing breast cancer. Furthermore, a high proportion of these older women (22%) had not had a clinical breast examination in the past 3 years, well beyond the recommended annual time interval.

Screening rates for mammography also decrease with age. Sixty-three percent of women fifty to fifty-nine years of age, 54 percent of women ages sixty to sixty-nine, and 49 percent of women over age seventy were screened within the past year (tab. 2.1). Older women also go longer without being screened. Nineteen percent of women ages fifty to fifty-nine years did not have a mammogram in the past 3 years, compared with 30 percent of women sixty to sixty-nine years and more than one-third of women (35%) age seventy or older.

Latinas have lower rates of annual clinical breast examination (56%) than either Anglo (68%) or African American (67%) women (tab. 2.1) and go for longer intervals without a clinical breast examination. One in four Latinas (26%) has not had a clinical breast exam in the past 3 years, compared with a much lower proportion of Anglo and African American women (16%).

As with cervical cancer screening, lower socioeconomic status is also associated with reduced access to breast cancer screening. Only 58 percent of women with lower incomes (household incomes less than $25,000) had an annual clinical breast examination, compared with 75 percent of women with household incomes over $25,000 (tab. 2.1). The pattern of reduced access to clinical breast examination is found for nonelderly and elderly women. Lower income is also associated with lower rates of mammography (tab. 2.1). Women with less education also have reduced access to clinical breast examination and mammography screening (tab. 2.1), paralleling the lower rates found among low-income women.

Blood Pressure Screening

Of the five clinical preventive services examined, rates of blood pressure screening are the highest (tab. 2.1) and include the fewest differences among subgroups of women. Eighty-nine percent of women had a blood pressure screening within the past year, with no statistical differences in screening rates by age. Latinas have lower screening rates (82%) than either Anglo (89%) or African American women (91%) (tab. 2.1). In contrast to the other clinical preventive services, poorer women do not have statistically lower rates of blood pressure screening; however, there is a slight trend toward higher screening rates among both nonelderly and elderly women with more education.

Blood Cholesterol Screening

The rates of blood cholesterol screening increase with age (tab. 2.1), unlike the trend seen for reproductive system cancer screening, where rates decrease for older women. Similar to all the clinical preventive services examined, Latinas are the least likely to have ever had a blood cholesterol screening, and there is a pattern of reduced rates of screening for disadvantaged women (tab. 2.1).

WOMEN WITHOUT COVERAGE FOR PREVENTIVE SERVICES OR UNCERTAIN ABOUT COVERAGE

A significant percentage of women lack coverage for basic preventive services. Lack of any health insurance coverage and, among those insured, lack of coverage for preventive services, leaves many women without adequate financial protection to cover the costs of clinical preventive services. Among women ages eighteen to sixty-four, four out of ten either do not have coverage for cervical cancer screening or are unsure whether they are covered: 15 percent are completely uninsured; 17 percent are insured, but are not covered for the Pap smear; and 7 percent are insured, but are not clear about coverage. Similarly, four out of ten women fifty to sixty-four years of age do not have coverage for mammography or are unsure whether they are covered: 14 percent are completely uninsured; 16 percent are insured but not covered for mammography; and another 11 percent do not know whether their policy covers this benefit. An even higher proportion of women lack coverage for blood cholesterol screening: slightly less than half of nonelderly women (46%) reported that they are covered for blood cholesterol screening; 17 percent of women are insured but are not covered; and 21 percent are not sure whether their policy covers this screening. Blood pressure screening and clinical breast examination are typically not covered as procedures, but are part of a physical examination. Fifty percent of women have coverage for a nondiagnostic-related physical examination.

Lack of coverage and lack of knowledge about what services are covered are barriers to access. Given the complexity of health insurance policies and the many deviations among plans in benefit coverage and cost-sharing arrangements, the lack of information about coverage is not surprising. This uncertainty about coverage for preventive services acts as a barrier to use because women may assume that their health plan will not pay for recommended services.

This problem applies to older women covered by Medicare and to younger women with private health insurance. Forty-five percent of female Medicare recipients over age sixty-five either reported that Medicare did not cover the Pap smear or were not sure if it was covered. However, in 1990, more than 2 years before this survey was conducted, Medicare coverage was extended to include Pap smear screening every 3 years. Before this time, Medicare only paid for diagnostic Pap smears. Similarly, one-third of elderly women (35%) were also not familiar with Medicare's coverage of biennial mammography screening. This lack of accurate information about Medicare coverage among recipients also leads to barriers to use even among women who are insured.

The lack of a consistent approach to covering preventive services and the delays in getting Medicare coverage for the Pap smear and mammography screening show the low priority that clinical preventive services have received. Over a 25-year period before the passage of coverage legislation in the 1990s, thirty-seven bills to cover mammography and thirty-six bills to cover the Pap smear were introduced in Congress (Schauffler 1993).

UNINSURED AND INSURED NONELDERLY WOMEN
WITH INADEQUATE COVERAGE

As other studies (Hayward et al. 1988; Woolhandler and Himmelstei ι 1988) have found, uninsured women have lower rates of using clinical preventive services than do insured women. Across each of the services examined, uninsured nonelderly women (who constitute 15% of women under age sixty-five) have much lower rates of using clinical preventive services than women who know what their coverage is (fig. 2.1). But being insured does not necessarily mean having adequate coverage. Women who are insured but do not have coverage for preventive services often have lower screening rates than do insured women whose insurance covers these benefits. This is seen for the Pap smear and mammography, two services for which specific benefit coverage is available.

Insured women with coverage for Pap smears have rates of annual screening (77%) 1.5 times that for uninsured women (52%). Screening rates fall in between these two groups for women who are insured but are not covered for the Pap smear (69%), demonstrating the advantage of insurance but also its limitations when specific services are not covered. Women who are not clear whether their coverage includes Pap smear screening had the lowest rates (36%). A similar pattern is seen for mammography screening among women ages fifty to sixty-four. Uninsured women are less likely to be screened (42%) than insured

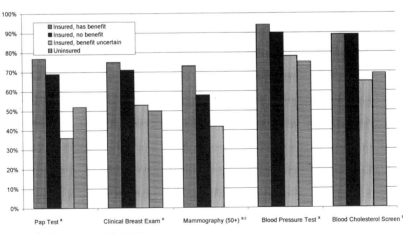

a   Criterion used: screen within past year.

[a] Criterion used: screen within past year.
[b] Criterion used: ever received a screen.
[c] Sample size too small to produce reliable estimates for "insured, benefit uncertain."
Note: For clinical breast examination and blood pressure screening, which typically are not covered as separate procedures, coverage for physical examination is used as a proxy indicator of benefit coverage.

Fig. 2.1. Percentage of Women Ages Eighteen to Sixty-four Years Who Received Clinical Preventive Services, by Insurance Status, 1993

Source: Analysis of The Commonwealth Fund survey on women's health, 1993.

women with mammography coverage (73%) and insured women without coverage for mammography (58%).[2]

Being uninsured also lowers the probability of having a clinical breast examination. Only one out of two uninsured women (50%) had a clinical breast examination during the past year, compared with 75 percent of insured women with a policy that covered physical examination and 71 percent of insured women without coverage for a physical examination.

The rates of blood pressure screening also vary by insurance status, but not to the same extent as other clinical preventive services. Uninsured women have lower rates (75%) of a recent screening than women with insurance. Among insured women there is a slight trend for those with policies that covered preventive services to have higher screening rates than for women whose policies did not cover these services (94% versus 90%).

For blood cholesterol screening within the past 5 years, insured women with and without benefit coverage have similar rates (89%); insured women without benefit coverage (65%) and uninsured women (69%) have the lowest rates.

THE HEALTH CARE DELIVERY SYSTEM AND WOMEN'S USE OF SERVICES

Women who do not have a usual place to go for medical care are less likely to receive clinical preventive services. Differences in use rates are found for all of the clinical preventive services examined, except for the blood cholesterol screening (tab. 2.2).[3] Even for blood pressure screening, where screening rates are almost universal, those without a usual source of care have lower rates of screening (79% versus 92%). The consequences of a lack of connection to the health care system are even more striking for access to other clinical preventive services (tab. 2.2).

A significant proportion of women—one out of five—lack a regular source of health care, a problem that affects equal proportions of nonelderly and elderly women. Even though uninsured women are more likely to lack a regular source of care (34%), it is not just lack of coverage that limits having a regular connection to the health care system. One out of five elderly and nonelderly insured women also has no regular connection to the health care system.

Another health care system determinant of the use of clinical pre-

Table 2.2. Percentage of Women Ages Eighteen Years and Older Who Received Clinical Preventive Service, by Health System Factors, 1993

	Pap Smear[a]	Clinical Breast Examination[a]	Mammography (50+ only)[a]	Blood Pressure Screening[a]	Blood Cholesterol Screening[b]
Source of care					
Regular source	68	71	60	92	83
No regular source	52	49	35	79	81
Physician type					
Internist/family practitioner/other	64	68	59	91	84
Ob/gyn	86	81	59	92	83
No regular physician	45	42	27	70	72

Source: Data from The Commonwealth Fund survey on women's health, 1993.

[a] Criterion used: screening within the past year.

[b] Criterion used: ever received a screening.

ventive services is the integration of these services into medical practice, which has been dominated by acute and curative care. One measure of this integration is how use rates differ by physician specialty. Among nonelderly women,[4] those whose regular provider is an obstetrician-gynecologist rather than an internist, family practitioner, or other type of provider have higher rates of Pap smear screening and clinical breast examination, but not of mammography, blood pressure screening, or blood cholesterol screening (tab. 2.2).

THE ROLE OF INSURANCE COVERAGE AND OTHER HEALTH CARE SYSTEM FACTORS

Multiple logistic regression analysis was used to examine the combined effects of several factors on the use of preventive services by nonelderly women ages eighteen to sixty-four (tab. 2.3).[5] After controlling for demographic differences (age, ethnicity, income, and education) and other health care system factors (having a usual source of care, having a usual physician, and that physician's specialty), uninsured women are more likely to have gone without a timely clinical preventive screening. This effect is found for each of the screenings—Pap smear (*OR* [odds ratio] = 2.6), clinical breast examination (*OR* = 1.6), mammography (*OR* = 3.6), blood pressure screening (*OR* = 3.0),

Table 2.3. Predictors of Not Receiving Clinical Preventive Screening among Women Ages Eighteen to Sixty-four Years, 1993

	Pap Smear[a]		Clinical Breast Examination[a]	
	OR[c]	p-value	OR[c]	p-value
Ethnicity				
Anglo[d]	1.00	—	1.00	—
Latina	1.22	NS	1.62	<0.05
African American	0.71	NS	1.12	NS
Income				
<$25,000	1.28	<0.05	1.58	<0.001
$25,000[d]	1.00	—	1.00	—
Education				
No college	1.53	<0.001	1.58	<0.001
Some college[d]	1.00	—	1.00	—
Health insurance				
Insured, benefit covered[d]	1.00	—	1.00	—
Insured, benefit not covered	2.14	<0.001	1.47	<0.05
Uninsured	2.58	<0.001	1.65	<0.05
Source of care				
Regular source[d]	1.00	—	1.00	—
No regular source	2.01	<0.001	2.23	<0.001
Physician type				
Ob/gyn[d]	1.00	—	1.00	—
Internist/family practitioner/other	2.92	<0.001	2.31	<0.001
No regular physician	3.80	<0.001	3.41	<0.001

Source: Analysis of The Commonwealth Fund survey on women's health, 1993

[a] Criterion used: screening within the past year.

[b] Criterion used: ever received a screening.

[c] Odds ratio.

[d] Reference group.

and blood cholesterol screening ($OR = 3.2$). Insured women who do not have preventive care coverage or are not sure about their coverage also have increased odds of being underscreened for each of the clinical preventive services—Pap smear ($OR = 2.1$), clinical breast examination ($OR = 1.4$), mammography ($OR = 3.9$), blood pressure screening ($OR = 2.1$), and blood cholesterol screening ($OR = 2.6$). These findings suggest that not only is insurance coverage important but also it must be comprehensive (covering needed benefits) and easy to understand.

Table 2.3. *(Continued)*

Mammography (50+ only)[a]		Blood Pressure Screening[a]		Blood Cholesterol Screening[b]	
OR^c	*p*-value	OR^c	*p*-value	OR^c	*p*-value
1.00	—	1.00	—	1.00	—
1.53	NS	1.48	NS	1.11	NS
1.42	NS	0.69	NS	0.71	NS
1.61	NS	1.24	NS	1.39	<0.05
1.00	—	1.00	—	1.00	—
1.61	NS	1.24	NS	1.39	<0.05
1.00	—	1.00	NS	1.00	—
1.00	—	1.00	—	1.00	—
3.87	<0.001	2.11	<0.001	2.65	<0.001
3.65	<0.001	3.02	<0.001	3.20	<0.001
1.00	—	1.00	—	1.00	—
3.10	<0.001	1.98	<0.001	0.78	NS
1.00	—	1.00	—	1.00	—
1.17	NS	1.38	NA	1.59	<0.05
1.36	NS	3.53	<0.001	2.35	<0.001

Other health care system factors also are associated with the use of clinical preventive services. Women without an established connection to the health care system are less likely to receive timely screenings. Having no regular source of care increases the odds of being under-screened from twofold to threefold for the Pap smear ($OR = 2.0$), clinical breast examination ($OR = 2.2$), mammography ($OR = 3.1$), and blood pressure screening ($OR = 2.0$).

Even among women with a regular physician, however, differences emerge based on the physician's specialty. Nonelderly women whose regular physician is a family practitioner or internist are more likely to be underscreened for a clinical breast examination ($OR = 2.3$), Pap smear ($OR = 2.9$), and, to a much lesser extent, blood cholesterol screening ($OR = 1.6$) than those women who see an obstetrician-gynecologist as their regular physician (tab. 2.3). Also, having no regular doctor increases the likelihood of being underscreened for all services except mammography.

Finally, even after health insurance coverage and other indicators of access are controlled for in the multivariate models, nonelderly women with lower incomes and less education are still more likely to be underscreened for the Pap smear and clinical breast examination. Women with family incomes of less than $25,000 have higher odds of not being screened at recommended intervals for the Pap smear ($OR = 1.3$) and clinical breast examination ($OR = 1.7$) than do women with incomes over this amount. Women with less education (less than a college education) also have higher odds of not receiving the Pap smear ($OR = 1.5$), clinical breast examination ($OR = 1.6$), or blood cholesterol screening ($OR = 1.4$) than do women with at least some college education. These findings demonstrate that, although health insurance coverage is important to increase the use of preventive services, social disadvantage remains a powerful determinant of access.

This analysis shows that, even when we control for the multiple factors that influence access to clinical preventive services, women who are disadvantaged in the health system or in their social condition are less likely to receive these services than are nondisadvantaged women. Examples of the effects of insurance coverage and education are provided to illustrate how women who are disadvantaged fare in the system. The comparison of two women—one insured and one uninsured—who are forty to sixty-four years of age and have a high school education, family income below $25,000, a regular source of care, and a physician who is an internist, clearly illustrates the differences in access. The woman with insurance coverage that includes the Pap smear has a 33 percent probability of not having a Pap smear in the past year; in comparison, the woman who is uninsured, but similar in other respects, has a 57 percent probability of not having the test. Similarly, by varying only education, and keeping all other characteristics the same, we can examine the effects of social conditions on the receipt of the Pap smear. An insured woman with the same demographic and health care system factors described above, and who has had at least some college education, has a 25 percent probability of not having a Pap smear in the past year; in comparison, an insured woman with all the same characteristics, except no college education, has a 33 percent probability of not being screened in the past year.

BARRIERS REPORTED BY UNDERSCREENED WOMEN

Women who are underscreened—that is, who did not receive at least one of the clinical preventive services in the past year or never received a blood cholesterol screening—reported several reasons for the lack of screening (tab. 2.4). The most frequently cited barrier is cost, which 33 percent of women reported as a reason for not being screened (tab. 2.4). Women under sixty-five are twice as likely as those over sixty-five to report an economic reason for not receiving services (38% versus 16%, respectively). The fact that cost is such an inhibiting factor in women's use of preventive care demonstrates how characteristics of the health care system (such as inadequate coverage) combine with many women's less-advantaged economic position to create an un-equal distribution of health care resources. Thirty-eight percent of low-er-income women (income less than $25,000) reported a cost problem, compared with 25 percent of women with incomes above $25,000. Cost is also a particularly strong barrier for uninsured women, 69 percent of whom reported it as a reason why they did not receive at least one of the screenings. Having insurance does not guarantee that preventive health services will be affordable, however. One out of three women (29%) with insurance coverage reported that cost is a barrier to use. High cost-sharing arrangements and the lack of coverage for specific services increase the financial risk for insured women, especially for those with limited resources.

The second most frequently cited reason for not obtaining a preventive service is lack of time, with one of four women (25%) reporting this as a factor. Nonelderly women are much more likely to experience time constraints than women sixty-five or older (29% versus 9%, respec-

Table 2.4. Percentage of Underscreened Women Ages Eighteen Years and Older Reporting Barriers to Health Care, 1993

Age	Cost	Time Constraints	Lack of MD Suggestion	Transportation Problems	Appointment Problems	Afraid of Results
18–64	38	29	21	8	6	9
65+	16	9	17	8	a	a
Total	33	25	20	8	5	8

Source: Data from The Commonwealth Fund survey on women's health, 1993.

a Sample size too small to produce reliable estimates.

tively). Women with multiple roles and responsibilities are the most affected. Women who work full-time reported the most time pressures. One-third of full-time workers (34%) who did not receive clinical preventive services reported that time is a barrier, compared with 26 percent of women who work part-time and 22 percent of women who do not work.

It is easy to dismiss time constraints as an individual problem for women. However, time constraints point to the multiple responsibilities that women have and the difficulties of balancing multiple commitments. Women are often responsible not just for their own health but also for the health of their family, and they often experience competing demands for time and have to make trade-offs to allocate the scarce resources available to them. The health care system can alleviate some of the time pressures women experience by improving the coordination of care offered to women and by providing on-site services, accessible either within a community or at the workplace.

The third most cited reason (by 20% of all women) for not receiving a preventive service is that it was not mentioned or suggested by a provider, a factor for 21 percent of nonelderly women and 17 percent of elderly women who did not receive services. Studies have shown the importance of physician suggestion or referral as a factor in receiving screenings (Romans et al. 1991). The high proportion of women who reported that they did not receive a recommendation or suggestion from their physician emphasizes the need for better training of physicians in preventive health care and adequate reimbursement and perhaps incentives to encourage the provision of such services.

Additional barriers to access reported by women are problems with transportation (8%) and an inability to obtain an appointment (5%). Although a relatively small percentage of women reported these as problems, they may reflect very entrenched features of the health care system. Lack of transportation may indicate not only a woman's inability to afford a car but also the maldistribution of health care providers. Physicians are less likely to practice in inner cities and rural areas, thus making transportation to a provider more difficult. Problems with obtaining an appointment may be related to insurance coverage inequities. Low provider reimbursement discourages physicians from accepting patients on Medicaid.

Eight percent of women reported that fear of the results of the screening was the reason they did not have a clinical preventive service. Some of this fear may be alleviated through appropriate and sensitive counseling by health care providers.

IMPLICATIONS FOR POLICY

Our study documented the powerful effects of financial barriers, other characteristics of the health system, and social and educational disadvantage on women's use of important clinical preventive services. We found, not surprisingly, that financial barriers have a profound effect on women's access to preventive care: women are more likely to use clinical preventive services if they have comprehensive insurance coverage and are adequately informed about their benefits. Although these findings accord with those of other research studies (Hayward et al. 1988; Woolhandler and Himmelstein 1988) and with common sense, our findings also demonstrate how many women remain uninsured and how many more have insurance coverage but do not have coverage for preventive services or are uncertain about whether they have such coverage. Only six in ten nonelderly women have insurance that clearly covers the Pap smear and mammography. Those who do not have such coverage are much less likely to receive essential clinical preventive services.

These findings argue strongly that full coverage for preventive health services at recommended intervals should be included in any benefits package if women are to have adequate financial access to these services. This requirement would ensure that women who have any health insurance coverage would be covered for these services, and it would facilitate efforts to inform women of these benefits. These steps would reduce the financial barriers that discourage women from obtaining preventive care.

Furthermore, the finding that cost remains a barrier to use even among insured women further suggests that catastrophic coverage, which imposes large deductibles and coinsurance on patients, would not increase the use of clinical preventive services to appropriate levels. If women must pay large out-of-pocket fees for preventive care, those who are economically disadvantaged will be much less likely to receive these services at recommended intervals. A recent study found that women ages fifteen to forty-four spend a larger proportion of their income on out-of-pocket medical costs than men the same ages because of the inadequacy of coverage for preventive and reproductive services. Furthermore, poor women assume a disproportionate share of this burden; 26 percent of poor women have out-of-pocket health expenditures exceeding 10 percent of their income, compared with 4.7 percent of high-income women (Women's Research and Education Institute 1994). Most of the major health care reform proposals prohibit cost sharing for a defined set of clinical preventive services, a provision that would reduce or eliminate the financial barriers that now discourage even women with coverage from receiving these services.

In addition to our findings concerning financial barriers, we found that nonfinancial barriers—including those related to the structure and process of the health system and those related to the social context of women's lives—are powerful deterrents to the use of clinical preventive services. Even after controlling for health insurance coverage, many women, particularly those who are economically and educationally disadvantaged, are still less likely to receive Pap smears and clinical breast examinations. Having a regular source of health care and a regular doctor at that source is important to women receiving these preventive services. Nearly one-third of women lack these facilitators of access. Moreover, having a gynecologist, as opposed to an internist or family practitioner, as the regular provider also greatly increases the odds of a woman receiving a Pap smear or clinical breast examination.

These findings suggest two important policy directions for organizing the delivery of health care. First, having a regular primary care practitioner should be viewed as an important component of women's health care. Simply providing geographic and financial access to health services will not sufficiently improve women's use of these clinical preventive services. The services themselves need to be organized to facilitate patients having a regular primary care provider.

Our findings suggest another policy consideration: that women may benefit from having a women's health specialist as their primary care provider, an area that requires additional research and consideration. Defining gynecologists as primary care providers would substantially increase the probability that women will receive Pap smears and clinical breast examinations. However, such a policy may pose problems for managed care plans, because they control use, in part, by limiting access to specialists. Even managed care plans that do not offer women's health specialists as primary care providers are well positioned to educate all of their practitioners about the value of preventive services and to offer incentives that encourage them to recommend or perform these services at appropriate intervals. Such steps may increase the use of clinical preventive services among women who have a generalist practitioner as their primary care provider.

Even after controlling for financial barriers and health system factors, however, women with lower incomes and/or less education have lower odds of receiving a Pap smear or a clinical breast examination. These findings suggest that special measures are necessary to promote access to and the use of services by disadvantaged women. Physicians, other health professionals, health plans, and public agencies should develop special outreach programs targeted to women at risk of not receiving preventive care to inform them about the need for particular preventive services, reduce barriers to their use, and bring services into the communities where disadvantaged women live (Lane and Burg 1993).

None of these proposals, however, would take direct steps to facilitate the use of preventive services by women whose competing social roles and responsibilities—paid employment, household work, and care of children and dependent parents—interfere with their own need for appropriate health care. A considerable portion of women who did not receive screening at appropriate intervals reported that time constraints were a deterrent to the use of services. These broader social conditions that affect women can also be addressed by public policy. For example, employers can provide women with paid time off to enable them to obtain preventive health care, just as most workers now receive sick leave. Health plans and public agencies can encourage and help women with family responsibilities to get the preventive care they need by educating husbands and other family members and by providing child care and transportation when needed. Health plans and employers also can coordinate joint efforts to provide preventive care at places where large numbers of women are employed.

Our study demonstrates that policy changes are needed to improve access to preventive health services. An effective strategy cannot be a simplistic, one-factor solution; it must involve changes on several fronts. Reducing or eliminating financial barriers by extending health insurance coverage more widely, ensuring that all plans include coverage for clinical preventive services at recommended intervals, and limiting or prohibiting patient cost sharing for these services are essential. An effective strategy, however, also requires organizing the delivery of care to facilitate access to these services, especially ensuring that women have a regular primary care practitioner who recognizes the importance of their receiving preventive care as recommended. Our analysis shows the importance of physician recommendation among a population-based sample; other studies have also shown the importance of the physician's role among women who use services (Burack et al. 1993). Finally, special educational and outreach efforts are needed for women whose own financial, educational, or social situations reduce their access to preventive care. Improving access to clinical preventive services is a critical component of women's health. An effective, feasible reform strategy is needed to achieve this goal.

IMPLICATIONS FOR RESEARCH

Our findings indicate several areas where additional research is warranted. First, a significant percentage of insured women are not clear about whether their insurance covers clinical preventive services. Research is needed on the most effective ways to inform women about their covered benefits. Clearly, having a standardized benefit package would reduce some of the confusion over coverage, but it would not entirely eliminate the lack of clarity. A significant portion of women on Medicare are not familiar with what clinical preventive services are covered.

Second, many women report that the lack of a physician suggesting a service also was a factor in their not being screened. More research is needed on the factors that promote a preventive orientation among providers. This would help structure professional and continuing education to encourage the integration of clinical preventive services into practice. This is of particular importance for physicians whose practice consists of a large proportion of underscreened women or women with multiple medical problems, whose preventive health needs may be perceived to be less salient.

Third, to ensure that special educational and outreach efforts are reaching their intended population, research analyzing the effectiveness of different educational and outreach programs is needed, especially analysis that focuses on how to effectively reach groups of women with the lowest rates of use, such as low-income, minority, and older women. Information about successful educational and outreach campaigns needs to be disseminated broadly to ensure that proven techniques can be replicated effectively.

Finally, facilitating access to clinical preventive services is only part of the process of improving the health of women through a reduction of preventable morbidity and mortality. Additional research is needed on the coordination and process of care once a woman has been screened and identified as needing further diagnostic work or treatment. Recent studies have shown that such factors as health insurance status and the site of care may affect the clinical outcomes of women diagnosed with breast cancer (Ayanian et al. 1993; Lee-Feldstein, Anton-Culver, and Feldstein 1994). Disparities in access to services, treatment approaches, and clinical outcomes among subgroups of women need to be investigated further to eliminate the causes of any inequities in the health care system.

NOTES

1. Data are not displayed for women obtaining screening over a 3-year interval or for those women who reported that they have never been tested.

2. The sample size was too small to report information about insured women who are unclear about their benefit coverage.

3. This was measured as ever having received a test. When rates of use in the past year are examined, women without a regular source of care have lower rates than women with a usual source.

4. The sample size was too small to conduct this analysis for women over sixty-five, because only 2 percent reported a gynecologist as their regular provider.

5. We used the following time intervals to define lack of timely screening or inadequate screening: Pap smear—not screened in the past year; clinical breast examination—not screened in the past year; blood pressure screening—not screened in the past year; and blood cholesterol screening—never screened. Sample sizes were too small to use this methodology for women sixty-five years or older.

REFERENCES

American College of Obstetricians and Gynecologists. 1992. State Legislative Fact Sheet: State Mammography Laws.
———. 1993. ACOG Committee Opinion: Routine Cancer Screening, no. 128.
Ayanian, J., Kohler, B., Abe, T., and Epstein, A. 1993. The relationship between health insurance coverage and clinical outcomes among women with breast cancer. *New England Journal of Medicine* 329:326–31.
Bal, D. G. 1992. Cancer in African Americans. *Ca-A Cancer Journal for Clinicians* 42:5–6.
Boring, C. C., Squires, T. S., and Heath C. W., Jr. 1992. Guest editorial: cancer statistics for African Americans. *Ca-A Cancer Journal for Clinicians* 42:7–17.

Boring, C. C., Squires, T. S., and Tong T. 1992. Cancer statistics, 1993. *Ca-A Cancer Journal for Clinicians* 43:7–26.

Burack, R., et al. 1993. Patterns of use of mammography among inner-city Detroit women: contrasts between a health department, HMO, and private hospital. *Medical Care* 31:322–34.

Burg, M. A., Lane, D. S., and Polednak, A. P. 1990. Age group differences in the use of breast cancer screening tests: the effects of health care utilization and socioeconomic variables. *Journal of Aging and Health* 2:514–30.

Calle, E. E., et al. 1993. Demographic predictors of mammography and Pap smear screening in US women. *American Journal of Public Health* 83:53–60.

Collins, K. S., et al. 1994. *Assessing and Improving Women's Health.* Washington, D.C.: Women's Research and Education Institute.

Dodd, G. 1992. American Cancer Society guidelines on screening for breast cancer: an overview. *Ca-A Cancer Journal for Clinicians* 42:177–80.

Farley, T. A., and Flannery, J. T. 1989. Late-stage diagnosis of breast cancer in women of lower socioeconomic status: public health implications. *American Journal of Public Health* 79:1508–12.

Fink, D. 1988. Change in American Cancer Society checkup guidelines for detection of cervical cancer. *Ca-A Cancer Journal for Clinicians* 38:127–28.

―――. 1991. *Guidelines for the Cancer-Related Checkup: Recommendations and Rationale,* American Cancer Society.

Franks, P., and Clancy, C. M. 1993. Physician gender bias in clinical decision-making: screening for cancer in primary care. *Medical Care* 31:213–18.

Harlan, L., Bernstein, A., and Kessler, L. 1991. Cervical cancer screening: who is not screened and why? *American Journal of Public Health* 81:885–90.

Hayward, R. A., et al. 1988. Who gets screened for cervical and breast cancer?: results from a new national study. *Archives of Internal Medicine* 148:1177–81.

Lane, D., and Burg, M. 1993. Strategies to increase mammography utilization among community health center visitors: improving awareness, accessibility, and affordability. *Medical Care* 31:175–81.

Lee-Feldstein, A., Anton-Culver, H., and Feldstein, P. 1994. Treatment differences and other prognostic factors related to breast cancer survival: delivery systems and medical outcomes. *Journal of the American Medical Association* 271:1163–68.

Longman, A. J., Saint-Germain, M. A., and Modiano, M. 1992. Use of breast cancer screening by older Hispanic women. *Public Health Nursing* 9:118–24.

Lurie, N., et al. 1993. Preventive care for women: does the sex of the physician matter? *New England Journal of Medicine* 329:478–82.

Makuc, D. M., Freid, V. M., and Kleiman, J. C. 1989. National trends in the use of preventive health care by women. *American Journal of Public Health* 79:21–26.

Mandelblatt, M., et al. 1993. Breast and cervical cancer screening for poor, elderly, black women: clinical results and implications. *American Journal of Preventive Medicine* 9:133–38.

Marchant, D. J., and Sutton, S. M. 1990. Use of mammography, United States, 1990. *Morbidity and Mortality Weekly Report* 39:621–30.

Muller, C., Mandelblatt, J., Schechter, C. B., Power, E. J., Duffy, B. M., and Wagner, J. L. 1990. Costs and effectiveness of cervical cancer screening in elderly women. Health program, Office of Technology Assessment. February.

National Cancer Institute. 1993a. Cancer screening summary: cervical cancer screening.

———. 1993b. Cancer facts: updating the guidelines for breast cancer screening.

———. 1991. Cancer Statistics Review, 1973–1988.

Piani, A., and Schoenborn, C. 1993. Health promotion and disease prevention, United States, 1990. National Center for Health Statistics. *Vital Health Statistics* 10.

Romans, M. C., et al. 1991. Utilization of screening mammography, 1990. *Women's Health Issues* 1:68–73.

Schauffler, H. H. 1993. Disease prevention policy under Medicare: a historical and political analysis. *American Journal of Preventive Medicine* 2:71–77.

U.S. Preventive Services Task Force. 1989. *Guide to Clinical Preventive Services: An Assessment of the Effectiveness of 169 Interventions.* Baltimore: Williams and Wilkins.

Volkers, N. 1993. Board recommends changes to draft breast cancer screening guidelines. *Journal of the National Cancer Institute* 85:1794–96.

Women's Research and Education Institute. 1994. *Women's Health Insurance Costs and Experiences.* Washington, D.C.

Woolhandler, S., and Himmelstein, D. U. 1988. Reverse targeting of preventive care due to lack of health insurance. *Journal of the American Medical Association* 259:2872.

3

Gender and Patterns of Physician-Patient Communication

Sherrie H. Kaplan, Ph.D., M.P.H.
Lisa M. Sullivan, Ph.D.
Dante Spetter, Ph.D.
Kimberly A. Dukes, M.A.
Amina Khan, M.A.
Sheldon Greenfield, M.D.

Considerable attention has recently been paid, in both the scientific community and the popular media, to the differences in conversational behavior between men and women. Men have been portrayed as more conversationally dominant, interrupting women more frequently than women interrupt them, more resistant to certain types of information seeking, more comfortable with "public" than with "private" speaking (Gilligan, 1982; Mattz and Borker, 1982; Carli, 1989; Tannen, 1990). Do these putative gender differences in general conversational behaviors and styles manifest themselves in the interpersonal aspects of health care, or, more specifically, in physician-patient communication? Women have frequently been found to have longer office visits than men (Meeuwesen, Schaap, and Van Der Staak, 1991; Roter, Lipkin, and Korsgaard, 1991; Bensing, van der Brink-Muinen, and de Bakker, 1993), talk more and present more complaints during those visits (Meeuwesen, Schaap, and Van Der Staak, 1991; Bensing, van der Brink-Muinen, and de Bakker, 1993), ask more questions (Wallen, Waitzkin, and Stoeckle, 1979; Kaplan and Greenfield, 1991; Roter, Lipkin, and Korsgaard, 1991), and get more information from both male and female physicians (Hooper et al., 1982; Waitzken, 1985; Kaplan and Greenfield, 1991). What implications, if any, do these paradoxical gender differences in communicating with physicians, which appear to favor women, have for patient outcomes?

Effective communication between physicians and patients has been shown to lead to improved patient health outcomes (Kaplan, Greenfield, and Ware, 1989a, 1989b). Patients who give lower ratings to physicians' interpersonal care are more likely to change physicians at least once, if not multiple times, over the period of a year (Marquis, Davies, and Ware, 1983; Ware and Davies, 1983; Louis Harris and Associates, 1985; Kaplan et al., 1996). Gender differences in interpersonal care and physician-patient communication may then confer differential experiences of health and other outcomes of care, by gender.

This chapter provides an overview of gender differences in interpersonal care (e.g., patterns and styles of communication) and their implications for provider-patient relationships. We also consider the degree to which methodological problems (e.g., bias in the measurement of health, appropriateness of study designs, etc.) might have led to exaggerated or spurious gender differences in interpersonal care. In the context of this overview, we present the results of a recent survey by The Commonwealth Fund on women's health and health care, which highlight a number of the problems inherent in conducting and interpreting gender research in interpersonal care.

DIFFERENCES IN INTERPERSONAL CARE

Physician Behavior

In several studies of interpersonal care, a substantial, if not the greatest proportion of variation has been attributed to the physician, rather than to patient, visit, or clinic characteristics in a number of variables, including patient satisfaction with care (PSQ Project Co-Investigators, 1989; Meeuwesen, Schaap, and Van Der Staak, 1991; Tamblyn et al., 1994), participatory decision-making style (propensity to involve patients in treatment) (Kaplan et al., 1996), and time spent waiting to see the physician (Tamblyn et al., 1994). Among the characteristics of physicians related in empirical studies to the interpersonal care process, the gender of the physician has been most consistently linked with variations in physician behavior. Women physicians spend on average approximately 2 minutes longer with patients in outpatient settings than do their male colleagues (Meeuwesen, Schaap, and Van Der Staak, 1991; Roter, Lipkin, and Korsgaard, 1991; Bensing, van der Brink-Muinen, and de Bakker, 1993). Women have been found to order more tests, prescribe more medications, order fewer procedures, and express more doubt than their male colleagues (Bensing, van der Brink-Muinen, and de Bakker, 1993).

In studies of physician-patient communication based on audiotaped conversations, women physicians have been noted to talk more during outpatient visits, exhibit more positive affect, and provide more information than men physicians (Kaplan and Greenfield, 1991; Roter, Lipkin, and Korsgaard, 1991). Women physicians have also been noted to be less controlling (Kaplan and Greenfield, 1991; Meeuwesen, Schaap, and Van Der Staak, 1991; Bensing, van der Brink-Muinen, and de Bakker, 1993), to have more egalitarian views (Heins et al., 1979), and to do more counseling than their male colleagues (Bensing, van der Brink-Muinen, and de Bakker, 1993). In a study using simulated patients, women physicians were reported to have a better interpersonal manner than their male colleagues (Colliver et al., 1993).

Some studies have shown that the gender of the patient is related to physicians' interpersonal behavior. Fewer physician-initiated interruptions have been observed for female than for male patients (Hooper et al., 1982). Men physicians have been noted to be more controlling with male versus female patients (Kaplan and Greenfield, 1991; Meeuwesen, Schaap, and Van Der Staak, 1991) and to give more objective information to female versus male patients (Meeuwesen, Schaap, and Van Der Staak, 1991). In a study using videotaped encounters with simulated patients, Lapp et al. (1983) found that in a predominantly male sample of physicians, women patients got 20 percent more prescriptions than men, but that the "vagueness of the complaint," versus patient gender, accounted for the difference. Physicians viewed women patients in this study who displayed demanding behavior as more attention-seeking than men patients displaying the same behavior.

Patient Behavior

Women appear to receive differentially better interpersonal care than men. The length of office visits with physicians is generally longer for women than for men (Meeuwesen, Schaap, and Van Der Staak, 1991; Roter, Lipkin, and Korsgaard, 1991). During these visits, women have been noted to talk more and to present more complaints (Verbrugge, 1980; Meeuwesen, Schaap, and Van Der Staak, 1991). Further, women differ from men in the ways they express complaints (Martin, Arnold, and Parker, 1988; Meeuwesen, Schaap, and Van Der Staak, 1991; Dawson et al., 1992). Women have been noted, for example, to express more psychosocial complaints than men (Meeuwesen, Schaap, and Van Der Staak, 1991). To the extent that the expression of such complaints influences physician behavior (e.g., psychosocial visits are longer than somatic visits [Meeuwesen, Schaap, and Van Der Staak, 1991] and may be more prevalent in certain primary care settings [Bowman and Gelbach, 1980]), women may receive qualitatively different care than men. Women patients ask more questions than men during office visits (Wallen, Waitzkin, and Stoeckle, 1979; Kaplan and Greenfield, 1991), get more information and explanations from their physicians (Wallen, Waitzkin, and Stoeckle, 1979; Hooper et al., 1982; Kaplan and Greenfield, 1991), and express more emotion than men during visits (Hooper et al., 1982; Kaplan and Greenfield, 1991). Some researchers in physician-patient communication note a tendency toward reciprocity in conversation (Roter, Lipkin, and Korsgaard, 1991). Greater affect expressed by physicians with women patients (Kaplan and Greenfield, 1991) may therefore in part reflect patient behavior. Women patients' ratings of interpersonal care reflect these differences, giving physicians higher ratings on information giving and empathy, compared with men patients (Hooper et al., 1982).

Physicians also appear to be less controlling with women than with men patients (Cleary, Burns, and Nyez, 1990), initiating fewer conversational interruptions with women than with men (Hooper et al., 1982). Some research suggests that physicians anticipate that women patients will be more demanding than men (Bernstein and Kane, 1981; Lapp et al., 1983).

To reflect physician bias, care would have to be delivered in a manner that is inconsistent with appropriate or needed service, and not reflect physicians' responses to patient preferences, or, for example, conservative treatment of women in the face of incomplete efficacy data. If women are more articulate, better informed, and better able to make their preferences known to physicians, as strongly suggested by the literature, it is difficult to assert that any superficially observed gender differences in health care are a product of physician bias versus shared decision making or appropriate care.

THE COMMONWEALTH FUND WOMEN'S HEALTH SURVEY

The Commonwealth Fund women's health survey is a recent national cross-sectional survey of 3,525 American men and women. It is presented in detail as an example of gender-related research on differences in interpersonal care. We present selected results and discuss them in the context of what is known and hypothesized about gender differences in health and health care and its relevance for current health policy.

Data Collection Methods

Data collection procedures have been described in detail elsewhere. Briefly, data were collected by telephone interview from a national cross-sectional sample of 2,525 women and 1,000 men in the United States, aged eighteen or older. To permit ethnic/racial comparisons, Hispanic ($N = 405$) and African American ($N = 439$) women were oversampled. Data were weighted based on age, race, education, insurance status, and Census region to ensure accuracy of inferences to the population of 94.6 million American women.

Sample Description

The age distributions of men and women in the sample were similar. Fifty-five percent and 59 percent of the women and men, respectively, were between the ages of eighteen and forty-four, while 18 percent and 14 percent of women and men, respectively, were aged sixty-five or older. The sample was predominantly white, accounting for 84 percent of the women and 81 percent of the men in the sample. The educational backgrounds of the respondents reflected a relatively well educated group and did not differ by gender—seventy-nine percent of both men and women had graduated from high school; 23 percent of women and 27 percent of men were college graduates or had postgraduate degrees. Income distributions were also similar by gender, with 27 percent of the women and 19 percent of men reporting annual incomes of $15,000 or less. A majority of the sample was married (55% of women and 64% of men).

Measures

All measures used in this analysis were based on interview data. No other data sources were used to validate responses. The primary outcome variable for the analysis presented below is provider switching due to dissatisfaction with care, dichotomized into groups—those who had ever switched physicians and those who had not. The gender of patients' current physician was used to classify patients by their physician gender. Switching therefore did not reflect switching *from* or *to* the present provider, but simply prior switching behavior. As independent variables and covariates, we included patients' current health status, measured using a single-item rating of health from excellent to poor; prior use of physician services, including the number of physician visits and number of different physicians seen in the prior year; characteristics of office visits, measured as the average time spent with the physician in minutes; patients' preferences for a specific gender of physician, measured on a scale ranging from strongly prefer a male to strongly prefer a female; patients' self-reported assessment of personal difficulty in communicating with physicians, measured on a scale ranging from finding it very difficult to talk to physicians to not difficult at all; and patients' overall ratings of interpersonal care, based on a multiple-item assessment of physicians' interpersonal care as well as specific aspects of physician-patient communication; and the primary reasons for switching physicians, measured among those who had ever changed physicians due to dissatisfaction with care.

Analytic Methods

The primary analytic objectives were to examine gender differences in physician-patient communication patterns, and to understand their relationship to disruptions of the physician-patient relationship, represented by switching providers. The first phase of the analysis involved the construction of a multiple-item measure of physicians' interpersonal care. Principal components analysis with a varimax rotation was used to identify the factor structure underlying seven candidate items addressing various aspects of physicians' interpersonal care (e.g., knowledgeable and competent to treat illness, cares about you and your health, spends enough time with you). This analysis revealed a single dimension, explaining 69.6 percent of the variation in the individual items. A multiple-item scale based on this analysis was constructed using cluster scoring. Internal consistency reliability of this scale was assessed using Cronbach's alpha and found to exceed standards for group comparisons (alpha = 0.93).

The second phase of the analysis involved a comparison of male and female patients for the dependent variable (switching) and independent variables and covariates (e.g., patients' health status, prior use of services, preference for specific provider gender, interpersonal care ratings, etc.), using two independent sample *t*-tests and chi-square tests. Two-way analysis of variance models was developed to test for patient and physician gender effects on the major study variables. Models with and without the interaction of patient and physician gender were evaluated. Separate logistic regression models were developed relating patient and physician gender to each reason for switching physician due to dissatisfaction. These analyses were restricted to the subsample of patients who reported ever switching physicians due to dissatisfaction.

The final phase of the analysis involved the development of a multiple logistic regression model relating all previously considered variables to provider switching, including patient and physician gender, patients' health status, prior use of health services, visit characteristics, overall ratings of interpersonal care, preference for specific gender provider, physician-patient communication, and specific reasons for switching. Both direct entry and backward elimination models were investigated. Parameter estimates, odds ratios, and 95 percent confidence limits on odds ratios were provided for the final model.

Results

Gender Differences in Major Study Variables. With the exception of overall health rating and self-reported difficulty in talking to physicians, there were significant differences between male and female respondents in most major study variables (tab. 3.1). Considerably more women than men had ever switched physicians due to dissatisfaction (41.0% versus 27.3%, respectively, $p < 0.0001$). Consistent with the literature on gender differences in the use of health care services described above, women in this study had made more visits to the physician in the prior year and had seen more physicians during that period. Although the average length of the visit did not differ significantly by gender, findings are in the hypothesized direction, with women reporting longer visits than men. Also consistent with the literature, women rated physicians' interpersonal care more favorably than men.

Patient Gender Differences in the Gender of the Provider Seen. The majority of respondents in this study saw male physicians (tab. 3.2). Despite the small proportion of respondents seeing female physicians, twice as many women as men saw a female physician. In assessing the characteristics of patients seeing same- versus opposite-gender physicians, we found that patients of male physicians were significantly older than

Table 3.1. Means and Standard Deviations of Major Study Variables, by Patient Gender

Study Variable	k of Items	Range of Scores	Meaning of a High Score	Male (N = 1,000)	Female (N = 2,525)	p^a
Overall health status rating[b]	1	1–5	Poorer health	2.3 (0.03)	2.4 (0.02)	0.1212
Percentage ever switching physicians due to dissatisfaction[c]	1	0–1	Switch physicians	27.3%	41.0%	0.0001[d]
Number of physician visits in past year[e]	1	1–99	More visits	5.1 (0.32)	6.3 (0.19)	0.0019
Number of different physicians seen in past year[f]	1	0–10	More physicians	1.8 (0.05)	2.0 (0.03)	0.0024
Average time spent with physician per visit (in minutes)[g]	1	1–240	Longer visits	24.7 (0.84)	26.6 (0.50)	0.0537
Rating of physician's interpersonal care[h]	7	2–10	Higher rating	8.3 (0.06)	8.5 (0.04)	0.0061
General difficulty talking to physicians[i]	1	1–5	Not difficult	4.3 (0.04)	4.3 (0.02)	0.5655

Source: Data from The Commonwealth Fund survey on women's health, 1993.

[a] Significance based on two independent samples' *t*-test.

[b] Health status was rated using a single item where 1 = excellent, 2 = very good, 3 = good, 4 = fair, and 5 = poor.

[c] Indicator variable denoting whether patients ever switched physicians due to dissatisfaction.

[d] Significance based on χ_1^2 test.

[e] Total number of visits to physicians in the previous year: 16.4 percent of respondents reported no visits; of those making any visits to physicians, 80.0 percent made 7 visits or fewer in the previous year; 2.7 percent made 30 or more visits.

[f] Total number of different physicians seen in the previous year: 11.9 percent of respondents had not seen a physician; 74.4 percent had seen 2 or fewer, 5.7 percent had seen 5 or more.

[g] Total time (in minutes) that physician spent with patient on the last visit.

[h] Multiple-item scale measure of physicians' interpersonal care style.

[i] Single item indicating patients' difficulty talking to their physician where 1 = very difficult, 5 = not difficult at all, and 3 = not sure.

Table 3.2. Proportions (and Numbers)
of Male and Female Patients Seeing Same-
and Opposite-Gender Physicians

	Patient Gender	
Physician Gender	Male ($N = 793$)	Female ($N = 2162$)
Male ($N = 2532$)	92.4% ($N = 733$)	83.2% ($N = 1,798$)
Female ($N = 423$)	7.6% ($N = 60$)	16.8% ($N = 363$)

Source: Data from The Commonwealth Fund survey on women's health, 1993.

Note: $\chi^2 = 40.47$, $p < 0.0001$.

those of female physicians (45.4 years versus 43.4 years, $F_{MD} = 23.47$, $p < 0.0001$), were less well educated (12.7 years versus 13.4 years, $p < 0.0001$), had lower annual incomes ($35,000 versus $40,000, $p < 0.0001$), and reported significantly lower overall health status (2.4 versus 2.2, $p < 0.01$, where a lower score indicates better health). Female patients of female physicians were significantly younger than any other patient-physician group (tab. 3.3). Male patients of female physicians were significantly better educated, had higher incomes, and were more healthy than any other patient-physician group.

With respect to the previous use of health care services, there were no differences between patients seeing male versus female physicians. There were differences between female and male patients, however, with females making more physician visits in the previous year. The most visits were made by male patients of female physicians. There were no significant patient or physician gender differences in the number of different physicians seen in the previous year.

Patients of male physicians were significantly more likely to report a preference for a male versus a female physician (see tab. 3.3). Female patients seeing female physicians also reported a preference for same-gender physicians. However, there were no differences in the preference of physician gender for those patients seeing opposite-gender physicians.

Physician Switching by Patient and Current Physician Gender. Female patients were roughly twice as likely as men to have ever switched physicians due to dissatisfaction. More patients of female physicians

Table 3.3. Characteristics of Male and Female Patients Seeing Male and Female Physicians

| Patient Characteristic | Physician Gender | Patient Gender | | $F_{MD}{}^a$ |
		Male (N = 1,000)	Female (N = 2,525)	
Age[b]	Male	44.6	46.3	23.47***
	Female	46.0	40.8	
		$F_{PT}{}^c = 2.38$		
Educational level[d]	Male	13.0	12.5	24.73***
	Female	13.4	13.3	
		$F_{PT} = 12.68$***		
Income[e]	Male	38.1	33.5	12.16***
	Female	42.8	38.2	
		$F_{PT} = 17.70$***		
Overall health status rating[f]	Male	2.3	2.4	6.91**
	Female	2.2	2.3	
		$F_{PT} = 3.87$*		
Number of physician visits in past year[g]	Male	5.2	6.6	0.06
	Female	7.5	6.0	
		$F_{PT} = 8.05$**		
Number of different physicians seen in past year[h]	Male	1.9	2.1	2.90
	Female	2.7	2.1	
		$F_{PT} = 1.98$		
Preference for gender of physician[i]	Male	2.6	2.9	242.15***
	Female	3.1	3.6	
		$F_{PT} = 98.75$**		

Source: Data from The Commonwealth Fund survey on women's health, 1993.

Note: Table entries are mean scores by patient and physician gender. $*p < 0.05$, $**p < 0.01$, $***p < 0.001$.

[a] F(1, 2969) statistic testing for physician gender effects in two-way analysis of variance.

[b] Patient age in years.

[c] F(1, 2969) statistic testing for patient gender effects in two-way analysis of variance.

[d] Educational level was reported as the highest level completed, from 1 = less than high school to 5 = postgraduate, with a score of 3 corresponding to some college, but no baccalaureate degree; midpoints were used for each level reflecting years of formal education.

[e] Income was reported as total 1992 household income, in 8 categories ranging from 1 = $7,500 or less to 8 = $100,000 or more; midpoints were used for each level reflecting income in thousands of dollars.

[f] Health status was rated using a single item where 1 = excellent, 2 = very good, 3 = good, 4 = fair, and 5 = poor.

[g] Total number of visits to physicians in the previous year: 16.4 percent of respondents reported no visits; of those making any visits to physicians, 80.0 percent made 7 visits or fewer in the previous year whereas 2.7 percent of respondents made 30 or more visits.

[h] Total number of different physicians seen in the previous year: 11.9 percent of respondents had not seen a physician; 74.4 percent had seen 2 or fewer; 5.7 percent had seen 5 or more.

[i] Gender preference of physician was reported on a scale ranging from 1 = strongly prefer a male to 5 = strongly prefer a female, with a score of 3 corresponding to a neutral response.

had ever switched than those of male physicians, although these differences were small (tab. 3.4).

Of the 37 percent of patients who had switched physicians, patients cited a variety of reasons for switching (tab. 3.5). The most frequently cited reasons were lack of trust in the physician's skills and poor physician communication skills. There were no significant differences in reasons for switching by patient or physician gender, with two exceptions. A significantly higher proportion of patients of male physicians reported lack of trust in their physicians' skills, compared with patients of female physicians (42.0% versus 31.9%, $p < 0.05$), and more patients of female physicians reported prior switching due to poor physician communication skills.

We found differences by patient and physician gender in three specific physician communication skills: whether physicians "talked down" to patients (treating them like a child), said it was "all in the patient's head," or had to deliver bad news. Twice as many female patients as male patients reported that their physicians had "talked down" to them or treated them like a child (25.4% versus 12.1%, $p < 0.001$; tab. 3.6). Patients of female physicians were significantly more likely to report that they had been "talked down to" by their physicians. As noted above, these data do not allow linking of reported physician behaviors to patients' current primary care physicians. It is possible that patients' reports of these incidents may relate to a prior physician versus the current physician, and may have prompted a switch to the current provider. More than twice as many female patients as male patients reported being told that a condition was "all in

Table 3.4. Proportions of Male and Female Patients Ever Changing Physicians Due to Dissatisfaction, by Physician Gender

	Patient Gender	
Physician Gender	Male ($N = 799$)	Female ($N = 2,177$)
Male ($N = 2,532$)	27%	41%
Female (N 423)	24%	49%

Source: Data from The Commonwealth Fund survey on women's health, 1993.

Note: $\chi^2_{MD} = 4.54$, $p < 0.05$; $\chi^2_{PT} = 42.43$, $p < 0.0001$.

Table 3.5. Primary Reasons for Switching Physicians, by Gender:
Results of Logistic Regression Analyses ($N = 1,304$)

Reason for Switching	Patient Gender			Physician Gender		
	Male ($N = 272$)	Female ($N = 1,032$)	Odds Ratio[a]	Male ($N = 956$)	Female ($N = 191$)	Odds Ratio[b]
Didn't like the physician	15.3%	15.7%	1.30	15.8%	14.5%	0.87
Physician didn't listen	8.3%	13.5%	1.59	12.7%	15.9%	1.22
Physician didn't spend enough time	5.1%	8.0%	1.50	7.9%	6.2%	0.73
Didn't trust physician's skills	47.0%	38.9%	0.86	42.0%	31.8%	0.66*
Poor physician communication skills	25.8%	34.1%	1.27	31.9%	42.2%	1.50*
Physician is unaccessible	8.8%	6.8%	0.72	7.4%	7.8%	1.12
Physician's costs are too high	1.9%	1.8%	0.63	1.6%	2.2%	1.51

Source: Data from The Commonwealth Fund survey on women's health, 1993.

Note: Table entries are proportions of male and female patients, and proportions of patients of male and female physicians, among subsample of patients who switched physicians due to dissatisfaction ($N = 1,304$), endorsing each item. *$p < 0.05$.

[a] Odds of endorsing item (i.e., individual reason for switching physicians) for female patients relative to male patients.

[b] Odds of endorsing item (i.e., individual reason for switching physicians) for patients of female physicians relative to patients of male physicians.

their heads" (16.9% versus 7.3%, respectively, $p < 0.001$), and more female than male patients' physicians had to deliver bad news. There were no significant differences in the proportions of patients of male and female physicians who were told a condition was "all in their heads" or who were told bad news.

Based on a multiple logistic regression of patient characteristics, patients' health status, prior use of health care services, characteristics of the office visit (i.e., length), overall ratings of physicians' interpersonal care, preferences for physician gender, personal difficulty in talking to physicians, and specific physician communication skills, only patient gender, overall rating of physicians' interpersonal skills, and the three physician communication skills were related to physician switching (tab. 3.7). The odds of switching physicians were 1.35 for

Table 3.6. Physician Communication Patterns, by Patient and Physician Gender: Results of Logistic Regression Analyses

	Patient Gender			Physician Gender		
Physician Communication	Male (N = 1,000)	Female (N = 2,525)	Odds Ratio[a]	Male (N = 2,532)	Female (N = 423)	Odds Ratio[b]
Physician "talked down," or treated me like a child	12.1%	25.4%	2.29***	20.6%	31.%	1.62***
Physician said it was "all in my head"	7.3%	16.9%	2.63***	13.6%	18.2%	1.27
Physician had to deliver bad news about a health condition	22.2%	32.7%	1.50***	30.8%	40.0%	1.09

Source: Data from The Commonwealth Fund survey on women's health, 1993.
Note: Table entries are proportions of male and female patients, and proportions of patients of male and female physicians reporting each experience. ***p < 0.001.
[a] Odds of reporting each experience for female patients relative to male patients.
[b] Odds of reporting each experience for patients of female physicians relative to patients of male physicians.

Table 3.7. Factors Related to Switching Physicians:
Results of Multiple Logistic Regression Analysis

Patient Characteristic	Parameter Estimate	Standard Error	Odds Ratio[a]	95% Confidence Interval for Odds Ratio[b]
Patient gender	0.301	0.114	1.35[c]**	(1.08, 1.69)
Physician gender	0.105	0.135	1.11[d]	(0.85, 1.45)
Age	−0.003	0.003	1.00[e]	(0.99, 1.01)
Education	0.001	0.019	1.00[f]	(0.96, 1.04)
Income	0.004	0.002	1.01[g]	(1.00, 1.01)
Overall health status rating	0.084	0.052	1.09	(0.98, 1.02)
Average time spent with physician/visit (in minutes)	0.002	0.002	1.00	(1.00, 1.01)
Rating of physician's interpersonal care	−0.080	0.032	0.92*	(0.87, 0.98)
General difficulty talking to physicians	−0.032	0.050	0.97	(0.88, 1.07)
Physician "talked down"/ treated me like a child	1.850	0.127	6.35***	(4.96, 8.16)
Physician said it was "all in my head"	1.193	0.157	3.30***	(2.42, 4.48)
Physician had to deliver bad news	0.600	0.106	1.82***	(1.48, 2.24)

Source: Data from The Commonwealth Fund survey on women's health, 1993.

Note: Table entries are parameter estimates, standard errors, significance levels of Wald χ^2 statistics, and odds ratios from multiple logistic regression model. $*p < 0.05$, $**p < 0.01$, $***p < 0.001$.

[a] Odds of switching physicians relative to a one-unit change in each independent variable.

[b] Ninety-five percent confidence limits on odds ratio.

[c] Odds that female patients switch physicians relative to male patients.

[d] Odds that patients of a female physician switch physicians relative to patients of male physicians.

[e] Odds of switching physicians relative to a 5-year age differential.

[f] Odds of switching physicians relative to a 2-year education differential.

[g] Odds of switching physicians relative to a $10,000 income differential.

female patients as compared to male patients ($p < 0.05$). The odds of switching were 6.35 ($p < 0.001$) for patients whose physicians had "talked down" or treated them like a child, 3.30 ($p < 0.001$) for patients whose physicians had said it was "all in their heads," and 1.82 ($p < 0.001$) for patients whose physicians had had to deliver bad news, as compared to patients whose physicians had not done any of the above.

DISCUSSION

Many of the findings from this study are consistent with the literature cited above. Female patients reported more office visits to physicians in the prior year and more visits to different physicians in the prior year. As observed in previous research, their ratings of physicians' interpersonal care were more favorable than those of male patients (Hooper et al., 1982). Although the findings did not reach statistical significance, the average time spent with physicians per visit was longer than that for men. This finding is also consistent with the literature indicating that women spend approximately 2 minutes per office visit longer with physicians than do men (Meeuwesen, Schaap, and Van Der Staak, 1991; Roter, Lipkin, and Korsgaard, 1991). Few studies in the literature have examined the prevalence of gender congruence or noncongruence between physician-patient pairs. Since women physicians represent only 15 percent of the total physician population (Klepke, Marder, and Silberger, 1987) and considerably less than half of the primary care providers, the proportions of patients seeing women physicians in this study (less than 15%) are not remarkable. It is intriguing that younger, healthier men of higher socioeconomic status were currently seeing women physicians. Those patients were also more likely to prefer a female physician, compared with male patients seeing male physicians. Although there are no data from this study indicating prior experience with same- and opposite-gender physicians, these cross-sectional findings are consistent with those of Fennema et al. (1990), who found that patients preferring a male physician had less experience with female physicians.

With respect to changing or "switching" physicians due to dissatisfaction with care, only 37 percent of the sample whose average age was approximately forty years had *ever* switched physicians for that reason. Among those who did switch physicians, the results of this study support findings in the literature that women, especially younger women, are more assertive, active patients (Wallen, Waitzkin, and Stoeckle, 1979; Lapp et al., 1983; Kaplan and Greenfield, 1991); changing physicians if their standards, are not met would not be inconsistent with their pattern of health care behavior. In contrast, men in this study were much less likely to have ever changed physicians due to dissatisfaction. It could be that men received better care than women patients. However, there is no empirical support for this hypothesis in the literature (Kaplan and Greenfield, 1991; Meeuwesen, Schaap, and

Van Der Staak, 1991; Roter, Lipkin, and Korsgaard, 1991). More likely, men may fail to perceive or may be more tolerant of less optimal interpersonal care than women, and may be less likely to change physicians in response to such care.

The most common reasons for changing physicians reported by respondents to The Commonwealth Fund women's health survey were lack of trust of the physician's skills and poor communication. Of those patients who had ever switched physicians, those currently seeing a male physician had switched because they did not trust the skills of the physician from whom they switched. Of those currently seeing a female physician, more patients switched due to poor physician communication skills. These findings may reflect patient preferences and perceptions of differing attributes of physicians by gender. Fennema et al. (1990) found that humaneness was perceived by patients to be more characteristic of female than male physicians. We found no empirical studies supporting the notion that male physicians are perceived to be more technically skillful than female physicians. Further research is needed to explore the extent to which patients actively choose providers based on assumptions about gender-specific behavior.

Finally, there were patient and physician gender differences in patients' reports of physicians' communication skills. Considerably more females than males reported that they had been "talked down to," told that their health problem was "all in their head," and told unfavorable news about a health condition. These data are somewhat inconsistent with the literature suggesting that physicians are more controlling with male than female patients (Kaplan and Greenfield, 1991; Meeuwesen, Schaap, and Van Der Staak, 1991). If male patients expect to be treated as subservient, deferential to the physician's greater authority (Johnson, 1994), they may expect to be "talked down to" and not regard such behavior as necessarily negative but consistent with the physician's role. Further, while substantially more women than men reported having been told by physicians that their health problem was "all in their head," a very small proportion of patients reported this behavior. Other studies indicate no gender differences in the extent to which patients' complaints are taken seriously by physicians (McCraine, Horowitz, and Martin, 1978; Colameco, Becker, and Simpson, 1983; Heaton and Marquez, 1990). Whether this finding again represents different standards against which women, versus men, evaluate physicians' behavior, requires further research into differences in such standards and their impact on patients' assessments of similar interpersonal care.

That more current patients of female physicians reported that they had been talked down to, compared with male physicians, is difficult to interpret. Given the cross-sectional nature of the study, it is very plausible that patients of female physicians switched to them because they had been talked down to by another, perhaps male physician. It is also possible, as noted above, that patients hold female physicians to a higher standard of behavior, assuming that their gender should confer greater sensitivity and more affiliation (Weisman and Zeitelman, 1985). When they exhibit behavior consistent with their roles as physicians, such as controlling the conversation or obtaining rather than providing information, they may be evaluated more negatively than their male colleagues. To sort out the gender in the assessment of physicians' behavior, further research is needed, exploring simultaneously physicians' conversational behavior, patients' interpersonal care ratings, and patients' subsequent health behavior, including health outcomes and changing providers.

In summary, data from this study suggest that, although proportionately few patients had ever changed physicians due to dissatisfaction, women were roughly twice as likely as men to have changed. Women were also more likely than men to report problems in communication with physicians. For both men and women, such communication problems were the most important contributors to the likelihood of ever changing physicians. A number of other studies also confirmed findings from this study, that patients who give less favorable ratings of physicians' interpersonal care will be more likely to "doctor-shop" (Marquis, Davies, and Ware, 1983; Ware and Davies, 1983; Louis Harris and Associates, 1985; Kaplan et al., 1996). Results from this study suggest that problems with physician-patient communication, versus other patient-rated attributes of physicians, such as technical skills, inaccessibility, costs of care, or spending enough time with patients, may be the primary contributor to terminations of the physician-patient relationship, for both men and women.

Recent research suggests that increased practice volume and decreased time spent per patient are associated with measurable decreases in physicians' interpersonal care, related to changing physicians over a one-year period (Kaplan et al., 1996). Other research also suggests a direct relationship between physician-patient communication and patient outcomes (Kaplan, Greenfield, and Ware, 1989a, 1989b). Current cost-containment initiatives that result in less time per patient may therefore adversely affect physician-patient communication and potentially result in disrupted physician-patient relationships. Such disruption reduces the continuity of care, may lead to duplication of service, and may adversely affect patient outcomes, particularly for women who have more and more severe comorbidities. Cost-containment efforts that may produce some immediate and narrow benefits in efficiency, therefore, must be more carefully scrutinized for their broader and more long-term consequences for costs and the quality of care.

Data from this study highlight many of the problems in conducting and interpreting gender-related research. The cross-sectional nature of the data limits causal inference. Whether and to what extent women physicians in this sample attracted patients with prior physician-patient communication problems, or had such problems (i.e., "talked down" to patients), could not be assessed, given the study design and nature of data collected. Questionnaire-based information does not permit an assessment of whether male and female patients evaluate the same physician behavior differently. Even with a large sample size, men in this study were underrepresented. Because men changed physicians considerably less frequently than women, and questions regarding physician switching were asked only of those who switched, a disproportionately larger number of women provided information on the reasons for switching. Finally, there were very few patients of female physicians in this sample. Even though the proportions observed, roughly 15 percent or approximately the proportion of female physicians in the total U.S. physician population (Klepke, Marder, and Silberger, 1987), it is difficult to make generalizations about important subgroups, such as the behavior of male patients with male and female physicians, without an adequate sample size.

These problems are not unique to this study, but are part of larger methodologic dilemmas associated with conducting gender-related research. To construct a meaningful research and policy agenda regarding gender, health, and health care, these methodological problems must be addressed.

REFERENCES

Bensing, J., van der Brink-Muinen, A., and de Bakker, D. 1993. Gender differences in practice style: A Dutch study of general practitioners. *Medical Care* 31(3):219–29.

Bernstein, B., and Kane, R. 1981. Physicians' attitudes toward female patients. *Medical Care* 19(6):600–608.

Bowman, M., and Gehlbach, S. 1980. Sex of physician as a determinant of psychosocial problem recognition. *Journal of Family Practice* 10(4):655–59.

Carli, L. 1989. Gender differences in interactional style and influence. *Journal of Personality and Social Psychology* 56:565–76.

Cleary, P., Burns, B., and Nycz, G. 1990. The identification of psychiatric illness by primary care physicians: The effect of patient gender. *Journal of General Internal Medicine* 5:355–60.

Colameco, S., Becker, L., and Simpson, M. 1983. Sex bias in the assessment of patient complaints. *Journal of Family Practice* 16(6):1117–21.

Colliver, J., et al. 1993. Effects of examinee gender, standardized-patient gender, and their interaction on standardized patients' ratings of examinees' interpersonal and communication skills. *Academic Medicine* 68(2):153–57.

Dawson, N., et al. 1992. The effect of patient gender on the prevalence and recognition of alcoholism on a general medicine inpatient service. *Journal of General Internal Medicine* 7:38–45.

Fennema, K., et al. 1990. Sex of physician: Patients' preferences and stereotypes. *Journal of Family Practice* 30:441–46.

Gilligan, C. 1982. *In a Different Voice: Psychological Theory and Women's Development*. Cambridge, Mass.: Harvard University Press.

Heaton, C., and Marquez, J. 1990. Patient preferences for physician gender in the male genital/rectal exam. *Family Practice Research Journal* 10(2):105–15.

Heins, M., et al. 1979. Attitudes of women and men physicians. *American Journal of Public Health* 69(11):1132–39.

Hooper, E., et al. 1982. Patient characteristics that influence physician behavior. *Medical Care* 20(6):630–37.

Johnson, C. 1994. Gender, legitimate authority, and leader–subordinate conversations. *American Social Review* 59:122–35.

Kaplan, S. H., and Greenfield, S. 1991. Gender differences in physician-patient communication for patients seeing the same and opposite gender physicians [Abstract]. *Society of General Internal Medicine*.

Kaplan, S., Greenfield, S., and Ware, J. J. 1989a. Assessing the effects of physician-patient interactions on the outcomes of chronic disease. *Medical Care* 27:S110–S127.

Kaplan, S., Greenfield, S., and Ware, J. J. 1989b. Impact of doctor–patient relationship on the outcomes of chronic disease. In M. Stewart and D. Roter, eds., *Communicating with Medical Patients*, pp. 228–45. Newbury Park: Sage.

Kaplan, S. H., Ware, J. E., Jr., Gandek, B., and Greenfield, S. 1996. Physician characteristics that predict an egalitarian patient involvement style. *Annals of Internal Medicine* [in press].

Klepke, P., Marder, W., and Silberger, A. 1987. *The Demographics of Physician Supply: Trends and Projections*. Chicago: American Medical Association.

Lapp, J., et al. 1983. Effect of patient demand for drugs on physician prescribing. *International Journal of Psychiatry in Medicine* 13(3):193–205.

Louis Harris and Associates. 1985. *Americans and Their Doctors*. 28th ed. New York: Louis Harris and Associates.

Marquis, M., Davies, A., and Ware, J. J. 1983. Patient satisfaction and change in medical care provider: A longitudinal study. *Medical Care* 21:821–29.

Martin, S., Arnold, R., and Parker, R. 1988. Gender and medical socialization. *Journal of Health and Social Behavior* 29:333–43.

Mattz, D., and Borker, R. 1982. A cultural approach to male–female miscommunication. In J. Gumperz, ed., *Language and Social Identity*, pp. 196–216. Cambridge: Cambridge University Press.

McCraine, E., Horowitz, A., and Martin, M. 1978. Alleged sex-role stereotyping in assessment of women's physical complaints: A study of general practitioners. *Social Science Medicine* 12:111.

Meeuwesen, L., Schaap, C., and Van Der Staak, C. 1991. Verbal analysis of doctor–patient communication. *Social Science Medicine* 32(10):1143–50.

PSQ Project Co-Investigators. 1989. Final report on the patient satisfaction questionnaire project. Washington, D.C.: American Board of Internal Medicine.

Roter, D., Lipkin, M., and Korsgaard, A. 1991. Sex differences in patients' and physicians' communication during primary care medical visits. *Medical Care* 29(11):1083–93.

Tamblyn, R., et al. 1994. The feasibility and value of using patient satisfaction ratings to evaluate internal medicine residents. *Journal of General Internal Medicine* 9:146–52.

Tannen, D. 1990. *You Just Don't Understand: Women and Men in Conversation*. New York: William Morrow.

Verbrugge, L. 1980. Sex differences in complaints and diagnoses. *Journal of Behavioral Medicine* 3:327.

Waitzken, H. 1985. Information giving in medical care. *Journal of Health and Social Behavior* 26:81.

Wallen, J., Waitzkin, H., and Stoeckle, J. 1979. Physician stereotypes about female health and illness: A study of patient's sex and the informative process during medical interviews. *Women and Health* 4:135.

Ware, J. J., and Davies, A. 1983. Behavioral consequences of consumer dissatisfaction with medical care. *Evaluating Program Planning* 6:291–97.

Weisman, C., and Zeitelman, M. 1985. Physician gender and the physician-patient relationship: recent evidence and relevant questions. *Social Science Medicine* 20:11–19.

Weissman, M., and Klerman, G. 1977. Sex differences in the epidemiology of depression. *Archives of Gender Psychiatry* 34:98–111.

II

Cultural and Life Span Perspectives

4

African American Women
Social Factors and the Use of Preventive Health Services

Marsha Lillie-Blanton, Dr.P.H.
Janice Bowie, M.P.H.
Marguerite Ro, M.P.H.

Despite advances in medical science, improvements in access to health care, and the elimination of legal forms of race and gender discrimination, African Americans, male and female, continue to experience disproportionately and unacceptably high rates of illness and premature mortality. Research specifically on racial differences in the health of women is limited, as is our understanding of the factors that contribute to the persistence of these differences (U.S. Department of Health and Human Services 1985; Williams, Lavizzo-Mourey, and Warren 1994). Disparities between African American and white women undoubtedly reflect, in part, African Americans' greater exposure to social environments (e.g., poverty, neighborhood pollutants, and unsafe working conditions) that place them at risk for illness and injury (Jaynes and Williams 1989; Lillie-Blanton et al. 1993). However, inequities in access to health care are also likely to contribute to racial disparities in health.

While considerable research has been conducted on financial barriers to health care and other individual-level determinants of the use of health services (e.g., age, health problems), little is known about the extent to which social experience with health providers influences the use of services. As policy makers strive to reform the U.S. system of financing and delivering health services, it is important to advance the understanding of a broad range of factors that might affect the use of health services. Social experience and the perceptions of that experience deserve further investigation. Of interest is whether the character of the social encounter between a provider and a client is a determining factor in the receipt of health services.

Findings from The Commonwealth Fund survey indicate that the portion of African American women who did not get needed medical care is small (about 14%) but not inconsequential. Moreover, although a smaller share of African Americans than whites did not have a physical exam within a year, a larger share of African Americans than whites did not have a mammogram within a year (54% compared with 37%). Analyzing data from The Commonwealth Fund survey, this study explores whether socially determined factors influence African American women's use of preventive health services. The importance of preventive services in reducing illness and premature death is well recognized. However, such services are also important to this investigation because care seeking or caregiving for preventive services may be more susceptible to socially determined factors than are acute care services.

The domain of social factors (circumstances, relationships, and attitudes) that are potential determinants of the use of health services is not well defined or easily measured. Nonetheless, they may be important determinants of who gets care and how much care is obtained. Population groups that have experienced some alienation from the health system may be particularly sensitive to social encounters that do not appear to genuinely invite access to the services (whether intended or unintended).

The socially determined factors investigated in this study are education and satisfaction with care. Education is used as an indicator of an individual's social status and serves as a marker for the degree of shared social bonds between a client and a health provider (individual or institutional setting). Satisfaction with care is used as an indicator of the quality of a provider-client relationship. It is expected that individuals with fewer years of formal education will have weaker provider-client social bonds. Similarly, individuals who are the least satisfied with their care should have weaker provider-client relationships. Data from The Commonwealth Fund survey are used to examine the hypothesis that weaker provider-client social bonds or relationships translate into less use of needed health services. It is recognized, however, that stronger social bonds could translate into either appropriate or excessive use of services.

This study seeks answers to several questions: (1) Do African American and white women differ in their use of four preventive health services (Pap smear, mammography, clinical breast examination, and blood pressure screening)? (2) To what extent do social factors (as measured by an individual's education and satisfaction with care) influence African American women's use of preventive health services? (3) Do these two social factors similarly influence the use of preventive health services by African American and white women?

PRIOR RESEARCH

Few studies provide information on the use of health services by race, gender, and a measure of socioeconomic status. Of the research conducted, conflicting evidence exists about whether racial differentials persist. Blendon et al. (1989) found significantly lower rates of use in 1986 for African Americans than whites, even after adjusting for differences in age, gender, health, income, and insurance. Analysis of data on ambulatory health care visits in 1988 provided evidence that white and African American women of similar income are approaching comparable levels of entry into the health care system; racial differences, however, persisted in the volume of care received among those who obtained care (Lillie-Blanton et al. 1993).

Social Factors and the Use of Health Services

An abundance of research has documented the consequences of financial barriers in access to health care (Davis and Rowland 1983; Aday 1993; Weissman and Epstein 1994). Less is known, however, about the extent to which education, independent of one's financial resources, influences the use of health services. Ries (1991) found that age-adjusted rates of physician contacts are highest for those with the most education, while hospital discharges per one hundred persons are highest for those with the least education. Because neither finding is adjusted for health needs, both must be interpreted with caution. However, the finding regarding the use of physician services suggests that access to primary care may be a problem for women with the least formal education, assuming that health needs are greater among this population.

Several studies also examine ways in which race and/or socioeconomic status affects the quality of the provider–client encounter. Waitzkin (1985) found that better-educated patients from higher socioeconomic levels receive more physician encounter time and more less technical explanations. Roter and Hall (1992) found that doctors give more information to patients in higher social class categories and that care is often influenced by patients' social class standing. Because of the larger share of minority populations who are poor or near-poor, Roter and Hall (1992) concluded that minority populations generally have more negative health experiences with providers than do whites.

Studies of racial differences in satisfaction with caregivers provide varying results. The 1986 Robert Wood Johnson Survey on Access found that African Americans are less satisfied than whites with the ambulatory care and hospital care they receive (Blendon et al. 1989). However, data from a 1993 Kaiser/Commonwealth Fund survey did not find evidence of racial differences in satisfaction with care; nevertheless, African Americans were more likely than whites to report that problems in the health system were serious enough to warrant a major restructuring of the system (Harris and Associates 1993).

Most studies analyze data on satisfaction as a so-called outcome of care rather than examining how it relates to other measures such as the use of services. From studies that have undertaken such analysis, there is no conclusive evidence that individuals' patterns of using health services are affected by their level of satisfaction. For example, while one study found that less satisfaction does not translate into large differences in use (Freund et al. 1989), another study of low-income families found that a relationship does exist, but it depends on the context in which the care is provided and the patient's background characteristics (Zastowny, Roghmann, and Cafferata 1989). A recent study, however, found that patients are less likely to remain with physicians who received lower overall satisfaction ratings (Rubin et al. 1993).

The Use of Preventive Health Services

Several national studies provide data on race-specific patterns of the receipt of one or more of the preventive services examined in this study (see tab. 4.1). Two of these studies examined trends over time and provide evidence that, since 1973, African American women experienced larger increases in screening rates than white women, resulting in rates of receipt of preventive services that are comparable in 1985 and 1990 (Makuc, Fried, and Kleinman 1989; Breen and Kessler 1994). None of the studies using national data sources provides evidence that African American women are at greater risk than white women of not

Table 4.1. Percentage of African American and White Women without Preventive Service

| | Preventive Service | | | | | | | |
| | Pap Smear | | Clinical Breast Exam | | Mammography | | Blood Pressure Screening | |
Study/Time Frame/Age	African American	White	African American	White	African American	White	African American	White
Woolhandler et al. 1982, NHIS[a]								
1 year or more than optimal[b]								
45–64	21	27	32	38	—	—	7	13
Makuc et al. 1985, NHIS[c]								
within past 2 years								
20–79	30	36	25	31	—	—	18	22
Breen and Kessler 1990, NHIS								
within past year								
40 and older	—	—	—	—	68	67	—	—
50–54	—	—	—	—	65	60	—	—
55–59	—	—	—	—	64	61	—	—
60–64	—	—	—	—	68	62	—	—

[a] National Health Interview Survey.
[b] Definition of optimal varied by specific service.
[c] Age-adjusted.

receiving preventive care. Although a larger percentage of African Americans than whites did not have a mammogram in 1990 (tab. 4.1), the estimates do not differ statistically.

All three studies cited (see tab. 4.1) provide strong evidence of socio-economic determinants of the receipt of preventive services by both racial groups. Woolhandler and Himmelstein (1988) found that the likelihood of being inadequately screened was greater for women who were poor, had 12 or fewer years of education, or were uninsured. Similarly, Makuc, Fried, and Kleinman (1989) found that poor women were less likely than nonpoor women to receive preventive care. Breen and Kessler (1994) also found that income and education were significant determinants of who gets mammography screening.

METHODS OF ANALYSIS

Analyzing survey data collected for The Commonwealth Fund survey, this study explores whether social factors influence African American women's use of preventive health services. The analysis is limited to women under age sixty-five. Including nonelderly and elderly women in the study population would have required resources beyond the scope of what was available for this study, because the age groups differ greatly in their health and insurance coverage.

Selection of Key Variables

Education is used as an indicator of social status. Although socio-economic status frequently is measured by income or some combination of income, education, and occupation, the merit of the varying indicators is subject to continuing debate (Krieger et al. 1993; Williams, Lavizzo-Mourey, and Warren 1994). Income was not considered the better indicator for this study because money buys access to health resources. It is conceivable that higher-income individuals (of either race) are more successful in negotiating access to health services even if they display less socially normative attributes (e.g., use of colloquialisms, nontraditional dress). Moreover, because financial returns on educational investments are less for African Americans than for whites (U.S. Bureau of the Census 1991), education was considered useful in measuring societal norms of social status that may value nonfinancial indicators of upward mobility. In the absence of empirical data showing one indicator to be superior to the other, education was considered a sufficiently valid, although not perfect, indicator.

Satisfaction with care is used as an indicator of the quality of a provider–client relationship. Women's experiences with providers and their perceptions of these experiences translate into positive and negative attitudes about providers (individuals and institutions). Research has shown that clients can evaluate dimensions of the care they receive reliably and accurately (Davies and Ware 1988). These measures of satisfaction often are used as indicators of the quality of medical care (Davies and Ware 1988; Rubin et al. 1993). However, subjective assessments of the care provided, as opposed to objective accounts of what occurred in a medical encounter, generally evaluate interpersonal rather than technical aspects of care.

Measurement of Key Variables

The Commonwealth Fund survey requested information on socio-demographic characteristics, physical and mental health, use of health services, and perceptions of experiences with providers. Information on the use of preventive health services was obtained from responses to the question: "In the last year have you received a [health service] or not?" Included among the specific services queried were Pap smear, mammogram, clinical breast examination, or blood pressure screening.

The respondent's race was defined based on the question: "Do you consider yourself white, black, African American, Asian, or ———?" Women who reported their race as black or African American were classified as African Americans. Women identifying their race as white were classified as white. Respondents who reported their ethnic origin as Hispanic were excluded from the analysis. Thus, the racial groups refer to non-Hispanic whites and non-Hispanic African Americans.

The social factors investigated in this study were defined based on two survey questionnaire items. Information on the years of school completed was used to construct an education variable consisting of three categories: fewer than 12 years of education, completed 12 years of education, and 13 or more years of education. Satisfaction with overall care was measured based on responses to the question: "Would you say your regular doctor provides you with good health care overall?" Responses of fair, poor, good, and excellent were used to construct a satisfaction variable with three categories: most concerns (combined ratings of fair and poor); average concerns (rating of good); and

Exhibit A. Key Definitions

Race
  African American   Responses of black or African American
  White American[a]   Responses of white
    (The survey question asked: Do you consider yourself white, black,
    African American, Asian, or _____? *Note:* Respondents who reported
    their ethnic origin as Hispanic were excluded from the analysis.)

Education
  < 12 years[a]
  12 years
  13+ years

Age
  18–49[a]
  50–64[a]

Satisfaction concerns
  Least   Responses of excellent
  Average   Responses of good
  Most[a]   Responses of fair or poor rating
    (The survey question asked: Would you say your regular doctor
    provides you with good health care overall?)

Insurance coverage
  Private   Private insurance includes health insurance or a health
               plan through an individual's or a spouse's employer or
               union. Also included is health insurance purchased
               directly or through some other source.
  Public   Public coverage includes those persons who have any
               Medicaid or Medicare coverage.
  Uninsured[a] Uninsured is defined as having no coverage at all.

Poverty
  Poor[a]   Income below 100% of poverty
  Near-poor   Income below 200% of poverty
  Nonpoor   All others
    (Information on household income and household size was used to
    construct a measure of poverty status based on the Census Bureau's
    1992 weighted average poverty thresholds.)

Health status
  Good   Good represents those persons who answered the survey
               question excellent, very good, or good.
  Fair[a]   Fair represents those who answered fair or poor.
    (The survey question asked: Would you say your health, in general, is
    excellent, very good, good, fair, or poor?)

(*continued*)

Exhibit A. (*Continued*)

Source of care
  Yes
  No[a]
    (The survey question asked: Is there one place in particular you usually
    go when you are sick or want advice about your health, or isn't there?
    The responses were yes or no.)

Source: The Commonwealth Fund survey on women's health, 1993.

[a] Reference group for multiple logistic regression analysis.

least concerns (rating of excellent). In the text, the term *dissatisfied* is used to describe women reporting the "most concerns" with the care provided by their regular physician.

Information on household income and household size was used to construct a measure of poverty status. Based on the Census Bureau's 1992 weighted average poverty thresholds, three categories were constructed: poor (income below 100% of the poverty level); near-poor (income below 200% of poverty level); and nonpoor (those remaining). By holding constant poverty and insurance status, the study attempted to examine the socially derived benefits of education independent of a woman's financial means. Other key variables included in this analysis are defined in Exhibit A.

Plan of Analysis

The use of preventive services was examined using bivariate analysis and multiple regression techniques. Estimates of use by race were weighted to reflect population estimates corresponding to the age, race, education, insurance status, and Census region distribution of women in the United States. The multiple regression, however, used unweighted data because the emphasis was on examining relationships among variables rather than on comparing population estimates.

Multiple logistic regression was used to assess racial differences in the use of preventive services while holding constant factors that might influence the use of health services, such as sociodemographics (age, poverty status), need (health status), and enabling characteristics (health coverage, usual source of care). The regression also was used to identify factors associated with the use of preventive services. Education and satisfaction were examined, holding constant poverty status as well as other factors potentially affecting the use of services. To test statistically whether the key variables of interest (education and satisfaction) varied by race, regression models including interaction terms for race and these factors were tested. The interaction terms assessed whether the relationship observed for the measures is consistent for both racial groups.

RESULTS

The modified study sample consists of 1,652 women ages eighteen to sixty-four, or two-thirds of the 2,525 women interviewed (tab. 4.2).

Table 4.2. Demographic and Socioeconomic Characteristics of the Study Population: Women Ages Eighteen to Sixty-four Years

	African American		White	
	N^a	Percentage	N	Percentage
All women 18–64	354	100.0	1,298	100.0
Age				
18–24	351	4.7	106	14.3
25–44	208	57.7	667	52.3
45–64	111	27.6	525	33.4
Education				
< 12 years	48	24.2	94	14.3
12 years	117	34.8	450	39.0
13+ years	188	41.0	753	46.6
Poverty status				
Poor	83	33.3	108	12.0
Near-poor	90	25.8	233	21.7
Nonpoor	161	40.9	890	66.2
Employment				
Working full- or part-time	252	66.5	918	68.8
Not working	102	33.4	372	31.1
Satisfaction concerns				
Most (fair/poor rating)	43	15.0	101	9.9
Average (good rating)	121	39.3	453	38.6
Least (excellent rating)	144	45.6	608	51.5

Source: Data from The Commonwealth Fund survey on women's health, 1993.

[a] Ns are unweighted; percentages are weighted.

Of the 1,652 women, 21 percent are African American. The age distribution of white and African American women is similar, with slightly more than half of the women in both groups being twenty-five to forty-four years of age. Thus, age differences are unlikely to be a major factor influencing racial differences in the use of preventive services.

Racial Differences in Income and Employment

Consistent with prior research, there are noticeable racial differences in the economic conditions of women. Poverty rates are higher among African Americans than whites (33% compared with 12%), and racial differences in the income distribution of the two populations are considerable. While more than half (59%) of African American women are either poor (33%) or near-poor (26%), more than half (66%) of white women are nonpoor.

Despite greater poverty among African American than white women, a similar proportion of African Americans (67%) and whites (69%) are working full- or part-time. These employment statistics challenge public perceptions that African American women are disproportionately poorer because they are unwilling to work. Higher poverty rates among African American women are likely a consequence of multiple factors, including racial differences in earnings from employment, family composition (i.e., number of children and income earners in the household), and family financial wealth.

Racial Differences in Education and Satisfaction with Health Care

African American women have less formal education than whites (tab. 4.2). About 70 percent more African Americans than whites did not graduate from high school (24% compared with 14%). Racial differences among high school graduates and those with 13 or more years of school are smaller but noteworthy. Fewer African Americans than whites were high school graduates (35% compared with 39%) or had some college education (41% compared with 47%). The measure of education shows that a larger share of African Americans than whites are in the bottom social stratum of society.

Overall, African American women are less satisfied with their regular physician than are white women. About 50 percent more African Americans than whites reported dissatisfaction with the care provided by their regular doctor (15% compared with 10%). Most of the racial difference in satisfaction is found among high school graduates. African Americans with a high school degree were twice as likely as whites to report dissatisfaction with the care provided (18% compared with 9%).

In sum, African American and white women are of similar age and are equally as likely to be working full- or part-time. African American women, however, have less formal education, are poorer, and are less satisfied with their care than whites. These population differences could affect the use of preventive health services and, thus, should be considered when seeking to identify differences in use that are race-specific, rather than largely a consequence of socioeconomic conditions.

Racial Differences in Other Correlates of the Use of Health Services

Data on potential barriers to care (i.e., being uninsured, being without a usual source of care, and using the emergency room as the usual source of care) are presented (tab. 4.3). To assess whether racial differ-

Table 4.3. Indicators of Potential Barriers to Care for Women Ages Eighteen to Sixty-four Years (weighted)

Potential Barrier	African American (%)	White (%)	Ratio of African American to White
Uninsured			
< 12 years	28.5	23.5	1.21
12 years	16.5	16.3	1.0
13+ years	10.4	10.8	1.0
Total	16.8	14.8	1.1
No usual source of care			
< 12 years	16.6	16.5	1.0
12 years	27.5	21.1	1.3
13+ years	20.5	20.0	1.0
Total	21.9	20.0	1.1
ER as usual source of care			
< 12 years	14.3	8.3	1.7
12 years	20.8	2.8	7.4
13+ years	8.2	3.0	2.7
Total	13.9	3.7	3.7

Source: Data from The Commonwealth Fund survey on women's health, 1993.

ences exist among women of similar social status, data on these factors are presented for three groups of African American and white women: non–high school graduates, high school graduates, and those with 13 or more years of education.

Despite considerable differences in economic circumstances, African American and white women ages eighteen to sixty-four are similar in terms of the proportion uninsured (17% compared with 15%) and without a usual source of care (22% compared with 20%). Racial differences are observed for two subgroups of women. About 20 percent more African Americans than whites who did not graduate from high school are uninsured (29% compared with 24%). Also, among women with a high school degree, about 30 percent more African Americans than whites are without a usual source of care (28% compared with 21%).

As expected based on prior research, there are large racial differences in use of the emergency room (ER) as a usual source of care. More than three times as many African Americans as whites identified the ER as a usual source of care (14% compared with 4%). Surprisingly, differences in using the ER as a usual source of care are most pronounced among African American and white high school graduates (21% compared with 3%). This finding may reflect racial differences in the benefits of education.

The Use of Preventive Health Services

About one in four African American women did not have a Pap smear (23%) or a clinical breast exam (30%) during the past year. Mammography screening is the preventive service least likely to be obtained by African American women ages fifty to sixty-four years, with more than half (54%) not having a mammogram during the past year. The proportion who did not have their blood pressure checked is considerably less, with fewer than one in ten African American women (8%) not being screened within the past year.

Differences among African American Women

The extent to which social influences affect who gets preventive care among African American women is assessed by their level of education and satisfaction with care (tab. 4.4). The ratios presented indicate how the use of preventive services in the subgroup presumed to be at great-

Table 4.4. Percentage of African American Women Ages Eighteen to Sixty-four Years without Preventive Service, by Social Factors (weighted)

	Education				
	Percentage			Ratio	
Service	<12 years	12 years	13+ years	<12 years: 13+ years	12 years: 13+ years
Pap smear	30.6	23.7	17.9	1.7	1.3
Mammogram[a]	59.1	54.5	44.5	1.3	1.2
Clinical breast exam	41.3	33.1	20.7	2.0	1.6
Blood pressure screening	6.2	11.4	5.0	1.2	2.3

	Satisfaction Concerns				
	Percentage			Ratio	
Service	Most	Average	Least	Most: Least	Average: Least
Pap smear	20.4	20.8	23.6	0.9	0.9
Mammogram[a]	62.8	55.2	45.4	1.4	1.2
Clinical breast exam	39.3	30.9	22.1	1.8	1.4
Blood pressure screening	5.0	9.5	3.3	1.5	2.9

Source: Analysis of The Commonwealth Fund survey on women's health, 1993.
[a] Ages 50–64 only.

est risk of not receiving the service (i.e., women without a high school degree or those who are the most dissatisfied with their caregivers) fared relative to the subgroup at lowest risk (i.e., women with 13 or more years of education or those who are the least dissatisfied with their caregivers). Ratios are also presented comparing the middle subgroup of women with the subgroup presumed to be at lowest risk.

As anticipated, striking differences are observed. When comparing African American women without a high school degree (fewer than 12 years) and those with some college education (13 years or more), notable differences are observed in the proportion without a Pap smear (31% compared with 18%), a mammogram (59% compared with 44%), and a clinical breast exam (41% compared with 21%). Moreover, differences are apparent, although they are not as large or consistent for each service, when comparing high school graduates and those with some college education. The exception is blood pressure screening, the preventive service that shows the highest rate of use by all women. Differences here between those with the most and the least education are small. However, twice as many high school graduates as those with some college failed to have their blood pressure taken in the past year (11% compared with 5%).

Who gets preventive care given women's level of satisfaction with care varies somewhat. With the exception of a Pap smear, dissatisfied African American women generally used fewer preventive services than those who were not dissatisfied. Differences are largest for the clinical breast exam, with nearly twice as many of the most dissatisfied women not getting the exam as the least dissatisfied women (39% compared with 22%, respectively). In addition, there is evidence that the middle subgroup of women fare worse in blood pressure screening than those presumed to be at greatest risk. About 10 percent of women who rated their providers as average had not had their blood pressure taken, compared with 5 percent of the most dissatisfied women and 3 percent of the least dissatisfied women.

Comparing White Women and African American Women

Of the four preventive services examined, African Americans appear to be disadvantaged in obtaining access to only one—mammography. More African Americans than whites ages fifty to sixty-four did not receive a mammogram in the past year (54% compared with 37%). Racial differences in mammography rates persisted when comparing women of similar education or satisfaction level. Furthermore, there is some indication that satisfaction with care differentially affects access to one preventive service—the Pap smear. While the proportion of African Americans and whites without a Pap smear is comparable for those who reported the least satisfaction concerns (rating of excellent), there are twofold racial differences in Pap smear testing among those who were dissatisfied. Whites who were dissatisfied were twice as likely as African Americans not to get a Pap smear.

Likelihood of Receipt of Service

When holding constant factors related to the use of health services, the likelihood of not getting three of the preventive services (i.e., clinical breast exam, blood pressure screening, mammography) is not statistically different for African Americans and whites (tab. 4.5). Racial

Table 4.5. Likelihood of Women Ages Eighteen to Sixty-four Years Being without a Preventive Health Visit, by Selected Respondent Characteristics (Logistic Regression Results)

	Adjusted Odds Ratio[a] (95% Confidence Interval)			
	Pap Smear	Clinical Breast Exam	Mammography[b]	Blood Pressure Screening
Race				
African American	0.69	0.84	1.47	0.62
	(0.58, 0.97)[c]	(0.61, 1.16)	(0.80, 2.73)	(0.35, 1.09)
White	Reference	Reference	Reference	Reference
Education				
13+ years	0.46	0.43	0.56	0.70
	(0.29, 0.75)[c]	(0.26, 0.70)[c]	(0.27, 1.19)	(0.33, 1.49)
12 years	0.75	0.78	1.00	1.18
	(0.47, 1.20)	(0.49, 1.26)	(0.49, 2.04)	(0.56, 2.46)
<12 years	Reference	Reference	Reference	Reference
Satisfaction concerns				
Least	0.66	0.53	0.92	0.91
	(0.43, 1.01)	(0.35, 0.80)[c]	(0.42, 2.01)	(0.47, 1.74)
Average	0.95	0.81	0.96	1.19
	(0.62, 1.46)	(0.53, 1.23)	(0.42, 2.17)	(0.63, 2.26)
Most	Reference	Reference	Reference	Reference

Source: Analysis of The Commonwealth Fund survey on women's health, 1993.

[a] Adjusted odds ratio was calculated holding constant age, insurance coverage, poverty, health status, and usual source of care.

[b] Women ages 50–64.

[c] $p < 0.05$.

differences are observed, however, in the likelihood of having a Pap smear. It is interesting to note that African Americans are less likely than whites not to have had a Pap smear. There is also suggestive evidence that African Americans are more likely than whites not to have had a mammogram. The unadjusted likelihood of not receiving a mammogram is nearly 50 percent higher for African Americans than for whites, and does not change appreciably when adjusted for factors related to the use of health services. Findings are only suggestive because the differences are not statistically significant; however, the relatively small number of observations for women ages fifty to sixty-four weakens the power of the model to detect significant differences.

When holding constant other factors related to the use of health services, education persists as a factor related to the receipt of two of the preventive services. Women with the most education are twice as likely as those with the least education to have had a Pap smear or a clinical breast exam. The analysis does not provide evidence of differences in the use of services by high school graduates and non–high school graduates. This finding is hardly encouraging, however, because non–high school graduates have the lowest rates of use of preventive services. The absence of a relationship between education and blood pressure screening is promising news because the vast majority of women had their blood pressure taken during the past year. However, since the rates of mammography screening are fairly low, the lack of a relationship is an indication that women are equally disadvantaged across levels of education.

Differences in the use of preventive care by the most and least dissatisfied women diminished when population characteristics (e.g., income and insurance) were held constant. Satisfaction with caregivers, however, persists as a factor related to the receipt of one of the four services—a clinical breast exam. Women who are dissatisfied are twice as likely not to have had a clinical breast exam as the least dissatisfied women. Since reasons for dissatisfaction are not assessed and the data are cross-sectional, a causal relationship cannot be inferred from this finding. Further research is warranted, however, because dissatisfaction appears to have some influence, although not a consistent impact, on the use of preventive health services.

In addition, the lack of a statistically significant interaction term for race and education or for race and satisfaction gives evidence that these relationships do not differ substantially for white and African American women. Other factors significantly associated with the use of preventive health care varied by service. Having a usual source of care, however, is associated with the receipt of each of the preventive services. Women without a usual source of care are at greater risk of not getting each of the services. Moreover, having no usual source of care is the only factor significantly associated with not getting a mammogram in the past year.

SUMMARY OF FINDINGS

Despite tremendous gains in improving access to health care in the past 25 years, sizable numbers of African American women do not receive the preventive care that could reduce their risk of disability and premature death from heart disease, stroke, breast cancer, and cervical cancer. About one-fourth of African American women did not have a Pap smear or clinical breast exam in the past year, and more than half of women ages fifty to sixty-four did not have a mammogram in the past year. This compares with only 8 percent of African American women not having their blood pressure taken within a year. While this study does not provide evidence that race-specific barriers account for the relatively low rates of use of preventive services, there is evidence that factors intertwined with race and other social considerations may affect access to certain types of preventive care.

Racial differences in the experiences of women who complete high school (i.e., the middle subgroup) warrant further study. A larger share of African Americans than whites with a high school degree were dissatisfied with their providers, had no usual source of care, used the emergency room as a usual source of care, and had not had their blood pressure tested. Although these findings were not adjusted for the multiple factors that could account for racial differences, they provide a consistent enough pattern to suggest that a subset of African American women—high school graduates—may be more vulnerable for poorer access than similarly educated whites.

There are many possible explanations for racial differences in the health care access indicators of high school graduates, including differences in the types of employment and in neighborhood health services. For example, a high school degree may afford African American women access to entry-level positions in the workforce; their earnings, however, disqualify them from Medicaid and, yet, are inadequate to purchase health care comparable to that of similarly educated whites. Or they may reflect differences in the availability of health services in the neighborhoods in which African Americans and whites with high school degrees live. To improve access to the most appropriate sources of care, these and other explanations deserve further research.

Does Race Affect Access to Preventive Care?

In contrast to the findings of Breen and Kessler (1994), this study provides evidence suggestive of racial differences in the likelihood of mammography screening after controlling for population differences in age, health, poverty, insurance, and having a usual source of care. One possible explanation for the varying findings is that Breen and Kessler's analysis included women age forty or older, while this study restricted the analysis to women ages fifty to sixty-four. Although estimates of mammography screening by race are not statistically different, they are cause for further investigation. If replicated in other study populations, factors accounting for the conflicting results should be sought.

The only other evidence of a racial difference in preventive health services use is in receipt of a Pap smear. African Americans' observed advantage in obtaining Pap smears may be related to racial differences in the validity of self-reported information on Pap smears or it may be a consequence of differences in sources of care or in a provider's perceptions of need. For example, African Americans are more likely than whites to identify usual sources of care (e.g., health clinics or community health centers as opposed to private physicians) that can provide a comprehensive range of family planning screening tests at lower cost. However, it is also conceivable that providers' assessment of risks or of presenting symptoms result in more African Americans than whites getting a Pap smear for diagnostic purposes.

Do Social Factors Affect Access to Preventive Care?

As hypothesized, women with the least formal education were at greatest risk of not having at least two of the preventive services: a Pap smear and a clinical breast exam. This finding did not vary significantly for African American and white women. Both groups of women appear to be equally disadvantaged by whatever social forces are operating in the culture of the health system. It is disturbing that women who have already missed an opportunity theoretically available to all, a high school education, are also most at risk of not getting the care needed for early diagnosis of a health problem. Factors that account for these differentials deserve further investigation.

Education is likely measuring a complex process. As a proxy for the individual's social status, it was intended to measure the shared social bonds that exist between a provider and a client. However, education could shape the provider–client interaction and ultimately the use of services in varying ways. It could affect one's trust in the provider, confidence in negotiating a specialized system of caregiving, influence (i.e., clout) with the provider, or ability to understand information. It also could affect a provider's thoroughness in taking a client's history, a client's openness in revealing information to a provider, and the courtesies or explanations afforded either party.

The finding that dissatisfaction with care is associated with the receipt of only one of the four screening exams—a clinical breast exam—was not as expected. Although it is conceivable that satisfaction affects the use of some services but not others, the varying patterns for two tests (i.e., Pap smear and clinical breast exam) that are similar in many respects appear inconsistent. Perhaps the findings are indicative of the options women perceive themselves to have or reflect the varying degrees of control women or providers exert regarding certain tests. For example, women may view breast self-exam as a substitute for clinical breast exam, whereas there is no substitute for a Pap smear.

Equally as perplexing is that women's satisfaction with care was not related to the patterns of use of the other preventive services. Is it good news that women's use of health services is not related to their level of satisfaction? The finding differs from consumer behavior generally, but it may be one more example of how the health care marketplace differs from other markets. It also may reflect learned behavior for a sector of society that has lacked alternatives when dissatisfied with a service. Much remains to be learned about the relationship between satisfaction and the use of health services, including whether a single measure of satisfaction is sufficiently sensitive to capture the complex pathways by which caregiving and care seeking occur.

IMPLICATIONS FOR POLICY AND RESEARCH

Encouraging individuals to accept greater responsibility for their health has been one of the primary objectives of federal health policy since 1980. *Healthy People Year 2000* (U.S. Department of Health and Human Services 1991) established goals for reducing unhealthy behaviors and increasing the use of preventive health services. To achieve these goals, the findings of this study suggest, attention must be devoted not only to ensuring financing for preventive care but also to developing interventions to reduce the extent to which social inequalities related to education influence the receipt of preventive care.

Assurance of Financing for Preventive Services

Perceptions that preventive services are of low cost, and thus affordable, have shaped policy proposals that exclude these services from health insurance plans. However, given the disproportionate number of African American women who are poor or near-poor, including these services in the scope of covered benefits will be essential to improving access. In addition, for preventive services that use costly technology, such as mammography, African American women will continue to face undue financial barriers in obtaining access if adequate financing is not available. The only service for which there is even suggestive evidence that African Americans are at a disadvantage in obtaining is the most technologically sophisticated one. This may be due to differences in the scope of health benefits available to African Americans compared with whites in employer- or state-based publicly financed health plans. Thus, factors related to race and health coverage may affect who gets preventive care.

Reduction of Social Inequalities in the Use of Preventive Services

This analysis provides evidence that socially determined factors influence the receipt of preventive services by women of both racial groups. Thus, in addition to financial and racial barriers facing underserved African American women, social inequalities measured by differences in education appear to influence care seeking and caregiving. Efforts are needed to identify and reduce practices that create a social environment that results in differentials in the use of services by social stratum. Providers may need to develop a more inclusive culture of operations (i.e., interpersonal skills, sensitivity to sociocultural differences) and women with less formal education may need to improve their skills in negotiating a complicated and what may sometimes appear to be alienating service delivery system.

Although more precise information about the nature of the problem is needed, systematically evaluated interventions can improve knowledge while also evaluating approaches to reduce inequalities in the use of services. An important first step in this process is to improve providers' and women's awareness of the differentials observed. For providers, this process should begin by including curricula on sociocultural competence and interpersonal relations in medical schools and residency training programs. Efforts to reach practicing physicians through journal articles and continuing medical education also should be pursued.

Increasing knowledge of the need for preventive services among all women is important, but it is particularly critical for women who did not complete high school. Targeted outreach and educational efforts should seek to empower women with the skills and confidence to demand needed services. Educational efforts such as these generally cost little relative to the benefits to be gained. The large share of women who had their blood pressure taken provides an instructive example. The nation's investment in educational campaigns about the risks of high blood pressure and in developing low-cost screening procedures likely account, in part, for the larger numbers of African American women obtaining this service, regardless of education. Obviously, policy efforts to increase the general educational level of women should be encouraged. These efforts would have broad societal benefits, while also reducing the potential for social inequalities to affect access to health services.

ACKNOWLEDGMENTS

We gratefully acknowledge Sally Schwartz and Nancy Breen for their thoughtful critique of and editorial suggestions concerning an earlier draft of this chapter.

REFERENCES

Aday, L. A. 1993. *At Risk in America: The Health and Health Care Needs of Vulnerable Populations in the United States.* San Francisco: Jossey-Bass.

Blendon, R. J., Aiken, L. H., Freeman, H. E., and Corey, C. R. 1989. Access to medical care for black and white Americans: a matter of continuing concern. *Journal of the American Medical Association* 261:278–81.

Breen, N., and Kessler, L. 1994. Changes in the use of screening mammography: evidence from the 1987 and 1990 National Health Interview Surveys. *American Journal of Public Health* 84:62–67.

Davies, A. R., and Ware, J. E., Jr. 1988. Involving consumers in quality of care assessment. *Health Affairs* 7:33–48.

Davis, K., and Rowland, D. 1983. Uninsured and underserved: inequities in health care in the United States. *Milbank Memorial Fund Quarterly* 61:149–76.

Freund, D., Hurley, R., Paul, J., Grubb, C., Rossiter, L., and Adamache, K. 1989. Interim findings from the Medicaid competition demonstrations. *Advances in Health Economics Research* 10.

Freund, D., Rossiter, L., Fox, P., Meyer, J., Hurley, R., Carey, T., and Paul, J. 1988. *Nationwide Evaluation of Medicaid Competition Demonstrations*, vol. 1, *Integrative Final Report.* Research Triangle Institute.

Harris, Louis, and Associates. 1993. The Kaiser/Commonwealth Fund Health Insurance Survey II, Study no. 932010. Unpublished data.

Hurley, R., and Freund, D. 1988. Determinants of provider selection or assignment in a mandatory case management program and their implications for utilization. *Inquiry* 25:402–10.

Hurley R., Freund, D., and Gage, B. 1991. Gatekeeper effect on patterns of physician use. *Journal of Family Practice* 32:167–74.

Jaynes, G. D., and Williams, R. M. 1989. *A Common Destiny: Blacks and American Society.* Washington, D.C.: National Academy Press.

Krieger, N., Rowley, D., Herman, A., Avery, B., and Phillips, M. 1993. Racism, sexism and social class: implications for studies of health, disease and well-being. *American Journal of Preventive Medicine* December:82–122.

Lillie-Blanton, M., Martinez, R. M., Taylor, A. K., and Robinson, B. G. 1993. Latina and African American women: continuing disparities in health. *International Journal of Health Services* 23:555–84.

McCall, N., Jay, D., and West, R. 1989. Access and satisfaction in the Arizona health care cost containment system. *Health Care Financing Review* 11:63–77.

Makuc, D. M., Fried, V. M., and Kleinman, J. C. 1989. National trends in the use of preventive health care by women. *American Journal of Public Health* 79:21–26.

Miller, R., and Luft, H. 1994. Managed care performance since 1980: a literature analysis. *Journal of the American Medical Association* 271:1512–18.

Neighbors, H. W., and Jackson, J. S. 1987. Barriers to medical care among adult blacks: what happens to the uninsured? *Journal of the National Medical Association* 79:489–93.

Ries, J. 1990. Medicaid maternal and child health care: prepaid versus private fee-for-service. *Research in Nursing and Health* 13:163–71.

———. 1991. Educational differences in health status and health care. National Center for Health Statistics. *Vital Health Statistics* 10.

Roter, D. L., and Hall, J. A. 1992. *Doctors Talking with Patients, Patients Talking with Doctors.* Westport, Conn.: Auburn House.

Rubin, H., Gandek, B., Rogers, W., Kosinski, M., McHorney, C., and Ware, J. 1993. Patients' ratings of outpatient visits in different practice settings. *Journal of the American Medical Association* 270:835–40.

Temkin-Greener, H. 1986. Medicaid families under managed care: anticipated behavior. *Medical Care* 24:721–32.

U.S. Bureau of the Census. 1991. *Poverty in the U.S., 1990.* Series P-60, no. 175. Washington, D.C.

U.S. Department of Health and Human Services. 1991. *Healthy People 2000: National Health Promotion and Disease Prevention Objectives.* Washington, D.C.: U.S. Government Printing Office.

———. 1985. *Report of the Secretary's Task Force on Black and Minority Health: Executive Summary.* Washington, D.C.: U.S. Government Printing Office.

Waitzkin, H. 1985. Information giving in medical care. *Journal of Health and Social Behavior* 26:81–101.

Ware, J. E., Davies, A. R., and Rubin, H. R. 1988. *The Quality of Medical Care:*

Information for Consumers. Washington, D.C.: Office of Technology Assessment.

Weissman, J., and Epstein, A. 1994. *Falling through the Safety Net: Insurance Status and Access to Health Care.* Baltimore: Johns Hopkins University Press.

Williams, D., Lavizzo-Mourey, R., and Warren, R. 1994. The concept of race and health status in America. *Public Health Reports* January–February.

Woodhandler, S., and Himmelstein, D. U. 1988. Reverse targeting of preventive care due to lack of health insurance. *Journal of the American Medical Association* 259:2872–74.

Zastowny, T., Roghmann, K., and Cafferata, G. 1989. Patient satisfaction and the use of health services. *Medical Care* 27:705–23.

5

Latino Women
Health Status and Access to Health Care

Annette B. Ramírez de Arellano, Dr.P.H.

A concern with the appropriate targeting of health care services has fueled the need to aggregate data in a variety of ways. As a result, generic "woman" has given way to women with specific characteristics, and ethnicity has joined age and race as an increasingly important variable around which health status and care seeking can be examined.

As the youngest and fastest-growing minority population in the United States, Latinos are beginning to emerge from the category of "other" to which they were formerly relegated. The findings of the Hispanic Health and Nutrition Examination Survey (HHANES) of 1982–84 uncovered an array of unmet needs, as well as interesting differences among various Latino subgroups. This chapter presents data produced by The Commonwealth Fund survey and updates previous data, focusing exclusively on Latino women.

METHODOLOGY

Subsample of Interest

The Commonwealth Fund survey oversampled Hispanic and African American women relative to their proportion in the population to allow a detailed analysis of these two groups (Louis Harris and Associates 1993). The Latino sample was identified by asking women whether they were "of Hispanic origin or descent." This chapter summarizes and interprets the data for the female Hispanic subgroups, a total of 405 women.

Caveats

Five percent of the women in the overall sample and 7 percent of the women in the Latino oversample chose to be interviewed in Spanish. Although the Spanish questionnaire is generally a close translation of the original, linguistic nuances may account for different responses to any given question. Therefore, the analysis that follows indicates whenever an answer may have been affected by the language in which it was asked.

The survey was conducted by telephone, which limited the pool of respondents; Census data indicate that 18.5 percent of Latino households do not have a telephone (Institute for Puerto Rican Policy 1990). Because those households that have telephones tend to have higher socioeconomic status and are more residentially stable than the rest, the sample may be biased toward better-off Latinas. Data on health status and behavior may therefore be somewhat more favorable than those for the Latino population as a whole.

The data are aggregated for all Latinas, and the small numbers involved do not permit a breakdown by specific subgroup (e.g., Cubans, Puerto Ricans, Mexican Americans). As a result, the data may be more representative of the largest group—Mexican Americans—than of the others. Persons of Mexican origin constitute 63 percent of the Latino population in the United States and 54 percent of the Latino respondents in this survey. Lumping all subgroups may therefore mask intragroup variation. Moreover, because Mexican American women have unusually favorable reproductive health indicators (National Center for Health Statistics 1993), the data may also underestimate some of the problems affecting other Latino women.

Because the Latino sample includes women of all races, Latinas are compared to the total of all women surveyed rather than to a race-specific group. The differences found are therefore smaller than would be the case if two mutually exclusive groups had been compared.

Measure of Significance

In the analyses that follow, a difference is considered statistically significant at the 0.05 level if the difference in the percentages for the two samples is at least twice as large as its standard error.

RESULTS OF ANALYSES

Demographic Data

The profile of Latino women emerging from this survey is one of a relatively young population, most of whom live in larger-than-average households with children under age eighteen and who work. Having less education and lower incomes than their non-Latina counterparts, they rely on welfare programs to a greater extent than other low-income women.

Women indicating that they are "of Hispanic origin or descent" were asked where they were from. Of those self-identifying as Hispanic, 54 percent were Mexican, 14 percent were Puerto Rican, 4 percent were Cuban, 4 percent were from Spain, and 14 percent were "other Hispanic." Some 65 percent had been born in the United States; the remaining 35 percent had been born in other countries. Because of the relatively small numbers involved, the remaining data sets are not broken down by national origin or place of birth.

Almost three-quarters of all Latinas surveyed (74%) said they are white; an additional 9 percent described themselves as black or African American, and one percent indicated they are American Indian. The remaining 16 percent answered "not sure," which suggests they are of mixed racial origin or did not want to identify themselves as members of a particular race.

Latino women tend to be younger than the total female population surveyed. While a similar proportion of both samples falls between the ages of eighteen and forty-four (68% of Latinas and 65% of all women), only 8 percent of the Latina subsample, in marked contrast with 18 percent of all women, are age sixty-five years and older.

The data on marital status indicate that the proportions of Latina women who are married, separated, or divorced are similar to those for all women interviewed. But Latinas are significantly more likely to be single (23% compared with 16%) and less likely to be widowed than women respondents as a whole. Data on household composition indicate that Latinas are significantly more likely to live with a family member other than a spouse, or with someone else, than the rest of the population. They are also less likely to live alone (16% compared with 22% of all women).

In keeping with the traditional image of large families and households, Latinas are also more likely to report being a parent or guardian of a child under age eighteen. Of those living with someone else, 59 percent (compared with 48% of all women) have children under age eighteen living with them. Household size reflects this; the median size for all Latino respondents is four (compared with two for all women). Fully one-fourth (25% compared with 13% of all women) live in homes with five or more persons.

The Latino respondents are much more likely to be urban residents than the sample as a whole. Almost 54 percent live in urban areas, compared with less than 33 percent of all women.

Latino women reported significantly less education than the total study sample. Among Latinas, 38 percent responded that they have less than a high school education, in contrast with 21 percent of all the women surveyed. Only 11 percent, compared with 18 percent of all women, are college graduates.

The data on employment status reveal similar rates of labor participation for Latinas as for U.S. women in general. Some 38 percent of Latinas (and 41% of all women) indicated that they work full-time for pay; 19 percent work part-time; and 40 percent do not work. A majority of the latter, however, expressed a desire to work: fully 68 percent of Latinas, in contrast to 47 percent of all women, would prefer to work, and 61 percent of these would be able to work if a suitable job were available in their area. Similar to women as a whole, those who are not currently working for pay but who want to gave "the need for money" (mentioned by 64% of Latinas and 54% of all women) as the major reason for their response.

The lower educational and occupational status of Latino women is reflected in the data on income. Latinas are significantly poorer than women as a whole. Almost one-third (33% compared with 27% of all women) reported annual family incomes of $15,000 or lower. Only 22 percent (compared with 33% of all women) have annual incomes above $35,000.

Among women with incomes under $25,000, Latinas are more likely to be receiving supplemental benefits than all poor women surveyed. Latinas tend to have higher rates of participation in most public assistance programs. This can be partly explained by the fact that they have larger households and more children; therefore, even within a given income level, Latinas are poorer than the rest. Moreover, the fact that a larger proportion avail themselves of certain programs (e.g., food stamps) may lessen the stigma associated with receiving such benefits.

Health Status

Self-reported health status has been found to be a reliable indicator of morbidity and mortality (Idler and Angel 1990). Surveys therefore often ask respondents how they rate their own health. The Commonwealth Fund survey found that Latinas are significantly less likely than women as a whole to give a positive report of their health (76% compared with 85%) and significantly more likely to report being in "fair/poor" health (24% compared with 15%). The perception of being in poor health is particularly marked, considering that Latinas tend to be younger and that negative self-appraisals increase with age.

The negative perception that Latinas have of their own health is consistent with data from the National Center for Health Statistics. These data show that, at all age levels, minorities are more likely to consider their health to be fair or poor, with Hispanics ranking approximately halfway between whites and African Americans in all cohorts (U.S. Department of Health and Human Services 1990). It also coincides with the findings of the HHANES, which showed that Mexican Americans and Puerto Ricans reported worse health status than that found by a physician's examination (Angel and Guarnaccia 1989). The lack of congruence in health assessments was particularly marked among respondents opting to take the interview in Spanish, a choice that was associated with poorer self-assessed health. The researchers therefore speculated that "these findings may reflect a culturally conditioned response pattern in addition to actual poorer overall health" (Angel and Guarnaccia 1989:1234).

The higher level of reported ill health cannot be attributed to a higher rate of functional disability: significantly fewer Latinas (11% in contrast with 16% of all women) reported in The Commonwealth Fund survey that a disability, handicap, or chronic condition restricts their full participation in school, work, housework, or other activities. Similarly, the number of sick days is lower for Latinas than for all women: 2.9 and 3.2 per year, respectively. Half (50%) of all Latinas, compared with 42 percent of all women, reported one or no sick days during the previous year. This lower rate of restricted activity and use of sick days may be a function of the different age compositions of the two groups.

When asked whether they require help with activities of daily living (e.g., eating, bathing), Latinas indicated a rate of impairment (2%) similar to that of the whole sample. But fewer Latino women (6%

compared with 9% of all women) indicated needing help with basic activities such as household chores and shopping.

Asked if a doctor had told them if they had one or more of sixteen specific conditions, Latinas answered affirmatively in proportions similar to or lower than all women in fifteen of the conditions. Diabetes is the only condition for which Latinas are more likely to be told by a physician that they are at risk: 12 percent (compared with 7% of all women) answered Yes to this question. This is consistent with epidemiological studies showing that diabetes is more prevalent in certain groups of Hispanics than in the rest of the population. The 1982–84 HHANES found that Mexican Americans and Puerto Ricans had a two to three times greater prevalence of type II (non–insulin-dependent) diabetes mellitus than non-Hispanic whites. Recent studies also show that Mexican Americans have a greater chance of developing diabetes and are at higher risk of suffering from the complications of the disease than non-Hispanic whites (Stern and Haffner 1992).

At the same time, Latinas are less likely to be told they have arthritis or bursitis, osteoporosis, or endometriosis. This can probably be attributed to the younger mean age of the Latino sample.

Emotional Well-Being

Reflecting the interplay between health and morale (Susser and Watson 1988), reports of emotional well-being mirror those of self-assessed health status. The survey found Latinas scoring lower on several indicators of life satisfaction and emotional well-being (tab. 5.1). They are significantly less likely to say that they are "very satisfied" or "somewhat satisfied" with life (85% compared with 94% of all women) and more than twice as likely to report that they are "not at all" or "not very" satisfied with life (13% compared with 6%). They also score lower on a self-esteem scale, with 42 percent (compared with 51% of all women) reporting high self-esteem and 27 percent (compared with 20% of all women) reporting low self-esteem. This is a consistent pattern of responses. Latinas are less likely than all women to agree with each of five positive statements about themselves. And they are more likely than women as a whole to agree with all five negative statements about themselves.

Latinas are also significantly more likely to report feelings of depression, with more than half (53% compared with 40% of all women) scoring high on a depression scale. Nevertheless, the proportion who

Table 5.1. Percentage of Women Agreeing Somewhat or Strongly with Specific Statements

	All Women	Latino Women
I feel that I have a number of good qualities	96	94
I feel that I am a person of worth, at least on an equal plane with others[a]	95	92
I am able to do things as well as most other people	91	88
I take a positive attitude toward myself[a]	92	88
On the whole, I am satisfied with myself	92	90
I wish I could have more respect for myself[a]	28	34
I certainly feel useless at times	31	35
I feel I do not have much to be proud of[a]	12	20
At times I think I am no good at all[a]	12	19
All in all, I am inclined to feel that I am a failure[a]	5	8

Source: Data from The Commonwealth Fund survey on women's health, 1993.

[a] Differences are significant; $p \leq 0.05$.

indicated having considered suicide is similar for both subgroups (6% and 7%).

The survey asked Latino women about sources of stress, experience with conflicts and violence, marital relations, and social supports, which provides a more precise picture of their emotional well-being. Women were asked about difficulties in coping with a key source of stress: combining work with family responsibilities. Latino responses do not vary much from those of all women: 47 percent and 44 percent, respectively, reported this to be somewhat or very difficult.

The extent to which Latinas are vulnerable to acts of violence was probed in a series of questions about whether they had been abused, assaulted, or raped, or were victims of other types of physical crimes (tab. 5.2). It is important to note that Latinas are less likely to discuss these incidents of abuse with a doctor than are women in general (10% and 21%, respectively). Furthermore, they expressed a greater interest than all respondents in talking to someone further about this topic (33% compared with 22%).

No significant differences are apparent in the proportion of Latinas answering that they had been verbally or emotionally abused, physically abused, or raped while they were growing up. Some 27 percent reported verbal abuse, 14 percent reported physical abuse, and 13 percent reported sexual abuse. The corresponding percentages for all

Table 5.2. Percentage of Women Who Have Been Victims of Crime in the Past 5 Years

Type of Crime	All Women	Latino Women
Mugging, robbery, or assault[a]	8	12
Burglary	9	11
Rape or sexual assault	2	3
Other kind of crime	3	3

Source: Data from The Commonwealth Fund survey on women's health, 1993.

[a] Differences are significant; $p \leq 0.05$.

women are 27 percent, 13 percent, and 10 percent, respectively. As in the case of women as a whole, those who suffered sexual abuse are most often the victim of someone they knew (87% and 85%, respectively). But Latinas are significantly more likely to be abused by a member of their immediate family (72% compared with 55%).

Although Latinas are more likely to live in poorer, more urban environments, they are not more likely than women in general to have been the victims of physical crime (tab. 5.2). The only type of crime for which they are significantly more at risk is mugging, robbery, or assault. Of those who had these experiences, Latinas are not more likely to have been hurt physically than all women (35% and 29%, respectively).

Marital relations are no different for Latinas than for the female population as a whole. Almost one-third of all Latino respondents (32% compared with 29% of all women) said they were the victims of verbal or psychological battering by their spouses. Five percent reported being physically assaulted by their spouses, a proportion similar to that for the population as a whole. One percent of Latinas responded that they had been held down or otherwise forced by their spouses to have sex (less than one percent of all women reported this).

Similarly, Latinas are equally likely to report that their spouses or partners resorted to violence when they had an argument. Although Latino women reported a slightly higher prevalence of each of eleven behaviors reflecting conflict, the differences are not statistically significant.

The importance of social supports has been increasingly recognized in the literature on health behaviors. Among other things, support networks have been found to enhance healthful practices, mitigate stress, and facilitate health seeking (Berkman and Breslow 1983). The literature on Latino families has often pointed out that Latinos are members of large families and have dense and extensive networks, which in turn cushion some of the problems associated with poverty and social marginalization (Bernal 1982; García-Prieto 1982; Hayes-Batista 1992).

The survey, however, found that significantly fewer Latina women (88% compared with 95% of all women) have someone to call on for help when they have a problem. The most frequently mentioned person is a parent (28%), followed by a sibling (22%) or a friend (18%). For all women, the modal source of social support is also a parent (26%) followed by a son or a daughter (23%) or a friend (18%). Latinas' greater reliance on siblings may be explained by their larger families.

Another source of social support is the extent to which household tasks are shared. More than three-fourths of married Latinas (76%) said that their partners share responsibility for housework, a proportion comparable to that reported by women as a whole. Also, 88 percent have spouses who take responsibility for child care, as similarly reported by all women (92%).

Health Behaviors

The behavioral aspects of health and disease have received increasing attention during the past two decades (Lalonde 1974; Knowles 1977). While some of this attention has focused too much on individual responsibility and led to "blaming the victim," this focus has also served to uncover new links in disease causality and thereby broadened the possible targets for health promotion and disease prevention. The Commonwealth Fund survey covers an array of health-related behaviors, including weight problems, exercise, smoking, substance abuse, and contraceptive practices.

Using body mass indexes, the survey shows significant differences between Latinas and all women. Fewer Latinas (13% compared with 18% of all women) are within the recommended range for weight or are underweight (9% compared with 14% of all women). More than three-quarters of all Latinas in the sample are overweight (77% compared with 67% of all women). The high prevalence of overweight Latino women was also found in the HHANES, although the measurements varied and the prevalence of weight problems was different in the two surveys. The HHANES found that 31.6 percent of Cuban women, 40.2 percent of Puerto Rican women, and 41.6 percent of Mexican American women were overweight (Fanelli-Kuczmarski and Woteki 1990). These rates were higher than the corresponding figures for non-Hispanic white women, but not as high as those for non-Hispanic African American women.

Given the extent of weight problems among Latinas, it is not surprising that half are dissatisfied with their weight, a proportion similar to that for all women (45%). There is no meaningful difference in the incidence of bulimia between the two groups, with 3 percent of Latinas and one percent of all women reporting having tried to control their weight by vomiting. Nor is there a difference in the proportion who said that a doctor had told them that they were underweight or had an eating disorder (7% of Latinas compared with 11% of all women).

While much of the problem of excess weight is probably due to diet, at least part of the problem can be explained by sedentary lifestyles. More Latinas (38% compared with 31% of all women) indicated that they never exercise strenuously. Similar proportions of Latinas and women in general (28% and 31%, respectively) exercise strenuously 3 or more days per week.

Smoking, long associated with a variety of health problems and therefore the target of behavior-modification campaigns, is one behavior for which Latinas appear to be at less risk (tab. 5.3). The proportion

Table 5.3. Percentage of Women Reporting Specific Health-Related Practices

	All Women	Latino Women
Exercising 3 or more days per week	31	28
Smoking[a]	25	14
Drinking alcoholic beverages[a]	49	36
Trying marijuana[a]	21	14
Trying crack or cocaine, heroin, speed, or downers[a]	5	3
Taking tranquilizers over past 12 months	8	10
Receiving counseling from doctor on smoking, drinking, drug use[a]	21	15
Not using contraception	70	73
Having had an abortion[a]	12	17
Currently taking calcium supplements[a]	29	24
Currently on hormone replacement therapy (age 40+)[a]	21	10

Source: Data from The Commonwealth Fund survey on women's health, 1993.

[a] Differences are significant; $p \leq 0.05$.

of current smokers among Latinas is significantly lower than that for the female population as a whole: 14 percent and 25 percent, respectively. Moreover, those who smoke tend to smoke less than women as a whole (a median of fifty compared with ninety-six cigarettes per week, respectively). Both of these findings confirm the data from the 1982–84 HHANES (Rogers 1991).

Latinas are also less likely to drink alcohol than the rest of the female population: 36 percent, in marked contrast to 49 percent of all females, reported drinking alcoholic beverages (tab. 5.3). For those who drink, however, their frequency is similar, with both drinking on 3 or fewer days during the past 2 weeks. Only 2 percent of Latinas (compared with 4% of all women) report drinking on a daily basis during the previous 2 weeks. The volume of drinking among Latinas who do drink is also similar to that for all women: most (82% of Latinas compared with 86% of all women) reported having had one to three drinks a day on the days they drank during the past 2 weeks.

A smaller portion of Latino women reported having used marijuana, crack or cocaine, heroin, speed, or downers (see tab. 5.3). Only 3 percent of Latino women, as opposed to 5 percent of all women, had tried these substances.

Possibly because they collectively appear to be less at risk than other women, Latinas who drink, smoke, or use drugs are less likely to report having been counseled by a doctor concerning these practices. Only 15 percent of Latinas, compared with 21 percent of all women engaging in one of these behaviors, said they had been counseled.

The survey also asked women about their contraceptive practices (tab. 5.3). The pattern for Latinas does not differ significantly from that for women in general: some 73 percent of Latinas and 70 percent of all women do not use a contraceptive method. This is a very low rate of nonuse of contraception, particularly in view of the fact that other surveys have found that 60 percent of U.S. women between the ages of fifteen and forty-four practice contraception by relying on surgical or reversible methods (Mosher 1990).

Of all birth control methods, oral contraception is the modal choice, mentioned by 15 percent of Latinas and 16 percent of all women. This is followed by condoms, used by 5 percent of Latinas and 7 percent of all women. Two percent of all Latino women use a diaphragm; not more than one percent of the Latina sample use other methods. The survey does not capture the extent to which women currently rely on sterilization, which has emerged as the most popular method of fertility control among ever-married women in the United States and is particularly prevalent among certain Latino subgroups (Mosher 1990).

Given the relatively low level of contraception practiced by all the women surveyed, it is not surprising that almost one in eight has had abortions. A significantly higher proportion of Latinas reported having had an abortion—17 percent, in contrast with 12 percent for women as a whole. This suggests that a sizable proportion of pregnancies are unwanted, and that religious beliefs and cultural taboos do not appear to deter abortion.

The survey also asked women if they were currently taking hormones and calcium supplements. The data suggest significant differences between Latinas and women in general with respect to both practices. Among those age forty or older, only 10 percent of Latino women, compared with 21 percent of all women, reported being on estrogen replacement therapy. Similarly, proportionately fewer Latinas take calcium supplements (24% compared with 29% of all women). This difference is smaller than expected in view of the fact that 46 percent of Latinas, in marked contrast to 25 percent of all women, reported not being familiar with osteoporosis.

Access to Health Care

Insurance coverage is key to facilitating access to health care. Lack of coverage, therefore, generally is associated with less use of services and a lower probability of having a regular source of care (Treviño et al. 1992). The Commonwealth Fund survey shows that Latinas are significantly more likely to lack health insurance than women in general (22% compared with 13%). In keeping with their lower income levels, Latinas are more likely to rely on Medicaid or public assistance (tab. 5.4). The relatively low portion of Latinas on Medicare can be explained by their lower mean age.

Proportionately as many Latinas as all women reported being enrolled in a health maintenance organization (16% and 17%, respectively). At least part of this near-parity may reflect the fact that a substantial portion of Latinos live in western states in which HMOs have made significant inroads.

Most of the Latinas surveyed (73%) have a regular source of care. This measure is significantly less than is the case for all women (79%). Moreover, having a regular source of care does not say much about the quality of care received; previous surveys have found that emergency

Table 5.4. Percentage of Women Covered by Health Plans or
Health Insurance, by Type of Coverage

Type of Coverage	All Women	Latino Women
Medicare[a]	22	12
Medicaid/public aid[a]	5	12
Employer-paid[a]	53	48
Self-paid/private insurance	7	6
None[a]	13	22

Source: Data from The Commonwealth Fund survey on women's health,
1993.
[a] Differences are significant; $p \leq 0.05$.

rooms may constitute a regular source of care for segments of the
population (Solís et al. 1990). Indeed, the Commonwealth Fund survey
shows that, of those Latino women who reported having a regular
source of care, 11 percent go to an emergency room, more than twice the
proportion for all the women surveyed (5%). Compared with all wom-
en, Latinas go to a doctor's office less frequently (74% and 63%, respectively) and to clinics more often (22% compared with 17% of all women).

Given their lower insurance coverage and different sources of care,
it is not surprising that more Latinas than women in general reported
not having seen a doctor during the past year (13% and 9%, respectively). Otherwise, the patterns of medical utilization are not very different between the two groups. The mean number of two different
doctors is the same for both populations. Latinas who reported visiting
a physician during the past year reported an average of seven visits a
year, somewhat higher than the six reported by all women. The proportion of high users of medical care (eleven or more visits per year)
was 13 percent for both groups.

Latinas are significantly more likely to indicate that, during the past
12 months, there was a time when they needed medical care but did
not get it (17% compared with 13%). Financial reasons clearly emerge
as a barrier to care. The main reason mentioned by Latinas for their
failure to receive needed care is that "it was not covered by insurance."
This is the answer of 43 percent of the Latino respondents, in marked
contrast to only 27 percent of all women. The second most frequently
mentioned reason is that the medical services "cost too much" (33%
compared with 57% of all women). Failure to get an appointment is the
third most frequently mentioned reason (10%).

The survey also asked all respondents if they had received specific services during the past year. Latinas are significantly less likely to have received four of seven preventive services when compared with all women (tab. 5.5). This suggests that, even when patterns of using health care are similar for both groups, the content of the care may vary.

The proportion of Latinas who never received each of the listed preventive services is higher than the proportion for all women (tab. 5.6). The differences are significant with respect to blood pressure screenings, mammograms, breast examinations, and pelvic examinations. It is obvious, therefore, that there is a great need for preventive care among Latino women.

Those who reported not receiving particular services during the past year were asked why. For Latinas, as for women as a whole, cost is the major reason, followed by lack of time. Significantly more Latinas are also deterred by a fear of what they might find out, lack of transportation, and failure to get an appointment (tab. 5.7).

Patterns of Physician Use and Interaction

In keeping with their greater reliance on emergency rooms and clinics, Latinas are significantly less likely than all women to have a regular physician. Eighteen percent do not have a regular physician, compared with only 10 percent of all women. Among those with a regular physician, more than half (53%) see a family practitioner; this is similar to the proportion of all women relying on a family doctor (56%).

Table 5.5. Percentage of Women Who Received Preventive Services in the Past Year, by Type of Service

Service	All Women	Latino Women
Complete physical examination	61	59
Blood pressure screening[a]	89	82
Blood cholesterol screening	53	50
Clinical breast examination[a]	67	56
Mammogram[a]	36	29
Pelvic examination[a]	63	52
Pap smear	64	60

Source: Data from The Commonwealth Fund survey on women's health, 1993.

[a] Differences are significant; $p \leq 0.05$.

Table 5.6. Percentage of Women Who Reported Never Having Received Certain Services, by Type of Service

Service	All Women	Latino Women
Complete physical examination	4	8
Blood pressure screening[a]	6	18
Blood cholesterol screening[a]	32	42
Clinical breast examination[a]	17	32
Mammogram[a]	60	67
Pelvic examination[a]	11	23
Pap smear	2	4

Source: Data from The Commonwealth Fund survey on women's health, 1993.
[a] Differences are significant; $p \leq 0.05$.

Table 5.7. Percentage of Women Who Gave Reasons for Failure to Receive Specific Services in the Past Year

Reason	All Women	Latino Women
Costs too much[a]	29	35
Could not get appointment[a]	5	10
Lack of transportation[a]	7	11
Doctor did not suggest/discuss it	23	21
No time/too much to do[a]	23	30
Afraid of what I'd find out[a]	11	17

Source: Data from The Commonwealth Fund survey on women's health, 1993.
[a] Differences are significant; $p \leq 0.05$.

Among both groups, 13 percent reported using an obstetrician-gynecologist as their regular source of medical care.

Of those who have a regular physician, 23 percent of Latinas see a female physician, compared with 17 percent of all women. Latinas are also more likely to express a preference for female physicians; 21 percent (compared with 14% of all women) indicated such a preference. Nevertheless, a majority of both groups (70% of Latinas and 74% of all women) answered that they had no preference between male and female physicians.

In addition to their regular physician, 47 percent of Latinas see another physician for female-related problems, a proportion comparable to that for all women (46%). This other physician is an obstetrician-gynecologist in most cases (93%). Latinas rely on female physicians for these types of problems more than women do as a whole (37% compared with 30 percent).

The survey also looked into the content of physician visits and the exchange that occurs between doctor and patient. Latinas reported that, on their last visit, the doctor spent 28 minutes with them on average, the same amount of time reported by all women. Eleven percent of Latinas and 10 percent of all women feel that the physicians' attitudes and treatment of them would have been different if they had been men.

Latinas are significantly less likely to report that a physician had talked down to them or treated them like a child; only 14 percent, in contrast to 25 percent of all women, say they had been treated in a condescending or patronizing manner. At least part of the difference may be attributed to the Spanish version of the survey instrument. "Talked down to" was translated *le habló de mala forma*, which means "rudely" or "roughly" and is therefore stronger and less subtle than the concept of "talking down to" someone. The proportion of Latinas saying that a physician had told them that their medical condition was "all in your head" is the same as that for all women: 17 percent.

Only 22 percent of the Latinas surveyed, in marked contrast to 32 percent of all women, responded that a doctor had given them bad news about a health problem. Among those who had this experience, Latinas tend to be more dissatisfied than all women, with 22 percent and 15 percent, respectively, reporting negative feelings.

The vast majority of Latina women (91%) revealed that their physicians listen to them somewhat or very well; this is comparable to the proportion of all women (93%). Nevertheless, more Latinas (22% in contrast with 15% of all women) find it difficult to talk to their doctor. Moreover, one out of every six Latinas (16% compared with 10% of all women) said they had not discussed particular problems or needs with their doctors because they felt uncomfortable about doing so. (Problems related to reproduction are mentioned most frequently in this category.) These levels of unease and discomfort in communications represent significant differences between Latinas and women as a whole, and can probably be ascribed to the less equal relationship between Latinas and their physicians. Class, gender, and language barriers may play a part, as may the environment within which care is provided.

Similarly, Latinas tend to rate their physicians lower in terms of specific aspects of care. A smaller portion of Latinas are positive about their physicians' performance in terms of eight items about which they were questioned. As a result, Latinas expressed significantly more dissatisfaction with their physicians than all women: 48 percent of Latinas and 39 percent of all women rated their physicians as fair or poor on one or more items.

This apparent dissatisfaction does not result in changing physicians. A significantly smaller proportion of Latinas (34% compared with 41% of all women) reported changing physicians because they are not satisfied with their care. This may be explained by fewer alternatives available to Latinas, or by their greater reliance on clinics or hospital emergency rooms, where patients do not see the same provider consistently.

Among those who switched, communication problems are the main reason for their decision; 34 percent of the respondents who had changed physicians mentioned this, a proportion similar to that for all women (32%). The next most frequently given reason is lack of trust, mentioned by 14 percent of the Latino sample.

The data on physician-patient interaction therefore reflects that, in addition to the problems of an unequal relationship faced by most women seeking health care, Latinas confront special problems related to fear and communication difficulties. Although this may not have any obvious overt manifestations (i.e., changing doctors), it may result in distrust, postponement of needed care, and failure to comply with a prescribed regimen.

IMPLICATIONS FOR POLICY AND RESEARCH

Latino women in the United States are younger, poorer, and less educated, and have larger households than the female population as a whole. These demographic realities condition their life chances and hence their perceptions of themselves and their access to care. The survey findings suggest policy issues that need to be addressed and areas that need further research.

Differences among Latinos are as wide as the differences between Latinos and the rest of the population. The HHANES highlighted the extent to which Latinos make up distinct ethnic groups, with different migration histories, socioeconomic characteristics, and health indicators (Stroup-Benham, Treviño, and Treviño 1990). This variation in turn implies the need for different strategies to meet the needs of different groups. While broad portraits provide the preliminary contours for a health agenda, subgroup-specific data are needed to design programmatic interventions.

Patterns of the use of health care show that, although Latinas are less likely to have health insurance and a regular source of care, they use medical services as frequently as other women. Nevertheless, where they go and what care they get vary significantly. Therefore, they are not so much *under*served as *ill* served.

In the area of prevention, the survey data show that Latinas are less likely than women as a whole to be informed, receive adequate counseling, or be screened for specific conditions. While Latinas are less likely to drink or smoke, they are more likely to be overweight and to lead sedentary lives. At the same time, Latinas are less likely to have been told that they have certain conditions and may therefore be unaware of specific health-related practices. The relatively high proportion of women who have never had a breast examination or mammogram is symptomatic of the failure of discrete, procedure-oriented preventive measures that are not integrated into primary care. The high prevalence of abortion also represents a glaring failure of prevention.

The greater reliance of Latino women on the emergency room as a regular source of care is another issue that should be addressed. If this results from a lack of prevention and the postponing of needed care until a condition becomes urgent, more aggressive outreach efforts and earlier interventions are likely to curtail the practice. Yet the emergency room may have advantages over other sources of care—for example, it provides accessible 24-hour service and so-called one-stop shopping for all conditions—that may offset the disadvantages of a system designed for episodic care. Policy makers must recognize that Latinas often live in residentially segregated areas in which major hospitals and medical centers are one of the few "mainstream" establishments with which they have contact. The challenge is to create lower-cost alternatives that ensure availability and convenience, on the one hand, and continuity of care, on the other.

With respect to physician-patient interaction, the survey uncovered a sizable proportion of disgruntled, medically demoralized women who appear to have nowhere to turn. Latinas reported greater dissatisfaction with physicians than did women in general, but are less likely to seek care elsewhere. This suggests that their alternatives are restricted or that they have low expectations concerning other options for care.

While unsatisfactory communication between physicians and women patients cuts across all groups, Latinas are differentially affected by barriers of language, class, and gender. Coming from a culture that is male-centered, patriarchal, and highly sensitive to hierarchical distinctions, Latinas are unlikely to challenge authority and ask for additional information. It is not surprising that they reported greater feelings of fear and distrust of physicians than women as a whole. Health education efforts need to take this into account when reaching out to Latino women, and practitioners must be made aware of the fact that silence does not mean comprehension or acquiescence.

The findings of the survey show that Latinas are disadvantaged socioeconomically, and this affects how they fare in the medical marketplace. They have less access to insurance, preventive measures, and information concerning specific conditions. They are also less likely to have a regular source of care, and are more likely to feel dissatisfied and uncomfortable when they do see a physician. Although lowering the financial barriers to care will increase accessibility to needed services, it will not automatically improve the health status and perceptions of Latino women. More fundamental changes in terms of how care is delivered, and by whom, are required if the health delivery system is to offset the disadvantages intrinsic to poverty and marginalization.

Despite their relative youth and lack of functional impairment, Latinas are more likely to rate their health status as fair or poor. This apparent disparity between functioning and self-perception deserves greater attention, because unfavorable ratings of health may be self-fulfilling. The phenomenon of underestimating one's health has been ascribed to an array of factors, including cultural differences in disease perception, different thresholds of complaints, and variations in the willingness to accept the "sick role" and hence be exempt from certain obligations and responsibilities (Susser and Watson 1988).

Latinas also reported significantly lower rates of satisfaction and self-esteem and higher rates of depression than women in general. While the material circumstances of Latinas' lives (i.e., lower income, less education, restricted opportunities) may have an effect on these reports of emotional health, a cultural tendency toward downplaying self-worth and well-being may also be at work. Expressions of high self-worth may be seen as boastful; as a result, Latino women may be reluctant to manifest self-confidence and high self-esteem.[1] Conversely, social rewards may accrue to those who report feeling less than happy.

Other surveys have found a tendency for a significant proportion of Latinas to report psychological distress (Moscick et al. 1987). This has been attributed to different factors. Some believe that it is a methodological artifact, the result of instruments that, having been designed for other populations, fail to capture Latina perceptions of well-being (Wrinkle, Andalzua, and Reed-Sanders 1992). Others have suggested that the presentation of somatic symptoms may facilitate access to limited health care resources (Canino et al. 1992). Yet others argue that the reported high prevalence of depression is rooted in the religious belief that suffering cleanses; Latinas may therefore find it self-edifying to express a degree of sadness and dissatisfaction. Indeed, the "tragic sentiment of life" has been seen as emblematic of the existential angst that characterizes Hispanic culture (Monk 1990). The interplay between self-assessed health status and morale is an area ripe for further research because it sheds light not only on health behavior but also on how Latinas function vis-à-vis their families and the broader community.

At the same time, research has to focus on the particularities of different Latino subgroups rather than on Latinas as a whole. Like other aggregates, the Latino population in the United States is a statistical construct rather than an identifiable group with a collective identity. Aggregating data may therefore mask epidemiological distinctions and preclude effective interventions.

NOTE

1. As in other cultures, expressing satisfaction or feelings of well-being is seen as a way of tempting fate and prompting the so-called evil eye to counteract good fortune.

REFERENCES

Angel, R., and Guarnaccia, P. J. 1989. Mind, body, and culture: somatization among Hispanics. *Social Science and Medicine* 28:1229–38.
Berkman, L. F., and Breslow, L. 1983. *Health and Ways of Living*. New York: Oxford University Press.
Bernal, G. 1982. Cuban families. In M. Goldrick, J. K. Pearce, and J. Giordano, eds., *Ethnicity and Family Therapy*. New York: Guilford Press.
Canino, I. A., et al. 1992. Functional somatic symptoms: a cross-ethnic comparison. *American Journal of Orthopsychiatry* 62:611.

Fanelli-Kuczmarski, M., and Woteki, C. E. 1990. Monitoring the nutritional status of the Hispanic population: selected findings for the Mexican-Americans, Cubans, and Puerto Ricans. *Nutrition Today* May–June:6–11.

García-Prieto, N. 1982. Puerto Rican families. In M. Goldrick, J. K. Pearce, and J. Giordano, eds., *Ethnicity and Family Therapy*. New York: Guilford Press.

Harris, Louis, and Associates, Inc. 1993. *The Health of American Women*. Conducted for The Commonwealth Fund.

Hayes-Bautista, D. 1992. Latino health indicators and the underclass model. In A. Furino, ed., *Health Policy and the Hispanic*. Boulder, Colo.: Westview Press.

Idler, I., and Angel, R. J. 1990. Self-rated health and mortality in the HHANES-I Epidemiologic follow-up study. *American Journal of Public Health* 80:446.

Institute for Puerto Rican Policy. 1990. Puerto Ricans and other Latinos in the United States, 1989. *Datanote* July.

Knowles, J. H., ed. 1977. *Doing Better and Feeling Worse: Health in the United States*. New York: W. W. Norton and Co.

Lalonde, M. 1974. *A New Perspective on the Health of Canadians*. Ottawa: Ministry of National Health and Welfare.

Monk, A. 1990. Caregivers of Black and Hispanic Dementia Patients: Their Use of Formal and Informal Services. Paper presented at the annual conference of the Council of Senior Center and Services, New York, June 13.

Moscick, E. K., et al. 1987. The Hispanic Health and Nutrition Examination Survey: depression among Mexican Americans, Cuban Americans, and Puerto Ricans. In M. Gaviria, ed., *Health and Behavior: Research Agenda for Hispanics*. The Simón Bolívar Hispanic-American Psychiatric Research and Training Program, University of Illinois.

Mosher, W. D. 1990. Contraceptive practice in the United States, 1982–88. *Family Planning Perspectives* 22:198–205.

National Center for Health Statistics. 1993. *Monthly Vital Statistics Report* 41:10–11.

Rogers, R. G. 1991. Health-related lifestyles among Mexican-Americans, Puerto Ricans, and Cubans in the United States. In I. Rosenwaike, ed., *Mortality of the Hispanic Populations: Mexicans, Puerto Ricans, and Cubans in the United States and in the Home Countries*. New York: Greenwood Press.

Rosenwaike, I. 1991. Mortality experience of Hispanic populations. In I. Rosenwaike, ed., *Mortality of Hispanic Populations: Mexicans, Puerto Ricans, and Cubans in the United States and in the Home Countries*. New York: Greenwood Press.

Solís, J. M., et al. 1990. Acculturation, access to care, and the use of preventive health services by Hispanics: findings from HHANES, 1982–84. *American Journal of Public Health* 80:27–31.

Stern, M. P., and Haffner, S. M. 1992. Type II diabetes in Mexican Americans: a public health challenge. In A. Furino, ed., *Health Policy and the Hispanic*. Boulder, Colo.: Westview Press.

Stroup-Benham, C. A., Treviño, F. M., and Treviño, D. B. 1990. Alcohol consumption patterns among Mexican American mothers and among children from single- and dual-headed households: findings from HHANES 192–84. *American Journal of Public Health* 80:36–41.

Susser, M. W., and Watson, W. 1988. *Sociology in Medicine.* Oxford: Oxford University Press.

Treviño, F. M., et al. 1992. Health coverage and utilization of services by Mexican-Americans, Puerto Ricans, and Cuban Americans. In A. Furino, ed., *Health Policy and the Hispanic.* Boulder, Colo.: Westview Press.

U.S. Department of Health and Human Services. 1990. *Health Status of the Disadvantaged Chartbook, 1990.* Washington, D.C.: U.S. Government Printing Office.

Wrinkle, R. D., Andalzua, H., and Reed-Sanders, D. 1988. Analysis of scales measuring self-esteem, life satisfaction, and mastery for Hispanic elderly populations. In M. Sotomayor and H. Curiel, eds., *Hispanic Elderly: A Cultural Signature.* Edinburg, Tex.: Pan American University Press.

6

Midlife Women
Health Care Patterns and Choices

Nancy Fugate Woods, R.N., Ph.D.

As the Baby Boomers enter their middle years, there has been a surge of interest in midlife. Because midlife women are one of the most rapidly growing population groups in the United States, popular media and scientific literature alike have focused increasingly on topics such as menopause and how to manage it (Greer 1992). Aside from menopause, researchers have devoted little attention to other aspects of midlife women's health and how to promote it. The consequences of ignoring the health of the largest group of midlife women in U.S. history could lead to significant demands for health services and escalating costs of care as this cohort of women ages.

One of the challenges confronting those who study midlife is demarcating that portion of a woman's life. Definitions based on women's reproductive capacity, using menopause as a marker, have become less useful because of the increasing number of women using hormone therapies that mask the occurrence of natural menopause. Those definitions based on women's work role patterns, such as when the last child leaves home and when women increase their workforce involvement, also have become problematic as adult children now stay at home and most women remain in the labor force throughout their childbearing years. Moreover, some midlife women choose to become pregnant in their forties, resulting in some Baby Boomers having small children at the same time others are trying to launch their adult children. Age boundaries such as forty to sixty-five may be the best indicator of midlife, because such boundaries generally differentiate women's reproductive years from their retirement years (Brooks-Gunn and Kirsch 1994).

Whatever the indicator, midlife women's health has become an exceedingly important topic, given the large segment of the population that will reach old age early in the next century. As contemporary midlife women age, their longevity is likely to strain the health care resources they need, and those in poor health may strain the entitlement programs that support living expenses and health care for elderly persons. The health of contemporary midlife women—the Baby Boomers—bears careful watching as an indicator of future needs for health services and mechanisms for financing them. Moreover, how midlife women currently use health services to promote their health and prevent disease becomes particularly important in anticipating future needs.

The Baby Boom cohort of women is unique in many respects. The majority remain employed throughout their lives, regardless of marital status or the ages of their children. In addition, they have lived alone more of their adult lives than have past cohorts, reflecting differences in marriage and divorce rates from their mothers' generation. As a result, Baby Boomer women are married for a smaller proportion of their lifetimes than their mothers were. They are also better educated and have lower fertility rates than their mothers' generation (McLaughlin et al. 1988). Although some of these features of their lifestyles, such as employment, have positive consequences for health, others, such as lack of a second income for their households, may have negative health consequences.

Because midlife women's health, health promotion, and use of health services have important consequences for women themselves, as well as for projecting future health care requirements, the following questions were addressed using data from The Commonwealth Fund survey. How healthy are midlife women of the Baby Boom cohort? How do they rate their health? What kinds of health problems do they experience? What do midlife women do to promote their own health? What kinds of health services do midlife women use for health promotion and the early detection of disease? What factors affect their use of health services—in particular, hormone therapy?

HEALTH STATUS AND THE USE OF HEALTH SERVICES

Although 80 percent of midlife women rate their health as good to excellent in the National Health Interview Survey, midlife is when women begin to experience their first chronic illness, such as high blood pressure, arthritis, heart disease, diabetes, or bronchitis. Midlife women are hospitalized most frequently for heart disease, cancer, gallbladder disease, diabetes, and psychoses, especially depression. The most common surgical procedures for this age group are hysterectomy and cholecystectomy. The leading cause of death during women's middle years is cancer, followed by heart disease (National Center for Health Statistics 1993a).

Women visit health care providers more frequently than men and practice more preventive care. Data from the National Health Interview Survey indicate that midlife women visit physicians' offices approximately 4.5 times a year. Although women frequently use physicians' services for prevention and early detection of disease, the increasing frequency with which midlife women use physicians' services is attributable to the need to monitor for certain chronic health problems such as heart disease and diabetes (National Center for Health Statistics 1982).

THE IMPACT OF WORK ON HEALTH

Because of the dramatic changes in the Baby Boomers' participation in the labor force, many studies of this cohort's health have emphasized the health consequences of employment (Nathanson 1975; Verbrugge 1986). More recently, investigators have examined the effects of women's continued employment in the context of their family roles and responsibilities. Longitudinal works indicate that employment generally has beneficial effects on health and that work may be health promoting in the face of the stress women experience from their nurturing roles as spouse, mother, and caregiver. The quality of women's experiences in employment and family contexts has important consequences for health that may be mediated by each role as a source of support or stress. Employment seems to buffer the consequences of stress generated by women's nurturing roles (McKinlay et al. 1990).

HORMONE THERAPY

As the Baby Boomers approach menopause, the use of hormones (estrogen and estrogen with a progestin) by middle-aged and older women has generated renewed scientific interest in the potential protective value of hormones as well as their efficacy in managing symptoms. Although estrogen was first approved for use by postmenopausal women in the 1940s, the prevalence of estrogen use did not increase substantially until the 1960s, when clinicians prescribed it for the relief of menopausal hot flashes and urogenital symptoms. During the early 1970s evidence of an increased incidence of endometrial cancer associated with estrogen therapy and concerns about possible associations with increased risk of vascular disease (as had occurred with the use of oral contraceptives) led to a decrease in the prescription of estrogen therapy (Bush 1991). In the 1980s the practice of adding a progestin to prescriptions of estrogen therapy to reduce the risk of endometrial cancer predated an increase in prescriptions for hormone therapy (Gambrell 1987; Hemminki et al. 1988).

Possible risks that have been associated with the use of estrogen and combined hormone therapy include (1) increased risk of endometrial cancer in women who have a uterus and who are using estrogen alone; (2) increased risk of breast cancer; (3) the resumption of menses or spotting related to progestin therapy; (4) increased risk of gallbladder disease; (5) the growth of uterine fibroids; and (6) the necessity to adhere to a medication regimen for an extended period of one's life (Grady et al. 1992). On the other hand, the increased monitoring by a health professional associated with hormone therapy may also contribute to the early detection of other treatable diseases, thereby having a net positive effect on women's health.

The U.S. Food and Drug Administration approved the use of postmenopausal estrogen to prevent and manage osteoporosis (*Physicians' Desk Reference* 1993) based on evidence supporting the effectiveness of estrogen in reducing hip and vertebral fractures (Lindsay et al. 1978; Weiss et al. 1980). Evidence linking the use of estrogen therapy to a reduction in the incidence of heart disease has introduced yet another indication for hormone therapy—to prevent heart disease (Stampfer et al. 1985; Bush et al. 1987; Henderson, Paganini-Hill, and Ross 1988).

Current Recommendations

Completed studies have indicated that hormone therapies offer both benefit and risk to women using them (Lindsay et al. 1978; Weiss et al. 1980). Despite the promise of new evidence of the protective effects of estrogen and combined hormone therapy, caution pervades recommendations for its use because the studies were retrospective, looking at women who self-selected themselves for hormone use and who may have had other underlying protective factors (e.g., better access to health care and good health practices like a heart-healthy diet and exercise regimen). Definitive estimates of benefits and risks will come only from randomized clinical trials (i.e., women have an equal chance of being assigned to a group receiving a placebo, estrogen, or a combination of estrogen and a progestin). In the face of this uncertainty, but recognizing the increasing number of women receiving hormone therapy, the American College of Physicians published "Guidelines for Counseling Postmenopausal Women about Preventive Hormone Therapy," in which they advocated careful and individual consideration of the benefits of short-term use of hormone therapy to manage menopausal symptoms and to prevent disease (American College of Physicians 1992).

In the absence of definitive data, the American College of Physicians recommends that women of all races consider preventive hormone therapy and advises a limited course of therapy (one to 5 years) for women seeking relief from symptoms such as hot flashes, night sweats, and urogenital symptoms. Women who have had a hysterectomy benefit from estrogen therapy and have no need for combined hormone therapy (estrogen and a progestin). Women who have or who are at increased risk of coronary disease are likely to benefit from hormone therapy and should receive combined therapy instead of estrogen if they still have a uterus. Using estrogen alone requires careful endometrial monitoring (e.g., endometrial biopsies, aspirations) for early diagnosis of endometrial cancer. The risks of hormone therapy may outweigh the benefits for women at increased risk of breast cancer. The American College of Physicians guidelines conclude that "for other women, the best course of action is not clear" (American College of Physicians 1992:1038). Thus, many women face the decision of whether to adopt hormone therapy with incomplete information.

More Definitive Clinical Trials

At this writing, two large randomized clinical trials, the Postmenopausal Estrogen and Progestin Intervention (PEPI) study and the Women's Health Initiative Trial, are both under way to clarify the effects of hormone therapy. The PEPI trial results have begun to provide data about the consequences of using estrogen or combined hormone therapy (estrogen with a progestin) for risk factors for heart disease

(National Center for Health Statistics 1982).[1] Estrogen alone or in combination with a progestin improved lipoproteins and lowered fibrinogen levels without adversely affecting insulin response or blood pressure levels. Unopposed estrogen was the optimal regimen for elevating high-density lipoprotein-cholesterol (HDL-C). A high rate of endometrial hyperplasia occurred among women with a uterus using unopposed estrogen, indicating that this would be risky therapy for women with a uterus. Of all the estrogen and progestin combinations, CEE with cyclic micronized progesterone had the most favorable effect of all the combined therapies on HDL-C (Writing Group for the PEPI Trial 1995). Further analysis of the data is necessary before policy recommendations will be forthcoming.

The Women's Health Initiative clinical trial will assess the long-term consequences of hormone therapy in postmenopausal women for heart disease, osteoporosis, and breast cancer. In addition, the use of a low-fat, high-fiber diet and calcium and vitamin D supplementation will be compared with the effects of hormone therapy on several disease endpoints. Among the many important contributions of this trial will be the comparison of interventions that women themselves can initiate—dietary modification and the use of vitamins and minerals—with or without the use of hormone therapies (National Institutes of Health 1992). This trial, however, is still in its early phase.

Life-Cycle Event or Disease

As the medical indications for the use and prescribing practices of hormones have changed, so has the tenor of feminist critique of hormone therapy. Early feminist critics of those advocating the use of estrogen for women from "womb to tomb" so that they could remain "feminine forever" (Wilson 1966) alleged that the use of hormones without long-term assessment of effects represented dangerous experimentation with women's health. Many asserted that the medicalization of women's health events, such as giving birth, menstruation, and menopause, transformed natural events into diseases needing treatment. To many, hormone therapy for menopausal symptoms and even current attempts to assess its benefits and risks represented additional evidence of medicalization of women's lives. Critics asserted that as an early focus on symptom management grew to include the prevention of osteoporosis and heart disease, these diseases became defined increasingly as part of menopause, and menopause was viewed increasingly as a disease (MacPherson 1981, 1992; Bell 1990).

Understanding women's beliefs about hormone therapy and their actual practices would be incomplete without considering the social and historical context in which these occur. Women who are part of the Baby Boom birth cohort are now sifting through the available information about hormone therapy. Women who once asked, "What is the risk of using hormone therapies?" are now asking, "What is the risk of not using hormone therapies?"

Making a Choice

Despite the flurry of research activity investigating the health consequences of hormone therapy, to date only one research team has studied how women decide to adopt hormone therapy. In responding to hypothetical case studies focusing on the use of estrogen, women were influenced largely by symptom distress associated with hot flashes and to a lesser extent by the risk of osteoporosis and side effects of estrogen therapy. Although health professionals tend to emphasize risk reduction, women themselves were concerned about the immediate effects of estrogen on symptoms they perceived as distressing (Rothert et al. 1990). In a later study of midlife women's decisions to use estrogen or combined hormone therapy to alleviate symptoms of menopause, again based on hypothetical cases, women's decision patterns fell into four distinct groups. One group's decision to take hormones was based on whether their hot flashes were severe. A second group of women decided they would use hormones if hot flashes were severe, but also would consider the risk of osteoporosis and cancer in making the decision. A third was most influenced by the unpleasant effects of adding progestin to the hormone therapy because its members did not want to resume menses or spotting. The fourth emphasized health risks in making decisions, particularly the risk of cancer. In all cases, the willingness to take estrogen was related to the perception that hormone treatment might be helpful in controlling symptoms of menopause and being informed about menopause and its effects on women. Expectations that menopause would be difficult were related to a lower likelihood of taking hormone therapy. Current comfort level, as indicated by hot flashes, was an overriding concern in women's decisions (Schmitt et al. 1991).

Studies of women who actually were given prescriptions for hormone therapy reveal that women use hormones sporadically. Women's primary reason for stopping treatment was the fear of cancer. Of those receiving their first hormone prescriptions, 20 percent stopped treatment within 9 months, 10 percent took the prescription sporadically, and 20 percent to 30 percent never had the prescription filled (Ravnikar 1987). The results of another survey indicated that women using estrogen were more likely to be aware that lower levels of estrogen were associated with osteoporosis, to perceive that menopause was a medical condition, to believe natural approaches to managing menopausal symptoms were less preferable, to receive care from a gynecologist, and to believe women should take hormones for hot flashes. Women using estrogen were also more than twice as likely to have had a hysterectomy and to have a Pap smear at least every 2 years. Those not using estrogen were more likely to have had relatives with uterine cancer. Women rated the resumption of menstrual periods as the most unfavorable aspect of using hormones (Ferguson, Hoegh, and Johnson 1989).

SURVEY FINDINGS

The Commonwealth Fund survey provides a unique opportunity to assess contemporary midlife women's health and to explore their patterns of health promotion and use of health services, including the use of hormones. The analyses presented here: (1) describe contemporary midlife women's health; (2) describe their health-promotion efforts and use of health services; and (3) compare women who are using hormone therapy with those who are not, with respect to demographic factors, access to health care, women's personal health practices, health status, use of preventive and diagnostic services, and characteristics of their health care providers. The data set for these analyses is 1,022 women between forty and sixty-five years of age.

Demographic Characteristics of the Study Population

The Commonwealth Fund survey included midlife women from a variety of ethnic groups among its respondents, with 10.9 percent of midlife women identifying themselves as black, 6 percent as African American, and 80.1 percent as white. Both Native American (0.4%) and Asian American (0.8%) women are underrepresented in the survey. Thirteen percent are of Hispanic descent, and, of these, over 60 percent are Mexican American. Most women have completed high school, but their education ranges from less than high school to postgraduate education. The majority (71%) live in a partnered relationship, and 39 percent have children under age eighteen living at home. Nine percent are widowed, and nearly 15 percent are divorced. Their household income for 1992 ranges from less than $7,500 to more than $100,000; the modal category is $35,000 to $50,000. Only 4 percent receive welfare. Women from across the country are represented in the survey, with 21 percent from New England and Middle Atlantic states, 33 percent from the Southeast or South Central states, 26 percent from the Upper Midwest and Bread Basket region, and 19 percent from the Mountain and Pacific regions (tab. 6.1).

Social Context

The social context for midlife women's lives is predictably complex, with most combining employment, parenting, and an adult partner relationship. Most women are employed, with 52.2 percent working full-time, 15.3 percent working part-time, and 31.5 percent not working for pay. Nearly 51 percent indicated that they preferred to be working, but 41.7 percent of those employed responded that they preferred not working. Of those who were not employed, 53 percent said that they would be able to work if a job were available in their area. Most (55%) want to be employed because they need the money.

Midlife women who are employed indicated that it is not very difficult (20%) or not difficult at all (39.6%) to balance the demands of work and family. The small portion of women with children under age eighteen living at home may account for the women's apparent ease in balancing work and family responsibilities. Moreover, their children are likely to be schoolaged or older. Although half of the midlife women missed less than 2 days of work this year because of sickness, sick days vary from 0 to 98 days.

Most women (95.6%) reported that someone in their life would be available to help them if they had a problem. The most common sources of support are: spouses (24%), children (23%), friends (19%), and parents (17%). Women living with a spouse or partner were asked if their spouse or partner shared the responsibility for housework and child care. Most reported sharing housework (74%) and child care (85%).

Although the midlife women participating in the survey had access

Table 6.1. Demographic Characteristics of Participants

Variable	N	Percentage
Age		
40–44	279	27.3
45–49	243	23.8
50–54	172	16.8
55–59	176	17.2
60–64	153	14.9
Race/ethnicity		
White	819	80.1
Black/African American	172	16.9
Asian/Pacific Islander	8	0.8
American or Alaskan Native	4	0.4
Education		
< High school	130	12.7
High school graduate	362	25.4
Some college	271	26.5
College graduate	155	15.2
Postgraduate	104	10.2
Income		
< $7,500	88	9.2
$7,501–$15,000	93	9.7
$15,001–$25,000	146	15.3
$25,001–$35,000	171	17.9
$35,001–$50,000	195	20.4
$50,001–$75,000	157	16.5
$75,001–$100,000	57	6.0
> $100,000	47	4.9
Marital status		
Single	57	5.6
Married	672	65.8
Widowed	94	9.2
Separated	47	4.6
Divorced	152	14.9
Parenting		
Dependent child	323	38.5
No dependent child	514	61.3

Source: Data from The Commonwealth Fund survey on women's health, 1993.

to support from their spouses and other members of their social networks, violence and abuse are part of everyday life for many. In their relationship with their spouse within the past year: 31 percent were insulted; 4 percent were threatened; 3 percent were pushed around, grabbed, shoved, or slapped; and one percent were kicked, bitten, or hit with a fist or some other object. Many women revealed a history of abuse while growing up: 30 percent indicated they had been verbally abused, 13 percent had been physically abused, and 10 percent had been sexually abused. Twenty percent were exposed to a crime in which they were injured in the past 5 years, with 7 percent having been mugged, robbed, or assaulted; 10 percent were victims of a burglary; one percent had been raped; and 2 percent had been victims of some other physical crime.

Health Status

Most midlife women surveyed described themselves as healthy despite the fact that 20 percent to 30 percent suffer from depression or a chronic illness or disability. On a scale of poor to excellent, most rated their health as very good (34.7%) or excellent (21.9%). Only 15 percent described themselves as being in fair or poor health. This is similar to the National Health Interview Survey results, in which 80 percent of midlife women rated their health as good to excellent (National Center for Health Statistics 1993a). Commonwealth Fund respondents also rated their satisfaction with life as positive, with 55 percent indicating they are very satisfied and only 6 percent indicating they are not satisfied. In general, midlife women have relatively high self-esteem, with half scoring above 28 on a scale with a maximal score of 40. Scores of 27 and higher indicate high self-esteem in the sample as a whole.

Despite concern about midlife depression, most women participating in this survey are not depressed. Scores for most are relatively low, with half scoring below 4 on a scale with a maximal score of 24. Nonetheless, a significant number of women are troubled. Approximately 29 percent of the midlife women scored above 6 on the depression scale in a range considered to be high for the sample as a whole. Strikingly, approximately 6 percent had thought about ending their lives within the past year.

Women were asked if a disability, handicap, or chronic disease kept them from participating fully in school, work, housework, or other activities. Eighteen percent of women indicated that such a problem did limit them in their daily activities. Nonetheless, only one percent required other people's help with personal care and activities of daily living. Approximately 8 percent needed help in handling routine activities, such as household chores, business, shopping, or getting around.

In the survey, women also indicated whether they had been diagnosed during the past 5 years with a variety of health problems common in midlife. The most frequently occurring problems are arthritis (31%), high blood pressure (25%), anxiety or depression (17%), urinary tract infections (18%), and incontinence (10%). In addition, 9 percent had been diagnosed with a heart attack, angina, chest pains, or any heart disease; 9 percent with cancer; 7 percent with diabetes; and 8 percent with emphysema, asthma, or chronic obstructive pulmonary disease. These findings resemble estimates from the National Health Interview Survey (1993a).

Patterns of Health Behavior

Women engage in a variety of health-promoting and health-damaging practices by the choices they make regarding exercise, diet, smoking, and alcohol consumption. Most midlife women in this study do not smoke and consume alcohol in modest amounts. Despite evidence on the hazards of smoking, approximately 23 percent still smoke. This is similar to national health survey findings that nearly 27 percent of adult women smoke. Nearly half of The Commonwealth Fund survey respondents (48.9%) reported drinking alcohol, with 83 percent of those who did consuming one or two drinks on appropriate occasions. Drug use is uncommon in this sample, with less than one percent using marijuana and only one woman using cocaine, heroin, speed, or downers within the past month. Nonetheless, 20 percent had been counseled by a health professional to cut down on smoking, drinking, or drug use.

Many women in this survey engage in a number of health-promoting activities, with nearly one-third exercising for 20 minutes or more at least three times a week; however, nearly one-third reported never exercising (31%). Other studies have found that nearly 40 percent of women exercise regularly (National Center for Health Statistics 1993b). Thirty-five percent of the women take a calcium supplement.

Other studies have found that nearly half of midlife women are overweight (National Center for Health Statistics 1993b), but only 12 percent of the midlife women in this survey are considered overweight based on a Body Mass Index (BMI) of greater than 32. (BMI is weight in kilograms/height in meters squared.)

At midlife, the prevalence of contraceptive use is low. Only 2 percent reported using a condom, and fewer than one percent used any one of the following methods: diaphragm, spermicide, sponge, IUD, birth control pills, rhythm, Depo Provera, or Norplant. Ten percent had had an abortion in the past. Because women were not asked whether they had completed menopause, it is unclear what proportion is at risk of unplanned pregnancy. Because data were not obtained about their sexual practices, their risk for exposure to HIV infection also remains uncertain.

Use of Health Services

Most women indicated that they have a source of health care (83%). Most (77.7%) receive their health care in a physician's office, but 15 percent reported receiving care in a clinic and 3.5 percent from a hospital emergency room. Only 1.5 percent receive care from an HMO. Nine percent of the midlife women have no health insurance.

Most women receive primary health care from a family practitioner (60%), 10 percent from a gynecologist, one percent from a nurse practitioner, and 0.5 percent from a midwife. More than 40 percent of the midlife women receive their care from a gynecologist in addition to another type of provider. Most women see a male provider (82%).

More than half of the women surveyed received some form of screening exam within the past year. More than 63 percent had received a physical exam, 91 percent a blood pressure screening, 62 percent a cholesterol screening, 71 percent a clinical breast exam, 57 percent mammography, 65 percent a pelvic exam, and 66 percent a Pap smear. Earlier surveys found that only about half of U.S. women had a breast exam by a health professional in the past year, and that less than half had a Pap smear (National Center for Health Statistics 1982).

Patterns of Hormone Therapy

Because of the increased interest in the use of estrogen or combined hormone therapy to prevent osteoporosis and possibly heart disease, women's patterns of using hormones are analyzed to determine how those who are using hormone therapy differ from those who do not with respect to several factors: the woman's demographic characteristics, health practices, health status, access to health care, and use of health services for prevention and early detection of disease, and characteristics of her health care provider. Tests of association include chi-square analyses for associations between the use of hormones and categorical variables and Pearson's correlation between the use of hormones (coded 1 for use, 0 for no use) and continuous variables. All reported associations are significant at the $p < 0.05$ level.

Of the midlife women surveyed, 24 percent use hormone replacement therapy. Of the women using hormone therapy, 80 percent use estrogen only, 13 percent use a combination of estrogen and progestin, 3 percent use oral contraceptives, and 4 percent are uncertain about their type of preparation. This estimate of hormone use is consistent with surveys of other North American and European samples, in which 12 percent to 32 percent of postmenopausal women reported using hormones and fewer than one-fourth of hormone users take combined therapy (Scalley and Henrich 1993; Johannes et al. 1994).

Although the dosage of hormones women used and their length of use are important to consider, these data are not available in The Commonwealth Fund survey database. Future studies should include these data as well as the reasons women give for using or not using hormone therapy. Furthermore, women participants in The Commonwealth Fund survey were not asked whether they had had a hysterectomy or oophorectomy. Thus, it is not possible to examine the effects of these procedures on the use of hormones. Among other populations studied, the use of hormone replacement therapy was more prevalent among women who had had a hysterectomy and oophorectomy, most likely due to their experience of estrogen-dependent symptoms such as hot flashes (Cauley et al. 1990; Logothetis 1991; Johannes et al. 1994). Of great concern is the large proportion of women in The Commonwealth Fund study using estrogen without progestin (80%). It is unlikely that all of these women have had a hysterectomy. This pattern of hormone use, also observed in the Massachusetts Women's Health Study, places women at risk of endometrial cancer in the future.

Demographic Characteristics and the Use of Hormones

Women in the age group most likely to be experiencing the transition to menopause (having irregular menstrual periods) or completing menopause (stopping menstruating) are more likely to be using hormone therapy than those who are either younger or older. Thirty-nine percent of those fifty to fifty-five years of age, 31 percent of those fifty-five to sixty, and 26 percent of those forty-five to fifty and sixty to sixty-five use hormone therapy. In contrast, among those forty to forty-five, only 8 percent use hormone therapy.

The relationship of the use of hormones to age probably reflects both women's menopausal status and providers' prescribing practices. Women in the United States begin the transition to menopause, a time when symptoms of hot flashes and night sweats peak, at about age forty-seven and experience menopause at about age fifty-one (McKinlay, Brambilla, and Posner 1992). Although women were not asked about whether they had noticed a change in the regularity of their periods or if they had completed menopause, the peak use of hormone therapy is among women fifty to fifty-nine years of age, consistent with a pattern seen in other populations (Harris et al. 1990; Topo et al. 1991; Johannes et al. 1994). Moreover, women most likely to be receiving prescriptions for hormone therapy are those most likely to be experiencing symptoms related to menopause, such as severe hot flashes. For women over sixty years of age, the use of hormone therapy declines, as seen in other samples. Whether a similar proportion of this birth cohort will continue to use hormone therapy to prevent osteoporosis or heart disease past their perimenopausal years remains to be seen (Egeland et al. 1988; Barrett-Connor, Wingard, and Criqui 1989; Cauley et al. 1990).

The use of hormones also varies with ethnicity. White women are more likely to be using hormone therapy (26%) than are black or African American women (17%). This pattern is consistent with that observed in other studies (Egeland et al. 1988; Barrett-Connor, Wingard, and Criqui 1989; Cauley et al. 1990) and may reflect differences in providers' assessment of greater risk for osteoporosis among white women than among black women. Of interest is that Hispanic women are less likely to use hormone therapy (14%) than non-Hispanic women (26%). The difference between ethnic groups' use of hormone therapy may also reflect differences in women's access to health care or belief systems about the appropriateness of using hormones.

The sexual discomfort resulting from vaginal dryness has been linked to waning levels of estrogen, and often prompts sexually active women to seek hormone therapy. Living in a coupled relationship did not influence women's use of hormone therapy in this survey.

The use of hormone therapy also varies slightly with the area of the country. A higher proportion of women living in the Southeast, South Central, and Upper and Central (Bread Basket) Midwest regions use hormone therapy than in the New England/Middle Atlantic and Mountain/Pacific regions. This finding is not consistent with the higher prevalence of estrogen use in the Western region and lower prevalence in New England reported in other studies (Harris et al. 1990; Derby et al. 1993; Johannes et al. 1994).

One hypothesis is that women who are employed may be less tolerant of hot flashes and night sweats, and the associated sleep deprivation, and thus request medication to manage their symptoms. In this survey, employment is not related to the use of hormones: 26 percent of women employed full-time, 20 percent of those employed part-time, and 25 percent of those not employed use hormone therapy.

Access to Health Care and the Use of Hormones

Access to health care is mediated by education, income, and insurance, and each of these is related to the use of hormones. Hormone use is more prevalent among women with more formal education. Those who had completed some college (31%) followed by those who had graduated from college (24%) or completed high school (25%) or postgraduate work (20%) are more likely to be using hormone therapy than those who had less formal education. Women who had less than a high school education are least likely to be using hormone therapy (12%). This trend is consistent with that seen in other studies (Egeland et al. 1988; Cauley et al. 1990; Topo et al. 1991) and probably reflects women's access to health information and health care.

Income is also associated with the use of hormones, with those who have annual incomes over $25,000 more likely to use hormone therapy than those with lower incomes. This finding is consistent with results of other studies indicating an association between social class and the use of hormones. Because of the absence of a national health plan in the United States, income may influence hormone use through enhancing access (Spector 1989; Draper and Roland 1990; Logothetis 1991).

Women who are insured through their spouses are most likely to be receiving hormone therapy (27%), while women who have Medicaid coverage are least likely to be receiving hormone therapy (13%). Of interest is that women who are uninsured are not less likely than those who are insured to be using hormone therapy. This finding may reflect the relatively high portion of women who have some type of insurance (only 90 of the 1,022 women were uninsured), or it may reflect some women's willingness and ability to pay for their therapy out of pocket.

Women's Health Awareness, Health Behavior Patterns, and the Use of Hormones

Women's own health awareness and health behavior patterns influence their use of hormone therapy. Consistent with earlier studies, women participating in The Commonwealth Fund study who believe they are well informed about osteoporosis are most likely to use hormone therapy. More than one-third (35%) of those who say they are very familiar with osteoporosis use hormone therapy, compared to 29 percent who are somewhat familiar, 9 percent who are not very familiar, and 7 percent who are not familiar at all with osteoporosis (Draper and Roland 1990; Egeland et al. 1991; Wren and Brown 1991).

Women who observe certain personal health-promoting practices are more likely to use hormone therapy. Women who exercise more frequently are somewhat more likely to use hormone therapy. Those who never exercise are less likely to use hormone therapy (22%) than those who exercise more than one day a month to twice a week (25%) or 3 or more days a week (25%). The relationship between exercise and the use of hormones is consistent with the finding from other studies that women who are more active are more likely to use hormones (Cauley et al. 1990; Harris et al. 1990; Logothetis 1991; Topo et al. 1991). In addition to exercising, many women use calcium supplements to augment a diet deficient in this mineral. The use of calcium is positively associated with the use of hormones, with 39 percent of those taking calcium also taking hormones, as compared to 17 percent of those who are not using calcium.

One would expect women with a small body frame and low body mass to be more likely to receive prescriptions for hormone therapy, because these women are perceived to be at risk for osteoporosis. More women with a small body frame (29%) than a medium frame (21%) or large frame (26%) use hormone therapy. The Body Mass Index (BMI) is related to the use of hormones, with women having small to medium values more likely to use hormones (25%) than those with large values (20%). The relationship between body frame and the use of hormones is consistent with results of other studies showing that thinner women were more likely to be using hormone therapy (Cauley et al. 1990; Harris et al. 1990; Egeland et al. 1991; Topo et al. 1991; Wren and Brown

1991), and may reflect providers' prescriptive practices for women they believe to be at high risk for osteoporosis.

Although women who engage in health-promoting practices are more likely to use hormone therapy, there is little association between health-damaging behaviors (such as smoking or alcohol use) and hormone therapy. Women who smoke experience menopause at a younger age than nonsmokers, resulting in an earlier drop in their estrogen levels than that experienced by nonsmokers; one might anticipate that they would be more troubled by hot flashes (McKinlay, Brambilla, and Posner 1992). Smoking is not related to the use of hormones in this study: 24 percent of smokers, compared with 26 percent of nonsmokers, use hormone therapy. Drinking alcoholic beverages, like smoking, is not related to the use of hormones. Twenty-four percent of women who use alcohol also use hormone therapy, as opposed to 25 percent of those who did not use alcohol. Moreover, there is no relationship between the amount of alcohol women consumed during the past 2 weeks and their use of hormone therapy.

Overall, these data reveal that women observing more health-promoting and preventive behaviors are more likely to use hormone therapy. Future studies should include data about other health practices (such as use of caffeine) and dietary practices (such as intake of fat and fiber), so their relationship to the use of hormones can be analyzed.

Women's Health Status and the Use of Hormones

Based on earlier work, one would expect healthier women to be more likely to use hormone therapy (Pettiti, Perlman, and Signey 1987). In The Commonwealth Fund survey, evidence is mixed. Women's perceptions of their own health, rated from poor to excellent, are not related to the use of hormones. Moreover, neither indicators of well-being, including self-esteem and life satisfaction, nor scoring high on the depression scale is related to hormone use. Perceived good health may dissuade women from using hormone therapy. Those who are in good health may believe they do not need therapy or may be averse to the risks associated with the therapy, such as the unknown long-term risk of breast cancer. Alternatively, some women may adopt hormone therapy because they are healthy and feel less at risk for some of the diseases that hormone therapy may prevent. The relationship between health perceptions and the use of hormones cannot be understood without longitudinal studies that follow women through the course of decision making about adopting hormone therapy. Future work should investigate how women's perceptions of their health influence their decision-making process and to what extent symptoms such as hot flashes cue women to consider hormone therapy.

In contrast to the perception of health and well-being, certain health problems, particularly those that resulted in women's contact with health professionals, are associated with the use of hormones. Women with a recent (within the past 5 years) diagnosis of anxiety or depression, arthritis or bursitis, osteoporosis or brittle bones, or urinary incontinence are significantly more likely to be using hormone therapy than those without such a diagnosis (tab. 6.2). Of interest is that only two women had experienced a hip fracture, and neither is using hormone therapy. The proportion of women using hormone therapy who had been diagnosed with cancer is similar to that for women without a cancer diagnosis.

The different relationship with hormone use of women's perceived health compared with diagnoses of disease is intriguing. Diagnosis reflects providers' judgments about health as well as women's perceptions that something is wrong. This suggests that women having access to providers who diagnose health problems increases their likeli-

Table 6.2. Percentage of Women Using Hormones, by Diagnosis within the Past 5 Years

Diagnosis	With Diagnosis	Without Diagnosis
Anxiety, depression	33	23
Arthritis, bursitis	31	21
Cancer	27	24
Diabetes	19	25
Emphysema, asthma, COPD	26	22
Endometriosis	36	24
Fractured hip	23	22
Heart attack, angina	22	25
Hypertension	24	24
Incontinence, urinary	38	23
Menstrual problems	19	25
Osteoporosis	38	24
Reproductive problems	26	24
Stroke	37	24
Urinary tract infection	28	24

Source: Data from The Commonwealth Fund survey on women's health, 1993.

hood of using hormones. Future studies of the use of hormones should not only address disease endpoints but also emphasize the influence of women's own perceptions of their health and symptoms on decisions to use hormones, a factor not included in The Commonwealth Fund survey.

The Use of Health Services for the Prevention and Early Detection of Disease and Hormone Therapy

Women's patterns of using health services for the prevention and early detection of disease are strongly related to their use of hormone therapy. Those who had a physical exam in the past year are more likely than those who had not to use hormone therapy. Moreover, those who had a blood pressure screening, blood cholesterol screening, clinical breast exam, mammogram, pelvic exam, or Pap smear in the past year are more likely than those who had not had these procedures to be using hormone therapy (tab. 6.3). These results are consistent with other studies linking access to health care with the use of hormones. They may also indicate that women who monitor their health more carefully are more likely to adopt hormone therapy as an additional option for safeguarding their health.

An additional finding supporting the link between the use of health services and hormone therapy is a positive association between the use of tranquilizers and hormone therapy. Women who are currently using

Table 6.3. Percentage of Women Using Hormones, by the Use of Preventive and Early Detection Services during the Past Year

Service	Service Used	Service Not Used
Physical exam	30	15
Blood pressure screening	26	9
Blood cholesterol screening	30	16
Clinical breast exam	29	12
Mammogram	31	16
Pelvic exam	31	11
Pap smear	30	14

Source: Data from The Commonwealth Fund survey on women's health, 1993.

tranquilizers are more likely to use hormone therapy (42%) than those who are not (23%), but only 16 percent of hormone therapy users are taking tranquilizers. This association is consistent with more prevalent use of hormone therapy among women who have been diagnosed with anxiety or depression in the past 5 years. It may be that women who use health services because of distressing symptoms subsequently receive hormone therapy in addition to a prescription for a tranquilizer if they are perimenopausal and distressed (Matthews et al. 1990; Palinkas and Barrett-Connor 1992). The association may also reflect prescribing practices of health professionals who see women's depression and anxiety as related to menopause (such as the outmoded diagnosis of involutional melancholia) rather than to the exigencies of women's daily life, such as financial distress and abuse. Future work on depression in midlife would benefit from consideration of the context of women's lives as well as menopausal status.

Provider Characteristics and the Use of Hormones

Provider specialty is related to the use of hormones. Women who see a gynecologist in addition to their regular care provider (29%) or as their primary care provider (28%) are more likely to use hormone therapy than those who do not see a gynecologist (21%). Women who use hormone therapy are not more likely to see a woman physician than those who do not use hormone therapy (26% of those seeing men versus 19% of those seeing women). These results linking screening to the specialty of the physician are in agreement with findings from other studies, although the gender differences noted in other studies are not apparent in The Commonwealth Fund population (Lurie et al. 1993).

Women who received their health care from a gynecologist rather than another type of provider do not differ with respect to the use of estrogen or combined hormone therapy. Those who saw a gynecologist received combined hormone therapy at the same rate (13% combined, 87% estrogen only) as those who received their care from a physician with another specialty emphasis. Thus, the use of progestin to reduce the risk of endometrial cancer is not widespread, regardless of the physician's specialty. Because it is unlikely that the majority of women responding to the survey have had a hysterectomy, many women may remain at increased risk of endometrial cancer from this prescriptive practice.

Summary of Findings

Overall, the profile of health for midlife women is that of a predominantly healthy population in which many have a sense of well-being and high self-esteem. Nevertheless, a significant proportion of women are troubled, if not depressed (approximately 29%), and live with some form of disability (18%). In addition, a significant portion are experiencing one or more chronic illnesses, such as high blood pressure, arthritis, cancer, or heart disease, with at least 30 percent having one or more chronic illness.

Although not designed as a study of patterns of hormone use, The Commonwealth Fund survey provides data about several correlates of hormone use that invite further reflection and study. Taken together, the following demographic and health practice profile suggests that current use of hormone therapy is a function of socioeconomic status as it mediates access to health care and a function of perceived risk for disease by clinicians and their patients. In the survey population of midlife and older women, the use of hormones is most prevalent among women of perimenopausal age who are well educated, have middle- to upper-range incomes, are white and non-Hispanic, have partners, and reside in the midwestern region of the United States.

Hormone users are aware of the risk of osteoporosis, observe health-promoting practices (exercise regularly, use calcium supplements), and have a small body frame relative to nonusers. Users of hormone therapy also are more likely to have had health problems diagnosed within the past 5 years that required health care. They are most likely to have health insurance, but uninsured women use hormones at rates similar to those of women who are insured. Women who use hormones also are more likely to engage in many screening, early detection, and preventive practices, such as mammography and Pap smears. Women using hormones are more likely to be using tranquilizers, probably because of the combined influence of their age, depression or anxiety, and access to medical care. Women who receive their regular care from a gynecologist or receive care from a gynecologist in addition to another provider are more likely to be using hormone therapy than women who do not see a gynecologist.

The rates of hormone use reported by this national sample of midlife women do not indicate widespread adoption of hormone therapy, even among women who are most likely to be perimenopausal. The peak rates of use are 39 percent for those fifty to fifty-five years and 31 percent for those fifty-five to sixty years. Whether these data reflect that risks of heart disease, osteoporotic fractures, or selected cancers will remain unchanged from that of earlier birth cohorts remains uncertain. The relatively large proportion of hormone users who are being treated with estrogen alone raises concern about increased risk of endometrial cancer among those who have not had a hysterectomy.

Although The Commonwealth Fund survey provided a rich database for studying women's health issues, some limitations in the study design must be considered in interpreting the results presented here. First, the study was not designed to include information important to understanding the dynamics of hormone use among U.S. women. Although interviewers asked women whether they were using hormone replacement therapy and what kind, they did not elicit information about the dosages women are using and the duration of their use. In addition, they did not ask women why they were given prescriptions for estrogen or estrogen/progestin therapy, such as for the management or prevention of symptoms. Women who are not using hormones were not asked whether they were ever given a prescription for therapy. Therefore, conclusions can be made only about women who received prescriptions and were using therapy at the time of the interview. Finally, one of the common indications for prescribing estrogen is oophorectomy. Data are unavailable about what proportion of the sample had experienced oophorectomy. Likewise, one of the risks of using unopposed estrogen is endometrial cancer. Because data about whether women had a hysterectomy are unavailable, the appropriateness of their use of estrogen alone or combined hormone therapy cannot be evaluated directly.

IMPLICATIONS FOR POLICY

Policy implications suggested by these data begin with recommendations for careful attention to young and midlife women's health as an indicator of future needs for health care and health care financing. As the Baby Boomers age, they will swell the numbers needing primary, home, and long-term health care services. In addition, the magnitude of this birth cohort will have significant consequences for health services financing. It is in the nation's best interest, and in the best interest of women themselves, to create a system of careful public health surveillance designed to detect emerging risks for health problems and to invest in health promotion and prevention strategies that could attenuate the human and economic cost of high morbidity among women as they age. These programmatic efforts should include health educational programs for women that emphasize enhancing nutrition and exercise patterns, smoking cessation, and the reduction of the incidence of alcohol and substance abuse. Given the high prevalence of violent crime and abusive relationships that contribute to psychosocial and physical morbidity, services for women who have been victimized should receive high priority, as should services to reduce the incidence of violence in communities. In addition, enhancing women's ability to gain access to health education programs through providing them in workplace settings and through community-based organizations will be important, given the complexity of contemporary women's roles.

Clinical services for midlife women should optimize access to a wide range of health care providers, given the scope of preventive strategies suggested in this chapter. What is clear from the foregoing discussion is the complexity of the decision process, one that women share with their health care providers. Simply providing a prescription without helping women weigh the benefits and risks carefully will be a disservice to women who may make and remake decisions about the use of hormones for the management and prevention of symptoms several times during their middle and older years. Sorting out the short-term benefits versus long-term benefits versus risks will require not only the provision of information but also an examination of how women weigh their current experiences of symptoms, long-term well-being, and risk of disease. Educational programs for women experiencing menopause have become increasingly prevalent, and women's concerns about using hormone therapy have motivated many questions. Access to a range of health providers, including those prepared to provide health education and counseling services, will be essential in helping women select the health promotion and disease prevention options that best suit them.

Should future research indicate that hormone therapy provides substantial benefits for women's health beyond those outlined in the American College of Physicians' guidelines, estrogen and estrogen/progestin therapy for postmenopausal women may need to be considered an essential dimension of health care, raising implications for health care financing for long-term use of prescribed medications (Gambrell 1987; Hemminki et al. 1988).

Current hormone users responding to this survey engage in health-promoting practices such as exercise, taking calcium supplements, and using health services for a variety of screening and disease prevention services. They are a health-conscious group. If hormone therapy proves to offer substantial reduction of morbidity and mortality in ongoing clinical trials, dissemination of information about its benefits to women who are not aware of health promotion and prevention strategies will require careful, community-based efforts. Likewise, surveillance of women for adverse effects of hormone use, such as endometrial cancer, will be essential. Women who use hormones are also more likely to have health problems requiring medical care and are least likely to have health benefits linked to Medicaid or public assistance. Financing mechanisms for the prevention and early detection of disease that ensure women access to endometrial aspiration or biopsy, transvaginal ultrasound, or dilatation and curettage, mammography, and clinical breast exams will take on added significance for screening for endometrial and breast cancer.

Finally, professional education to prepare health care providers to counsel women about promoting their health during midlife is an essential step in safeguarding this population's health. Providers of health care need a vision of midlife as more than menopause.

IMPLICATIONS FOR RESEARCH

Midlife women's health clearly warrants attention to issues beyond menopause and hormone therapy. Indeed, a survey devoted solely to the health of midlife women could provide important data regarding health concerns that could guide health education and service delivery programs.

Currently, data support the short-term use of estrogen therapy for women who have severe menopausal symptoms, such as hot flashes. To prevent osteoporosis and heart disease, estrogen alone is recommended for women who no longer have a uterus. For women who have, or who are at increased risk for, heart disease, the American College of Physicians recommends using estrogen or estrogen and progestin (depending on whether the woman still has a uterus). What remains unclear is the best approach for the majority of women: those who still have a uterus, do not yet have heart disease, and are not at high risk for breast cancer. In addition to understanding the therapeutic, preventive, and harmful effects of ovarian hormones with limited and prolonged use of estrogen and estrogen/progestin combined therapy, we need to learn how these effects occur. Challenges for further research include clarifying the molecular and physiologic mechanisms that are involved in mediating the health-related effects of ovarian steroids, particularly for women using estrogen and combined hormone therapy over several years.

Of equal importance is further inquiry into women's own experiences with decision making about adopting a preventive strategy under conditions of uncertain risk. Studies examining the decision-making processes women use should focus on how and what information women consider, including the results of biomedical research, information provided by their social networks and the media, and their own prior experiences with the use of ovarian hormones, such as oral contraceptives. Values and beliefs about menopause, aging, and the significance of bodily changes and how they relate to women's adoption of health promotion and preventive self-care strategies as well as the use of hormones also need further analysis. Women's beliefs about the risk of cancer, especially breast cancer, figure prominently in earlier studies. Studies of the relative importance of menopausal symptoms, knowledge of therapeutic alternatives and the risks associated with each, and the human and financial costs associated with hormone therapy would complement the work to date, most of which focuses on women's decisions in response to theoretical scenarios rather than in response to their own circumstances.

In addition, studies of lifestyle changes (such as exercise programs), dietary changes (such as reducing fat, adding fiber, and including calcium supplements), and their effectiveness in reducing osteoporosis and heart disease risk will enhance our knowledge of health preservation for an aging population. Moreover, women's use of alternative strategies to manage the symptoms of hot flashes and disturbed sleep, such as meditation and herbal preparations, bears examination.

Finally, studies of the human and financial costs and benefits of hormone therapy as compared to dietary modification and exercise patterns would help determine whether health promotion programs or prescriptions for hormones reflect the optimal use of limited health care dollars. Such work will be valuable not only in understanding issues related to hormone therapy but also in structuring future public health programs for risk reduction and health promotion of midlife and older women.

NOTE

1. The PEPI trial included 875 healthy postmenopausal women aged forty-five to sixty-four years who had no known contraindication to hormone therapy. They were randomly placed in groups to receive: (1) placebo; (2) conjugated equine estrogen only, 0.625 mg; (3) conjugated equine estrogen 0.625 mg plus consecutive MPA 2.5 mg per day; or (4) conjugated equine estrogen 0.625 mg plus cyclic micronized progesterone 200 mg per day for 12 days per month.

REFERENCES

American College of Physicians. 1992. Guidelines for counseling post-menopausal women about preventive hormone therapy. *Annals of Internal Medicine* 117:1038–41.

Barrett-Connor, E., Wingard, D., and Criqui, M. 1989. Postmenopausal estrogen use and heart disease risk factors in the 1980's. *Journal of the American Medical Association* 261:2095–2100.

Bell, S. 1990. Sociological perspectives on the medicalization of menopause. In M. Flint, F. Kronenberg, and W. Utian, eds., *Multidisciplinary Perspectives on Menopause*. New York: New York Academy of Sciences.

Brooks-Gunn, J., and Kirsch, B. 1984. Life events and the boundaries of mid-life for women. In G. Baruch and J. Brooks-Gunn, eds., *Women in Mid-life*. New York: Plenum.

Bush, T. 1991. Feminine forever revisited: menopausal hormone therapy in the 1990's. *Journal of Women's Health* 1:1–4.

Bush, T., et al. 1987. Cardiovascular mortality and noncontraceptive use of estrogen in women: results from the Lipid Research Clinics Program Follow-up Study. *Circulation* 75:1102–9.

Cauley, J., Cummings, S., Black, D., Mascioli, S., and Seeley, D. 1990. Prevalence and determinants of estrogen replacement therapy in elderly women. *American Journal of Obstetrics and Gynecology* 163:1438–44.

Derby, C., Hume, A., Barbour, M., Phillips, J., Lasater, T., and Carleton, R. 1993. Correlates of postmenopausal estrogen use and trends through the 1980's in two southeastern New England communities. *American Journal of Epidemiology* 137:1125–35.

Draper, J., and Roland, M. 1990. Perimenopausal women's views on taking hormone replacement therapy to prevent osteoporosis. *British Medical Journal* 300:786–88.

Egeland, G., Kuller, L., Matthews, K., Kelsey, S., Cauley, J., and Guzick, D. 1991. Premenopausal determinants of estrogen use. *Preventive Medicine* 20:343–49.

Egeland, G., Matthews, K., Kuller, L., and Kelsey, J. 1988. Characteristics of noncontraceptive hormone users. *Preventive Medicine* 17:403–11.

Ferguson, K., Hoegh, C., and Johnson, S. 1989. Estrogen replacement therapy:

a survey of women's knowledge and attitudes. *Archives of Internal Medicine* 149:133–36.

Gambrell, R. 1987. Use of progesterone therapy. *American Journal of Obstetrics and Gynecology* 256:1304–13.

Grady, D., Rubin, S., Petitti, D., Fox, C., Black, D., Ettinger, B., Ernster, V., and Cummings, S. 1992. Hormone therapy to prevent disease and prolong life in postmenopausal women. *Annals of Internal Medicine* 117:1016–37.

Greer, G. 1992. *The Change: Women, Aging, and the Menopause*. New York: Knopf.

Harris, R., Laws, A., Reddy, V., King, A., and Haskell, W. 1990. Are women using postmenopausal estrogens?: a community survey. *American Journal of Public Health* 80:1266–68.

Hemminki, E., Kennedy, D., Baum, C., and McKinlay, M. 1988. Prescribing of noncontraceptive estrogens and progestins in the United States, 1974–1986. *American Journal of Public Health* 78:1479–81.

Henderson, B., Paganini-Hill, A., and Ross, R. 1988. Estrogen replacement therapy and protection from acute myocardial infarction. *American Journal of Obstetrics and Gynecology* 59:312–17.

Johannes, C., Crawford, S., Posner, J., and McKinlay, S. 1994. Longitudinal patterns and correlates of hormone replacement therapy use in middle aged women. *American Journal of Epidemiology* 140:439–52.

Kennedy, D., Baum, C., and Forbes, M. 1985. Noncontraceptive estrogens and progestins: use patterns over time. *Obstetrics and Gynecology* 65:441–46.

Lindsay, R., Hart, D., MacLean, A., Clark, A., Kraszewski, A., and Garwood, J. 1978. Bone response to termination of estrogen treatment. *Lancet* 1:13225–27.

Logothetis, M. 1991. Women's decisions about estrogen replacement therapy. *Western Journal of Nursing Research* 13:458–74.

Lurie, N, Slater, J., Mc Govern, P., Ekstrum, J., Quam, L., and Margolis, K. 1993. Preventive care for women: does the sex of the physician matter? *New England Journal of Medicine* 329:478–82.

MacPherson, K. 1981. Menopause as disease: the social construction of a metaphor. *Advances in Nursing Science* 3:95–114.

———. 1985. Osteoporosis and menopause: a feminist analysis of the social construction of a syndrome. *Advances in Nursing Science* 7:11–22.

———. 1992. Cardiovascular disease in women and noncontraceptive use of hormones: a feminist analysis. *Advances in Nursing Science* 14:34–49.

Matthews, K., Wing, R., Kuller, L., Meilahn, E., Kelsey, S., Costello, E., and Caggiula, A. 1990. Influences of natural menopause on psychological characteristics and symptoms of middle-aged healthy women. *Journal of Consulting and Clinical Psychology* 58:345–51.

McKinlay, S., Brambilla, D., and Posner, J. 1992. The normal menopause transition. *Maturitas* 14:103–15.

McKinlay, S., Triant, R., McLinlay, J., Brambilla, D., and Ferdock, M. 1990. Multiple roles for middle-aged women and their impact on health. In M. Ory and H. Warner, eds., *Gender, Health, and Longevity: Multidisciplinary Perspectives*. New York: Springer.

McLaughlin, S., Melber, B., Billy, J., Zimmerle, D., Winges, L., and Johnson, T.

1988. *The Changing Lives of American Women*. Chapel Hill, N.C.: University of North Carolina Press.

Nathanson, C. 1975. Illness and the feminine role: a theoretical review. *Social Science and Medicine* 9:57–62.

National Center for Health Statistics. 1993a. Current Estimates from the National Health Interview Survey, 1992. Series 10. Hyattsville, Md.: U.S. Department of Health and Human Services.

———. 1993b. United States Health and Prevention Profile, 1992. Hyattsville, Md.: U.S. Department of Health and Human Services.

———. 1982. Use of Selected Preventive Care Procedures, United States, 1982. Series 10, no. 157. Hyattsville, Md.: U.S. Department of Health and Human Services.

National Institute on Aging. 1993. Workshop on Menopause. Bethesda: National Institutes of Health.

National Institutes of Health. 1992. Opportunities for Research on Women's Health. Bethesda, Md.: National Institutes of Health.

Palinkas, L., and Barrett-Connor, E. 1992. Estrogen use and depressive symptoms in postmenopausal women. *Obstetrics and Gynecology* 80:30–36.

Pettiti, D., Perlman, J., and Signey, S. 1987. Noncontraceptive estrogens and mortality: long-term follow-up of women in the Walnut Creek Study. *Obstetrics and Gynecology* 70:854–59.

Physicians' Desk Reference. 1993. 47th ed. Montvale: Medical Economics Data.

Ravnikar, V. 1987. Compliance with hormone therapy. *American Journal of Obstetrics and Gynecology* 156:1332–34.

Rothert, M., Rover, D., Holmen, M., Schmitt, N., Talarczyk, G., Knoll, J. and Gogato, J. 1990. Women's use of information regarding hormone replacement therapy. *Research in Nursing and Health* 13:355–66.

Scalley, E., and Henrich, J. 1993. An overview of estrogen replacement therapy in postmenopausal women. *Journal of Women's Health* 2:289–94.

Schmitt, N., Gogate, J., Rothert, M., Rovner, D., Holmes, M., Talarczyk, G., Given, B., and Kroll, J. 1991. Capturing and clustering women's judgment policies: the case of hormonal therapy for menopause. *Journal of Gerontology, Psychological Sciences* 46:92–101.

Spector, T. 1989. Use of estrogen replacement therapy in high risk groups in the United Kingdom. *British Medical Journal* 299:1434–35.

Stampfer, M., et al. 1985. A prospective study of postmenopausal estrogen therapy and coronary heart disease. *New England Journal of Medicine* 313:1044–49.

Topo, P., Klaukka, R., Hemminki, E., and Uutela, A. 1991. Use of hormone replacement therapy in 1976–1989 by 45 to 64 year old Finnish women. *Journal of Epidemiology and Community Health* 45:277–80.

Verbrugge, L. 1986. Role burdens and physical health of women and men. *Women and Health* 11:47–77.

Wallace, R., Heiss, G., Burrows, B., and Graves, K. 1987. Contrasting diet and body mass among users and nonusers of oral contraceptives and exogenous estrogens: the Lipid Research Clinics Program prevalence study. *American Journal of Epidemiology* 125:854–59.

Weiss, N., Ure, C., Ballard, J., Williams, A., and Daling J. 1980. Decreased risk of fractures of the hip and lower forearm with postmenopausal use of estrogen. *New England Journal of Medicine* 303:1195–98.

Wilson, R. 1966. *Feminine Forever.* New York: M. Evans.

Wren, B., and Brown, L. 1991. Compliance with hormonal replacement therapy. *Maturitas* 13:17–21.

7

Older Women
Health Status, Knowledge, and Behavior

Linda P. Fried, M.D., M.P.H.

The health status and health care of older women is an issue of substantial import when considering women's health specifically and the health of older adults in general. Older women, defined here as women sixty-five years or older, currently constitute 14 percent of all females in the U.S. population (National Center for Health Statistics et al. 1987); it is anticipated that by 2020, this cohort will comprise 20 percent of all females (Rabin and Stockton 1987). As a result of substantially greater changes in life expectancy since the early 1900s (Wingard 1982), women also constitute the vast majority of all persons sixty-five or older. Women sixty-five to seventy-four comprised 53 percent of all persons in that over-sixty-five age group in 1985, and the proportion increased to 68 percent at ages eighty-five or older. There are now 17 million older women in the U.S. population (National Center for Health Statistics et al. 1987).

The high proportion of women in the upper age ranges is a consequence of major demographic shifts in this century. Life expectancy has increased substantially over the past 90 years. In 1900 women could expect to live forty-eight years (forty-nine years for Caucasian women and thirty-four for African American women); by 1987 life expectancy at birth had increased to seventy-eight years (by race, seventy-nine and seventy-four years, respectively) (U.S. Senate Special Committee on Aging 1991). While changes in life expectancy for those who reach age sixty-five have not been as dramatic, they are not insubstantial; years of life expectancy have increased from 12.2 years for sixty-five-year-old women in 1900 to 18.7 years in 1987 (U.S. Senate Special Committee on Aging 1991). This gain has meant that an increasing proportion of the population is living to old age. As a result, those sixty-five years or older increased from 4 percent of the U.S. population in 1900 to 12 percent in 1989 (Rabin and Stockton 1987). A further increase to 21.8 percent is expected by 2030 (U.S. Senate Special Committee on Aging 1991).

A significant issue in policy and health care for elderly persons is to define how to improve health and the quality of life in the many years of life after age sixty-five. Given that the use of health care by older adults is a major component of the substantial health care costs in the United States, a secondary benefit of decreasing the illness burden currently associated with aging would be resulting decreases in the needs for and costs of health care. The first steps toward accomplishing such a "compression of morbidity" (Fries 1980)—that is, a decrease in the disease and disability associated with aging to the latest points in the human life span—are to define the causes of this morbidity and the areas where prevention, improved treatment, or access to care may be needed.

Prevention in older adults used to be seen as a contradiction in terms, running counter to patients' and practitioners' fatalistic attitudes about old age. However, we now know that many of the chronic diseases associated with aging such as cardiovascular disease (Fried and Bush 1988) are not inevitable and that disability can improve as well as progress (Guralnik 1987). Health habits continue to be important modifiers of health status and well-being in old age, whether it is the role of exercise in preventing cardiovascular disease (Wagner and LaCroix 1992), frailty (Fiatarone et al. 1994) and disability (Hamdorf et al. 1992; Wagner and LaCroix 1992; Fiatarone et al. 1994; Simonsick et al. 1993), or the role of cigarette smoking in progressive lung disease (Higgins et al. 1993) and atherosclerosis (Jajich, Ostfeld, and Freeman 1984). Established components of preventive health care appear important in older as well as young and middle-aged adults. Thus, clinical preventive health care is highly relevant to the health status and health care needs of older adults. Evidence exists that older adults have high rates of compliance with health-related recommendations (German et al. 1978; German and Fried 1989), thus suggesting a high likelihood of success for effective preventive strategies.

There may also be modifiers of health status associated with aging that could be addressed in a broad, societal approach to maximizing well-being and minimizing health care costs. These may include the effects on health and functioning of living alone, losing opportunities for productivity and income with retirement, or becoming a widow.

These issues may lend themselves to population-based preventive interventions that may maximize the health status of older women.

This chapter describes the components of health status in older women, addresses a range of issues associated with access to and use of health care for both illness and prevention, and seeks to identify the dimensions of these issues that are of particular importance to older women. It concludes with a discussion of the implications of these findings for policy and research.

THE HEALTH STATUS OF OLDER WOMEN

Chronic Disease

Chronic diseases are the major causes of death and ill health for older persons; this reflects the shift from acute illnesses that has occurred in this century (Fried and Bush 1988). Currently, the major causes of death are the same for older women and older men: heart disease, cancer, and stroke (National Center for Health Statistics et al. 1987). However, older men are more likely to die at an earlier age from major chronic diseases, especially cardiovascular diseases, than are older women (Wingard 1982). Older women, on the other hand, are more likely to live many years longer with these chronic diseases and their consequences than are men.

The Commonwealth Fund survey identifies many of the major health problems of older women between the ages of sixty-five and eighty-five. Major chronic diseases that older women reported include arthritis and hypertension, each in approximately 50 percent of women over age sixty-five, followed by heart disease, depression or anxiety, cancer, emphysema and asthma, hip fracture, and stroke. These data are generally consistent with prevalence rates for women sixty-five or older, by self-report, in the U.S. National Health Interview Survey (National Center for Health Statistics et al. 1986). In addition, 0.5 percent of the older women surveyed reported HIV infection or AIDS, despite popular assumptions that older women are not at risk for HIV. In addition to diseases, several conditions associated with aging are also prevalent in older women. In The Commonwealth Fund survey, 15 percent of older women reported urinary incontinence and 13 percent reported being told by their physician that they have osteoporosis.

The high prevalence of heart disease in older women deserves special note. Fifteen percent of women sixty-five or older reported that their doctor told them that they have heart disease (Commonwealth Fund survey); similarly, 11 percent of women sixty-five or older reported ischemic heart disease in the National Health Interview Survey (National Center for Health Statistics et al. 1986). This high prevalence belies the frequent perception that heart disease is not a serious public health problem for women—including older women. In fact, women get heart disease at the same rate as men, but approximately 7 to 10 years later, so that by age seventy-five rates for women and men are similar (Wenger, Speroff, and Packard 1993). Heart disease is the leading cause of death in older women (National Center for Health Statistics et al. 1987). Thus, heart disease is a major health concern for older women, and its prevention should be a major focus.

A number of specific chronic diseases are highly prevalent in older women. Adding to this health burden, 51 percent of older women indicated having two or more chronic diseases among the nine assessed in the survey, and 24 percent have three or more diseases (tab. 7.1). The presence of these chronic diseases, individually and in combi-

Table 7.1. Health Status, Women Ages Sixty-five to Eighty-five Years ($N = 459$)

Health Status	%	(N)
Self-assessed health		
Excellent	18	(81)
Good	31	(139)
Fair	30	(134)
Poor	15	(69)
Not sure	7	(31)
Number of chronic diseases present		
0	18	(84)
1	31	(143)
2	27	(123)
≥ 3	24	(109)
Disability, handicap, or chronic disease precludes from full participation in work, housework, etc.	28	(129)
Due to impairment or health problem		
Needs help with IADLs, transport	16.3	(75)
Needs help with ADLs	2.7	(12)

Source: Data from The Commonwealth Fund survey on women's health, 1993.

nation, is associated with high morbidity, mortality, and a range of adverse outcomes, including falling, fractures, disability, and dependency. Some diseases, such as congestive heart failure, are linked with recurrent hospitalizations and high costs of health care (Zook and Moore 1980). Others, such as stroke and hip fracture, are tied to the need for long-term care. Many of these prevalent chronic diseases are associated with the development of physical disability, individually and in combination (Pinsky, Leaverton, and Stokes 1987; Mor et al. 1989; Fried et al. 1994).

The proportion of women reporting disability or dependency rises dramatically with the number of chronic diseases present (fig. 7.1). These findings are consistent with those of other studies, indicating that chronic disability or dependency is primarily a result of chronic disease and that the number of chronic diseases present in an individual is associated with the presence and severity of disability (Verbrugge 1984; Guralnik et al. 1989; Verbrugge, Lepkowski, and Imanaka 1989).

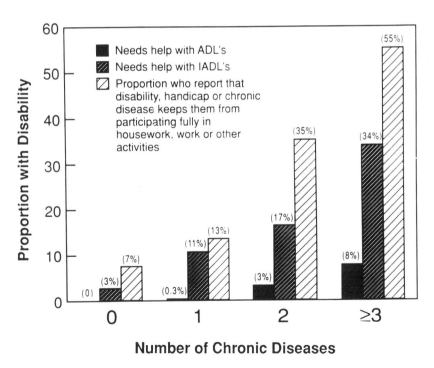

Fig. 7.1. Association of Comorbidity and the Number of Chronic Diseases Present with Disability

Source: Analysis of The Commonwealth Fund survey on women's health, 1993.

Disability

A major adverse consequence of these chronic diseases is physical disability, a substantial problem that affects older women at higher rates and for longer periods of time than older men. At any age over sixty-five, women have an expectation of living more years in a disabled state than do men (Katz et al. 1983; U.S. Senate Special Committee on Aging 1991). Twenty-eight percent of the women surveyed reported that they are unable to participate fully in work or housework as a result of disability or chronic disease (tab. 7.1). This is similar to the responses in the Health Interview Survey Supplement on Aging, in which 23 percent of women over sixty-five reported limitations in their ability to carry on their daily activities (National Center for Health Statistics, Kovar, and LaCroix 1987). The proportion in this survey who indicated that they need hel¹ ⁾ with instrumental activities of daily living (IADL: housework, m .al preparation, shopping, or transportation) is 16.3 percent overall (tab. 7.1), including 10.6 percent of those age sixty-five to seventy-four and 25.1 percent of those seventy-five or older ($p = 0.0001$). In addition, 2.7 percent of the women over sixty-five reported needing help with activities of daily living (ADL: bathing, dressing, walking across a small room, eating, toileting, transferring from bed to chair), ranging from one percent of those age sixty-five to seventy-four to 5 percent of those seventy-five or older ($p = 0.02$).

Major consequences of disability, as well as disease, are high use of outpatient and inpatient health care (Fried and Bush 1988; Leville et al. 1992), increased risk for acute illnesses and injuries (Fried and Bush 1988), and dependency and institutionalization (Rabin and Stockton 1987; U.S. Senate Committee on Aging 1991). Because of the high rates of disability in older women, coupled with longer lives and more widowhood compared with men, nursing home residents are primarily older women (Rabin and Stockton 1987).

Among those women sixty-five to eighty-five years who needed help with ADLs in the survey, 84 percent said that a person is available to help when they have a problem; this is a significantly lower proportion than for the women who did not need help with ADLs, of whom 96 percent reported having help when needed ($p < 0.0001$). This suggests that as many as 16 percent of those needing help with ADLs are not able to get assistance when needed. Prior reports indicated that most home-based care for disabled women is provided by relatives (primarily female) (Kaplan 1992; Leville et al. 1992; LaCroix et al. 1992;

Wenger, Speroff, and Packard 1993). In this study, women who needed help with problems and have help indicated that 89 percent of the helpers are children; only 11 percent turn to a spouse for help.

The presence of disability (self-reported) is associated with the presence of multiple chronic diseases, being in fair or poor health (self-assessed), feeling depressed, and age over seventy-five years ($p \leq 0.03$), in multiple logistic regression analyses. Other socio-demographic characteristics are not associated with such disability in this survey; these include race, income, education, and living alone, although each of these has been associated with disability in other studies (Pinksy, Leaverton, and Stokes 1987; Guralnik et al. 1989; Mor et al. 1989). These data support the conclusion that the prevention of chronic disease is critical to decreasing the rates of disability and dependency in older women.

Psychological Well-Being

The older women interviewed in The Commonwealth Fund survey reported a high prevalence of psychological symptoms. Twenty-eight percent stated that they felt depressed some or most of the time in the past week; this differs substantially by race, with 26 percent of white women and 39 percent of women of other races reporting feeling depressed in the past week. In contrast, in this survey only 10 percent said that they had been given a diagnosis of anxiety or depression in the past 5 years; this frequency did not vary by age group or race. Twenty-two percent of those who felt depressed said they have had a diagnosis of anxiety or depression in the past 5 years (compared with only 5% of those who did not feel depressed in the past week; $p < 0.00001$) suggesting that those with depressive symptomatology are at increased risk of clinical depression. Notably, those who reported disability are 50 percent more likely to have been depressed in the past 2 weeks than were women without disability.

In general, those who felt depressed are more likely to report fair or poor health (31% compared with 18% for those with no depressive symptoms) and more chronic diseases (1.9% compared with 1.6% chronic diseases, $p = 0.03$). However, they did not report more physician visits in the past year than those who were not depressed. Finally, 2 percent of these older women indicated they had suicidal thoughts in the past year. This finding is associated with having relatively higher incomes, with 4 percent of women with incomes greater than $15,000 reporting suicidal thoughts, compared with one percent with lower incomes ($p = 0.02$).

A high proportion of these older women reported poor self-esteem or low self-efficacy across a variety of measures (tab. 7.2). Thirty-four percent said they felt useless at times; this is significantly associated with health status, with 52 percent of women in fair or poor health feeling useless, compared with 29 percent of those in excellent or good health ($p = 0.00003$). Those feeling useless are more likely to be African American or Hispanic (46% compared with 33% of Caucasians; $p = 0.05$) with incomes less than \$15,000 (35% compared with 26% of those with incomes $\geq$ \$15,000; $p < 0.05$). Thirty-one percent stated that they wished they could have more respect for themselves, 6 percent stated they did not take a positive attitude toward themselves, and 14 percent stated that they felt they were not able to do things as well as most other people (tab. 7.2). These last three measures of self-esteem and self-efficacy are all associated with income (i.e., the higher the income, the better the self-assessment), while self-assessed health status was associated with two of the three questions (tab. 7.2).

These data indicate a high prevalence of poor self-esteem among older women and depressive symptoms in one-quarter to one-third of older women. This is consistent with other findings that 20 percent of those sixty-five or older experience depressive symptoms that require treatment (NIH Consensus Panel 1992). Overall, these data indicate an underreporting of depressive symptoms by older women and/or underrecognition, undertreatment, or inappropriate treatment by health care providers. This is especially the case for African American and Hispanic women. These depressive symptoms and signs are strongly associated with poorer physical health and with disability in these data as well as others, and with high rates of use of health care (Wells et al. 1989).

The association of depressive symptoms with low socioeconomic status and poorer health and disability suggests the need to target screening and the development of interventions in these groups. While women who are sicker or of low socioeconomic status appear at increased risk of depressive symptoms and low self-esteem, indicators of poor self-esteem are also present for women reporting excellent to good health and higher incomes. Suicidal ideation is most prevalent in women with incomes above \$15,000 (tab. 7.2).

The apparent underdiagnosis of depression and the poor psychological status of many older women indicate a need for increased

Table 7.2. Mental Health Characteristics, Women Ages Sixty-five to Eighty-five Years ($N = 459$)

| | | Self-Assessed Health | | | Association[a] with Race | | | Income | | |
		Excellent to Good	Fair or Poor	p	White	African American or Hispanic	p	≤$15,000	>$15,000	p
I feel useless at times	34%	29%	52%	0.00003	33%	46%	0.05	35%	26%	0.05
I wish I could have more respect for myself	31%	31%	33%	0.67	29%	46%	0.02	36%	23%	0.01
I take a positive attitude toward myself	94%	96%	89%	0.067	95%	86%	0.008	94%	98%	0.03
I am able to do things as well as most other people	86%	91%	68%	0.00001	88%	77%	0.04	84%	92%	0.02
I had suicidal thoughts in the past year	2%	2%	1%	0.48	2%	2%	0.98	1%	4%	0.02

Source: Data from The Commonwealth Fund survey on women's health, 1993.

[a] Chi-square.

awareness. More educational programs about the benefits of effective treatment and insurance coverage for mental health care needs to be targeted to older women. Finally, the finding of feelings of uselessness in one-third of older women, especially African American, Hispanic, and lower-income women, may suggest opportunities for social interventions in terms of employment or other activities, as will be discussed later in this chapter.

OLDER WOMEN'S USE OF HEALTH CARE

Sociodemographic Influence

The major differences in life expectancy between older women and older men have a number of consequences for women's social and economic status. Older women are much more likely to be widowed, to be living alone, and to have low incomes than are older men. Specifically, 65 percent of women age sixty-five years or older are not married and 57 percent live alone, compared with 26 percent and 23 percent of men sixty-five or older, respectively ($p < 0.0001$ for both). In this study, 8 percent of those community-dwelling older women who are not married are living with others, perhaps because of poor health. Prior studies indicated that older adults who live with persons who are not their spouse are likely to be in worse health than those who live alone (Magaziner et al. 1988).

The incomes of older women are significantly lower than those of older men. Forty-nine percent of women sixty-five or older reported annual incomes of $15,000 or less, compared with 28 percent of men the same age ($p = 0.00005$). This gender difference is thought to be a consequence of the long-term difference in earning power between men and women, the high rate and financial impact of widowhood, and spousal impoverishment resulting from the costs of long-term care for an ill spouse (Lewis 1985). In fact, the incomes of older women who are not married are significantly lower than those of women who are married: 49 percent of those women with incomes above $15,000 per year are married, compared with 26 percent of those with incomes below $15,000 ($p < 0.00001$). Income is also associated with education in this cohort of older women: 13 percent of women with incomes above $15,000 per year have less than a high school education, compared with 43 percent of women with incomes less than $15,000. Thus, widowhood and educational level are correlated with the financial well-being of older women.

Notably, the income differential between men and women is not explained by differences in current work; similar proportions of men and women at different income levels work. However, the proportion who are working is lower among lower-income than among higher-income older adults: only 10 percent of those with incomes of $15,000 or less reported working for pay, while 20 percent of those with incomes above $15,000 are working for pay. This suggests an important role in boosting income levels for full- or part-time work, for both women and men at older ages. In terms of other income supplementation, while only 4 percent of older women overall use food stamps, 16 percent of the African American and Hispanic women surveyed use them compared with 2 percent of white women ($p = 0.00001$).

The Impact of Insurance

Despite the major differences in socioeconomic status between older men and older women, there is not a substantial difference in health care coverage by gender (tab. 7.3). For those sixty-five or older, 93.2 percent of women and 90.5 percent of men reported Medicare coverage, with or without supplemental coverage. Among these, 13 percent of women and 12 percent of men reported Medicare without supplemental coverage.

Older women are generally satisfied with their usual health care: 93 percent stated that their doctor provides them with excellent or good health care, overall. Three-quarters of the women surveyed said that their doctor keeps their medical fees reasonable (tab. 7.3). More than 80 percent of older women with a usual source of care indicated that such care was from an internist or family practitioner. This varies primarily by race, with 81 percent of white women and 68 percent of other races receiving their care in a physician's office, while the proportions receiving care in a hospital emergency room are 2 percent and 12 percent, respectively.

Although insurance coverage is similar, 5 percent more men (84%) than women (79%) reported a usual source of care (tab. 7.3). One would expect to find the opposite—higher use of outpatient health care by women—because women are known to have comparable rates of many chronic diseases to men while living longer with chronic diseases and having more associated disability (Verbrugge 1984). There is

Table 7.3. Health Care Coverage and Use by Persons Ages Sixty-five Years or Older

Type of Coverage	Women (N = 459)	Men (N = 142)
Medicare only	13.0%	11.8%
Medicare plus private insurance or HMO	68.3%	63.7%
Medicare and Medicaid	11.9%	15.0%
None of above	6.8%	9.4%
Has a usual source of care	79.0%	84.0%
In addition to regular doctor, sees a separate doctor for female problems	18.1%	N/A
Doctor provides excellent or good health care, overall	92.5%	86.6%
Doctor keeps medical fees reasonable	74.3%	67.5%
Number of doctor visits per year		
Mean, SD	5.9 ± 6.9	6.8 ± 8.2
Range	1–52	1–50
Different doctors seen in the past year		
Mean, SD	2.0 ± 1.7	2.8 ± 3.7
Range	0–16	0–24

Source: Data from The Commonwealth Fund survey on women's health, 1993.

also no significant difference in the use of physicians by gender, with women in this survey reporting slightly fewer doctor visits per year and fewer different doctors seen per year than men, on average (tab. 7.3; $p > 0.05$).

This finding of no higher use of health care by women raises the question of whether older women are getting needed care. It is known that health care reimbursement currently meets only 50 percent to 60 percent of older women's medical expenses, and provides a low proportion of the costs of chronic outpatient care (Lewis 1985; Cornelius, Beauregard, and Cohen 1991; Lefkowitz and Monheit 1991). Given women's lower incomes, out-of-pocket expenses for health care are likely to consume a higher proportion of their incomes, compared with men. The gender effect of financial status relative to health care coverage in the use of health care needs to be understood better.

To address this issue, the characteristics associated with having a usual source of care were evaluated in multiple logistic regression analyses, for men and women. The results suggest that women in poorer health have access to physicians, but that having health care coverage is a significant modifier of this. In these analyses, a usual source of health care was defined as seeing a practitioner in a doctor's office, clinic, or HMO, or being seen regularly by a nurse practitioner. Because of the large proportion of the study population who did not report their income, this variable could not be evaluated in these analyses. However, marital status (married versus other), race, and education (more than high school versus high school or less) were evaluated in its stead.

For men and women age sixty-five or over, having a usual source of care is associated with having health care coverage, having two or more chronic diseases, being female, and being in fair or poor health, and there is a borderline relationship with education (tab. 7.4). In models with an interaction term, being a woman in poor health is associated with having a usual source of care (tab. 7.4). It is interesting to note that in these analyses the indicators of socioeconomic status had either borderline significance or no association with having a usual source of care.

In contrast, the number of physician visits a year (four or more

Table 7.4. Characteristics Associated with Having a Usual, Regular Source of Medical Care,[a] Women and Men Ages Sixty-five Years or Older

Characteristic[b]	B	p	Odds Ratio
Having health care coverage[c]	−1.2643	0.0004	0.28
Education[d]	−0.2292	0.06	0.80
Race[e]	0.2541	0.09	1.29
Self-assessed health	−0.0544	0.83	0.94
One chronic disease	−0.2277	0.10	0.80
Two chronic diseases	−0.4754	0.002	0.62
Three chronic diseases	−0.8194	0.0001	0.44
Interaction of female gender with poor health	0.4932	0.07	1.64

Source: Analysis of The Commonwealth Fund survey on women's health, 1993.

[a] Defined as in a physician's office, clinic, or HMO, or by a nurse practitioner; 340/448 persons, or 76 percent, reported such a usual source of care.

[b] Variables that did not enter the model were age and marital status. Gender and health were significant ($p < 0.05$) before interaction terms were entered.

[c] Any insurance = 1; no insurance or not sure = 2.

[d] ≤ high school = 1; > high school = 2.

[e] White = 1; other races = 2.

versus less than four) by older women is significantly associated with the number of chronic diseases present and with disability in multivariate analysis, while health care insurance coverage is not. Similarly, the number of physicians seen in a year is associated with the number of chronic diseases present and with education ($p \leq 0.05$), but not insurance status. Those with a usual source of care are more likely to see multiple physicians than those without a usual source of care. These data suggest that older women needing care for illness are likely to receive health care, especially if they have health care coverage.

U.S. data show that 76 percent of people sixty-five years or older who reported having no usual source of care stated that they seldom or never get sick (Cornelius, Beauregard, and Cohen 1991). These findings are also suggested by The Commonwealth Fund survey, if one considers the converse of the results above. However, they raise the question of whether women who are in good health are receiving appropriate care, especially preventive health care; this is discussed further below.

Employment

There has been increasing interest in the contributions that older adults might make to the nation's economy, skills, and social needs if they were provided with job opportunities (Commonwealth Fund 1993). In addition, there is increasing evidence that remaining physically, and perhaps cognitively, active confers health benefits through prevention of disease and disability (Larson and Bruce 1987; Hamdorf et al. 1992; Fiatarone et al. 1994); it is possible that working may be associated with such patterns of higher activity, although this remains to be evaluated. In the survey, 4 percent of the women work full-time and 8.7 percent work part-time; the proportion declines in those seventy-five or older, but does not differ by race. These rates are consistent with those of other national surveys (Leville et al. 1992). The proportions of women who are working do not differ by health status (excellent or good versus fair or poor) or the presence of disability (tab. 7.5), compared with those who are not working.

Some of those who are not working for pay (22% of all women surveyed) reported that they would prefer to work for pay; this includes 23 percent of white women and 47 percent of women of other races. The interest in working for pay decreases only slightly with increasing age: from 27 percent of women sixty-five to seventy-four

Table 7.5. Work Status of Women Ages Sixty-five to Eighty-five Years, and Associated Health Characteristics

| Working Status | Overall ($n = 454$) | Health Status | | | Disability | | |
		Excellent/ Good ($n = 354$)	Fair/Poor ($n = 100$)	p	Present ($n = 129$)	Absent ($n = 330$)	p
Working full- or part-time	13% (57/454)	13%	11%	0.66	12%	13%	0.62
Among those not working							
Prefer to work, not working now	22% (102/459)	25%	27%		28%	25%	
Prefer not to work	59% (269/459)	69%	66%	0.85	64%	69%	0.55
If prefer to work and suitable job were available in your area (% of those prefer to work; $n = 102$):							
Able to work	46% (47/102)	50%	34%		26%	55%	
Not able to work	48% (49/102)	44%	64%	0.23	67%	41%	0.03

Source: Data from The Commonwealth Fund survey on women's health, 1993.

years, down to 24 percent of those seventy-five or older. Those who preferred to work are significantly more likely to have lower income (less than $14,000; $p = 0.003$) or less education (high school or less; $p = 0.04$).

Although 22 percent among those not working for pay would prefer to be working, less than half of this group (46%) stated that they would be able to work for pay if a suitable job were available. Notably, current work status, preferring to work for pay (if not working currently), and ability to work are not associated with self-assessed health status ($p > 0.2$). However, not being able to work is associated with being disabled (tab. 7.5; $p = 0.03$).

The major reasons cited for wanting to work differ by income level, but not as much by education (tab. 7.6). Those with lower incomes (< $15,000) who wanted to work primarily cited needing the money or being bored, while those with incomes above $15,000 are most likely to

Table 7.6. Interest in Working for Pay, Women Ages Sixty-five Years or Older Who Are Not Working

	% of Total Population	(*n*/*N*)
Would prefer to work for pay	22	(102/459)
Among those preferring to work (*n* = 102)		
Reasons wish to work		
Need the money	26	(24/93)
To do something useful	13	(12/93)
Bored	23	(21/93)
To keep active	35	(35/93)
Friends working	3	(3/93)

Source: Data from The Commonwealth Fund survey on women's health, 1993.
Note: N = total population; *n* = subset of population.

say that they want to keep active or do something useful. Both income groups see wanting to do something useful as a major reason to work. Regardless of education, both groups cited wanting to keep active as the primary reason for wanting to work.

Thus, 13 percent of older women are working for pay and another 10 percent prefer to be working and feel they are able to work. Interest in working is motivated by a desire to improve income, to keep active, and to make a contribution to society. While one-quarter of older women would like to be working, only half of this group feel they are able to work. While data previously discussed suggest that maintaining activity, perhaps through work, may prevent disability, these findings indicate that disability is the major characteristic that makes older women feel they are not able to work. Both of these areas appear to be important aspects of preventive strategies for older women. If disability and other factors did not make women feel they are unable to work, 35 percent of older women either would be working or would prefer to be working.

Use of Health Care

Sixty-four percent of the women age sixty-five or older had physical exams in the past year; 36 percent had not. Those who had an exam reported being in worse health than those who did not. This is supportive of findings from U.S. studies that those not receiving medical

Table 7.6. (*Continued*)

Education			Income		
≤ HS (n = 286)	> HS (n = 105)	p	≤ $15,000 (n = 195)	> $15,000 (n = 120)	p
29%	18%	0.04	28%	17%	0.003
(n = 76)	(n = 17)		(n = 48)	(n = 19)	
28%	17%		37%	0%	
11%	21%		10%	25%	
27%	4%		27%	6%	
32%	52%		21%	65%	
2%	1%	0.14	4%	4%	0.001

care are likely to be in better health. Notably, the same proportion (64%) thought that their health care coverage paid for a physical examination (tab. 7.7).

Seventy-five percent of women age sixty-five or older had not had either a physical exam or one of the preventive screening procedures (recommended by current guidelines) in the past year. Among this group, 15 percent said they had not used health care or preventive services in the past year because they cost too much, and 17 percent indicated their physician had never suggested it; another 10 percent reported they were afraid of what they might find out. Others reported that they had too much to do (10%), lacked transportation (7.4%), or could not get an appointment (2.7%). In addition, 4 percent of the women surveyed stated that they had needed health care in the past year and had not gotten it; for half of these women, it is because it was too expensive or because they did not have health insurance coverage for what they needed.

Primary Prevention

Over the past 20 years, several groups have offered recommendations on preventive health care for older women, including the U.S. Preventive Services Task Force (1989) and others (Breslow and Sommers 1977; Canadian Task Force on the Periodic Health Examination 1979; American Cancer Society 1980). These guidelines indicate that health habits,

Table 7.7. Self-Report of Health Care Coverage, Women Ages Sixty-five Years or Older

Health Insurance Pays for	Percentage of Women 65–85 Thinking Care Is Covered by Insurance	Actual Medicare Coverage
Complete physical exam	64.4[a, b]	Not for screening
Blood cholesterol screening, preventive	66.7[a, d]	Not for screening
Mammogram, preventive	65.0[b, c]	Every 2 years
Pap smear, preventive	55.5[b, c]	Every 3 years

Source: Data from The Commonwealth Fund survey on women's health, 1993.

[a] No association with age: 65–74 versus ≥75.

[b] No association with race.

[c] $p < 0.05$: higher proportion of women 65–74 report health care coverage than those ≥75.

[d] $p < 0.05$: higher proportion of whites report coverage than other races.

such as regular exercise and not smoking, remain important aspects of primary preventive health care for older, as well as younger, women.

Despite such recommendations, while almost half of the older women surveyed reported being in excellent, very good, or good health, only 21 percent exercise regularly (4 or more days a week, the frequency recommended for cardiovascular health). An additional 12 percent exercise 2 or 3 days a week, while 67 percent reported exercising once a week or less, or never. In addition, 16 percent of older women are cigarette smokers. Smokers are primarily women sixty-five to seventy-four years. Otherwise, the rates of exercise and smoking do not vary significantly by age, race, or education. Overall, there is substantial opportunity to improve the exercise and smoking status of older women.

Remarkably, 85 percent of the older women reported that their blood cholesterol had been checked within the past 3 years; only 5 percent had never had their cholesterol checked. There is no difference in these statistics by age group or race. These high rates are despite the lack of Medicare coverage for such screening tests.

These women were also asked whether they were familiar with osteoporosis; 73 percent answered affirmatively. Those who are familiar with osteoporosis are almost twice as likely to use calcium supplements as those who are not familiar (46% of those familiar versus 26% of those not familiar; $p = 0.0002$). Furthermore, the group familiar with osteoporosis is ten times more likely to use hormone therapy (22% of those familiar versus 2% of those who were not; $p < 0.00001$). Whether familiarity leads to the use of these agents or results from physician counseling cannot be determined from these data. Recent data indicate that supplementation with calcium and vitamin D reduces the risk of fractures in older women (Chapuy et al. 1992).

In this survey population, lack of familiarity with osteoporosis is associated with being over seventy-five years, with lower education (87% of those not familiar had less than a high school education; $p = 0.00002$), and with incomes less than $15,000 (73% of those not familiar; $p = 0.006$). Familiarity is also associated with race: 61 percent of nonwhites and 23 percent of whites are not familiar with osteoporosis ($p < 0.00001$). While the difference by race may be associated with socioeconomic status and access to care, differentials by race may also be a result of what studies suggest is a lower risk for hip fracture in African American women, and less physician counseling as a result. Despite this perception, both African American and white women are at risk for osteoporosis.

Secondary Prevention

Current recommendations for secondary preventive health care for older women include blood pressure screenings at least biennially for women sixty-five or older (U.S. Preventive Services Task Force 1989; Breslow and Sommers 1977). Annual physical examinations are recommended for women seventy-five years or older and biennial ones for women sixty-five to seventy-four years by the Canadian Task Force on the Periodic Health Examination (1979); the U.S. Preventive Services Task Force (1989) recommended these be done annually. The proportions of women who received blood pressure screenings and physical examinations in the past 2 years are 94.5 percent and 71 percent, respectively (tab. 7.8). Those who had a physical examination in the past year are significantly more likely to have health problems than those who did not have an exam; specifically, 68 percent of those with one or more chronic diseases (of nine assessed) had a physical exam in the past year, compared with 46 percent of those with no chronic diseases ($p = 0.009$).

Current recommendations for secondary prevention also include screening for cancer of the reproductive organs in older women. This should include annual breast examinations and mammograms every

Table 7.8. Screening for Secondary Prevention, Women Ages Sixty-five Years or Older

	Percentage Who Received Screening				
	In Past Year	Past 1–2 Years	Past 2–3 Years	>3 Years	Never
Recommended annually					
Physical exam, persons ≥75 years	63.9	9.4	5.4	19.3	2.0
Clinical breast examination	59.0	9.9	7.1	15.4	8.6
Mammogram	50.3	10.2	5.4	16.3	17.7
Recommended biennially					
Physical exam, persons 65–74 years	64.3	7.1	7.8	18.4	2.4
Blood pressure screening	90.3	4.2	0.6	3.7	1.2
Pap smear[a]	44.4	7.9	6.7	33.5	7.5

Source: Data from The Commonwealth Fund survey on women's health, 1993.

[a] Every 1–3 years, if results normal with regular, repeated screening; additional screening may be necessary after age 65 in those with average risk.

one to 2 years (Breslow and Sommers 1977; American Cancer Society 1980; U.S. Preventive Services Task Force 1989), and Pap smears every one to 3 years (American Cancer Society 1980; U.S. Preventive Services Task Force 1989). One-half to two-thirds of women reported receiving at least one component of this recommended screening in the past 2 years (tab. 7.8). Eighteen percent of these older women never had a mammogram, and 9 percent never had a breast exam (tab. 7.8). Overall, one-third of older women are not receiving one or more components (among the five evaluated) of the recommended preventive health care screening.

Characteristics Associated with the Use of Preventive and General Health Care

Those who received preventive health care in the past 2 years are more likely to have a usual source of health care, to have seen more physicians in the past year, to have more chronic disease, and to think that their insurance paid for physical examinations and preventive screening (tab. 7.9). Such individuals are also more likely to be married, be better educated, and not live alone. Perceptions—or misperceptions—as to health care coverage thus play an important role in using health care. One-third of older women say that they have no health care coverage for physical examinations (tab. 7.7). Medicare does not pay for physical examinations for preventive purposes, although physical examinations to evaluate a health problem are likely to be covered. In addition, 35 percent and 44 percent, respectively, indicated that they do not have coverage for mammograms or Pap smears, although Medicare does pay for these to be done every 2 and every 3 years, respectively (tab. 7.7). Thinking a service is paid for by insurance is significantly associated with the use of mammograms (tab. 7.9; $p < 0.0001$), as well as obtaining a physical exam ($p = 0.02$) in bivariate analyses, while there is no association with obtaining a blood cholesterol screening ($p > 0.05$). These associations hold for all women when stratified by health status.

In multivariate analyses, the only characteristics significantly associated with having a physical examination in the past 2 years are having a usual source of care (odds ratio = 1.39; $p = 0.01$) and thinking that insurance paid for a physical examination (odds ratio = 0.60; $p < 0.0001$). In additional models in which the dependent variable was having a physical examination or other preventive screening according to current recommendations, self-assessed health status is also associated with this outcome (odds ratio = 1.36; $p = 0.05$). In contrast, characteristics associated with receiving just preventive screening are more education (odds ratio = 1.30; $p = 0.02$) and not living alone (odds ratio = 1.30; $p = 0.01$), as well as thinking insurance paid for such care (odds ratio = 1.86; $p < 0.0001$). These analyses are adjusted for self-rated health, education, age, marital status, having a usual source of care, and number of chronic diseases (zero, one, two, or three or more).

Overall, receiving preventive screening is strongly associated with having a physical examination. For example, 74 percent of women who had a physical in the past 2 years had a Pap smear, compared with 26 percent of those who had not had a physical examination ($p < 0.0001$). Thus, accessing care through a physical examination is generally the path to receiving additional preventive health care.

These analyses suggest that women with poorer health, health care coverage, or a regular health care provider (who may also have poorer health) are the most likely to use health care and to receive preventive

Table 7.9. Characteristics Associated with Having a Clinical Breast Exam or Mammogram in the Past 2 Years or a Pap Smear in the Past 3 Years, Compared with Having It Longer Ago or Never

Characteristic	Received Preventive Screening ($n = 424$)	Haven't Received Preventive Screening ($n = 23$)	p
Age			
65–74	64.3%	58.0%	
≥75	35.7%	42.0%	0.17
Marital status			
Not married	58.2%	70.7%	
Married	41.8%	29.3%	0.005
Education			
High school or less	64.1%	76.6%	
College or higher	35.9%	23.4%	0.003
Health care coverage			
Medicare only	11.0%	14.8%	
Medicare plus health insurance or HMO	74.2%	62.9%	
Medicare plus Medicaid	8.7%	14.8%	
None of the above	2.9%	4.0%	0.07
Living alone	49.0%	63.8%	0.001
Number of chronic diseases			
0	13.2%	23.2%	
1	33.5%	28.3%	
2	28.3%	25.8%	
≥3	25.0%	22.7%	0.06
Can't participate fully in work, housework, or other activities due to disability or chronic disease	30.5%	26.1%	0.30
Self-assessed health			
Excellent/very good	5.2%	51.0%	
Good	33.4%	26.4%	
Fair/poor	21.4%	22.5%	0.26
Has usual source of health care			
Yes	85.1%	74.5%	
No	14.9%	25.5%	0.005
Number of physician visits in past year (mean, SD)	6.27 ± 6.49	05.51 ± 7.38	0.29

(*continued*)

Table 7.9. (*Continued*)

Characteristic	Received Preventive Screening (*n* = 424)	Haven't Received Preventive Screening (*n* = 23)	*p*
Number of physicians seen in past year (mean, SD)	2.36 ± 1.7	11.73 ± 1.60	<0.001
Specialty of regular physician			
Family practitioner	59.1%	58.4%	
Internist	29.7%	18.8%	
Ob/Gyn	2.6%	1.5%	
Other	0.9%	1.8%	
No regular physician	3.0%	14.0%	
Not sure	4.7%	5.5%	0.0006
Insurance pays for			
Physical exam	69.6%	59.3%	0.02
Blood cholesterol screening	70.7%	62.7%	0.07
Mammogram	79.6%	51.4%	<0.00001
Pap smear	72.2%	39.6%	<0.00001

Source: Data from The Commonwealth Fund survey on women's health, 1993.

services. They also indicate that one-third of the older women surveyed had not received one or more components of recommended preventive care in the previous 2 years. Finally, they suggest that healthier women are less likely to be receiving preventive health care than are women with poor health, perhaps because they are not seeing physicians for chronic health problems. This subset of healthier women has a great likelihood of benefiting from primary prevention and preventive screening and is, in fact, supposed to be the targeted group for the current prevention recommendations. These data indicate a need for increased public education as to the importance of prevention for healthy older women.

IMPLICATIONS FOR POLICY

Several areas of concern for older women identified in this study— health care coverage, access to services, and public education needs— warrant attention in the public policy arena.

Health Care Coverage and Access to Health Care

This study suggests that lack of insurance coverage is a significant, independent factor in whether an older woman has a regular health care provider and whether she receives a physical examination or preventive health care services currently recommended for her age group. In addition, the cost of health care is a reason for not getting needed health care or preventive services, according to 15 percent of women who did not get needed care. It also appears that there is a substantial need for mental health care in older women, and the data suggest that a great many mental health problems are underdiagnosed and/or undertreated; this may result, in part, from current undercoverage of mental health needs. Because out-of-pocket costs are likely to be higher relative to income for women compared with men (given the income differences by gender), and the number of years lived with chronic disease and disability and the resulting chronic health care needs are greater for older women than older men, health care coverage and costs are highly salient issues for older women.

In each of these areas, it should be determined to what degree the underuse is a result of misinformation as to what care is covered, and to what degree it is a consequence of inadequate coverage, limited access, or underrecognition of need by the patient or provider. Improved health care coverage could make a substantial difference in the use of needed care by older women. This coverage particularly needs to include outpatient, chronic care, preventive care, and mental health services.

Public Education

Efforts at public education appear warranted in a number of areas. The target groups are, first, older women, their families, and health care providers; and, second, the girls and younger women who will make up the future generations of elderly women. For both groups, the importance of prevention needs to be emphasized.

Education for older women should make it clear that there is an important role for prevention as one ages, to prevent unnecessary disease and disability. It is noteworthy, in this regard, that 75 percent of the older women surveyed had not received one or more of the recommended preventive screening evaluations. An important target group for education is the healthier older women who are not seeing a physician regularly—as much as one-third of older women. In addition, all older women would benefit from accurate information about current Medicare and other insurance coverage for physical examinations, mammograms, and Pap smears. Finally, basic health habits are extremely important in health status and the risk for disease and disability; women need to be educated, in particular, as to the importance of regular physical exercise (at least four times a week) and the benefits of smoking cessation.

Public health education for older women should also target the prevention of specific diseases. For example, it is now recognized that cardiovascular diseases affect a substantial proportion of older women, and that they are not inevitable parts of the aging process. The treatment of hypertension, exercise, smoking cessation, and heart-healthy diets remain important parts of preventing cardiovascular disease in older, and younger, women. In addition, new information on cardiovascular risk factors for older women must be disseminated to the public as it becomes available from ongoing studies, such as the Cardiovascular Health Study. Other diseases and conditions amenable to prevention and/or treatment that were identified in the older women surveyed include HIV infection, cancers (reproductive, colonic, and skin, in particular), depression, osteoporosis, and urinary incontinence. Public education is warranted for these diseases, directed at both older women and their health care providers.

Targeting Care and Services

Several issues highlighted by these data suggest potential benefits from targeting education, screening, treatment or services, and education. For example, African American, Hispanic, lower-income, and sicker older women appear particularly at risk for depressive symptomatology. Increased alertness to this risk through screening in such groups may well be indicated. As mentioned, healthy older women who have not seen a physician in the past 2 years should be educated to use preventive health care services. This is also true for those who have less education or who are living alone.

Younger women, who will become the future generations of elderly women, are a target audience. These data demonstrate that education makes a substantial difference in health status, self-esteem, and self-efficacy among elderly women. The level of education among the current cohort of girls and young women is, therefore, likely to be a major force in the well-being of elderly women in the next century. This warrants major emphasis. As stated by the U.N. Non-Governmental Organization for Women (Smyke 1991), the most important thing a country can do to improve its public health is to educate its women. From education flow better health habits and better health and economic status of its women, and improved health of their children.

In addition, health habits such as exercise, nutrition, and smoking are extremely important predictors of the chronic disease status of young women as they age. Smoking rates among young women now exceed those among young men or any other age group in the United States. Public education should start by targeting these risk factors for improvement.

IMPLICATIONS FOR RESEARCH

Issues warranting further research complement, in large degree, the areas that warrant policy action. The overarching question that would make the greatest difference for future generations of elderly women is how to prevent the disability and dependency that now result from the chronic diseases of aging. For older women, methods of preventing disability are a priority. These include identifying how to prevent the onset of chronic diseases in older women; the major disabling diseases include ischemic heart disease, stroke, arthritis and other musculoskeletal disease, emphysema, and asthma. In addition, whether interventions in persons with chronic disease should also be directed to the prevention of comorbidity (multiple chronic diseases) as a strategy for preventing disability remains to be clarified. Finally, among the large portion of older women who are already disabled, opportunities for minimizing this disability and preventing progression are called for. A first step in this will come from research under way in the Women's Health and Aging Study, now in progress.

One outcome of such research would be the development of medical and public health approaches to the treatment of disability in older women. One explanation for why women report similar rates of health care use and not higher ones than men may be that the medical community currently offers little to treat chronically progressive disability. Developing and testing interventions are essential to assist disabled individuals to regain function, maintain independence, and prevent dependency. The most promising area at this time is in the potential for various exercise interventions to have such an effect (Fiatarone et al. 1994). However, additional approaches should be developed.

One area that deserves particular research attention is the psychological distress expressed by a large portion of the older women surveyed. In these women, depressive symptomatology, low self-esteem, and low self-efficacy are common. Additional research would define the causes of this, and develop effective screening and interventions to assist women who experience these symptoms. Understanding the etiology of these issues would provide a basis for strategies to prevent this in younger women.

The high frequency of feelings of uselessness in these women, as well as their interest in working as a way to be useful to others, suggests that one potential preventive strategy would be to create more opportunities for older adults to work. Creating opportunities for older women to have a productive outlet and improved self-esteem, to remain physically and socially active, and to increase their income while making contributions to society appears to be an approach that could benefit all concerned. Potential outcomes could include improved functioning and mental health, as well as improved financial status and health care coverage. However, research would clarify more fully which subsets of older women would be interested, and what the appropriate jobs, training, and compensation should be. There appear to be opportunities to recruit older women into the workforce, and with careful matching of skills and abilities to jobs, such opportunities could be created. Addressing these questions in a rigorous manner, with carefully developed jobs and appropriate training and evaluations of outcomes, would help determine the approaches that are effective and provide a definitive assessment of the costs and benefits of improving job opportunities for older women—and all older adults.

REFERENCES

American Cancer Society. 1980. *1980 Report on the Cancer-related Health Checkup. Cancer* 30:194–240.

Breslow, L., and Sommers, A. R. 1977. The lifetime health-monitoring program: a practical approach to preventive medicine. *New England Journal of Medicine* 292:601–8.

Canadian Task Force on the Periodic Health Examination. 1979. The periodic health examination. *Canadian Medical Association Journal* 121:1194–1254.

Chapuy, M. C., et al. 1992. Vitamin D_3 and calcium to prevent hip fractures in elderly women. *New England Journal of Medicine* 327:1637–42.

Commonwealth Fund. 1993. The Untapped Resource: The Final Report of the Americans over 55 at Work Program. New York: Commonwealth Fund.

Cornelius, L., Beauregard, K., and Cohen, J. 1991. Usual sources of medical care and their characteristics. AHCPR pub. no. 91–0042. National Medical Expenditure Survey Research Findings 11, Agency for Health Care Policy and Research. Rockville, Md.: Public Health Service.

Fiatarone, M. A., et al. 1994. Exercise training and nutritional supplementation for physical frailty in very elderly people. *New England Journal of Medicine* 330:1769–75.

Frame, P. S., and Carlson, S. J. 1975. A critical review of periodic health screening using specific screening criteria. *Journal of Family Practice* 2:283–89.

Fried, L. P., and Bush, T. L. 1988. Morbidity as a focus of preventive health care in the elderly. *Epidemiologic Reviews* 10:48–64.

Fried, L. P., et al., for the Cardiovascular Health Study (CHS) Collaborative Research Group. 1994. Physical disability in older adults: a physiological approach. *Journal of Clinical Epidemiology* 42:895–904.

Fries, J. F. 1980. Aging, natural death, and the compression of morbidity. *New England Journal of Medicine* 303:130–35.

German, P. S., and Fried, L. P. 1989. Prevention and the elderly: public health issues and strategies. *Annual Review of Public Health* 10:319–32.

German, P. S., et al. 1978. Health care of the elderly in medically disadvantaged populations. *The Gerontologist* 18:547–55.

Guralnik, J. M. 1987. Capturing the full range of physical functioning in older populations. *Proceedings of the 1987 Public Health Conference on Records and Statistics* National Center for Health Statistics, National Institute on Aging, U.S. Bureau of the Census.

Guralnik, J. M., et al. 1989. Aging in the eighties: the prevalence of comorbidity and its association with disability. Advance Data from Vital and Health Statistics, no. 170. Hyattsville, Md.: National Center for Health Statistics.

Hamdorf, P. A., et al. 1992. Physical training effects on the fitness and habitual activity patterns of elderly women. *Archives of Physical Medicine and Rehabilitation* 73:603–8.

Higgins, M. W., et al., for the Cardiovascular Health Study Research Group. 1993. Smoking and lung function in elderly men and women: the Cardiovascular Health Study. *Journal of the American Medical Association* 269: 2741–48.

Jajich, C., Ostfeld, A. M., and Freeman, D. H., Jr. 1984. Smoking and coronary heart disease mortality in the elderly. *Journal of the American Medical Association* 252:2831–34.

Kaplan, G. A. 1992. Maintenance of functioning in the elderly. *Annals of Epidemiology* 2:823–34.

Katz, S., et al. 1983. Active life expectancy. *New England Journal of Medicine* 309:1218–24.

LaCroix, A. Z., et al. 1992. The cost of disability in older women and opportunities for prevention. *Journal of Women's Health* 1:52–62.

Larson, E. B. 1991. Exercise, functional decline and frailty. *Journal of the American Geriatrics Society* 39:635–36.

Larson, E. B., and Bruce, R. A. 1987. Health benefits of exercise in an aging society. *Archives of Internal Medicine* 147:353–56.

Lefkowitz, D., and Monheit, A. 1991. Health insurance, use of health services, and health care expenditures. AHCPR pub. no. 92–0017. National Medical Expenditure Survey Research Findings 12. Rockville, Md.: Agency for Health Care Policy and Research.

Leville, S. G., et al. 1992. The cost of disability in older women and opportunities for prevention. *Journal of Women's Health* 1:53–62.

Lewis, M. 1985. Older women and health: an overview. *Women and Health* 10:1–16.

Magaziner, J., et al. 1988. Health and living arrangements among older women: does living alone increase the risk of illness? *Journal of Gerontology, Medical Sciences* 43:127–33.

Mor, V., et al. 1989. Risk of functional decline among well elders. *Journal of Clinical Epidemology* 42:895–904.

Morey, M. C., et al. 1991. Two-year trends in physical performance following supervised exercise among community dwelling older veterans. *Journal of the American Geriatrics Society* 39:549–54.

National Center for Health Statistics et al. 1987. Health Statistics on Older Persons, United States, 1986. *Vital and Health Statistic*, series 3, no. 25, DHHS pub. no. (PHS) 87–1409. Washington, D.C.: U.S. Government Printing Office.

National Center for Health Statistics, Kovar, M. G., and LaCroix, A. Z. 1987. Aging in the eighties, Ability to perform work-related activities. Data from the Supplement on Aging to the National Health Interview Survey, U.S., 1984. Advance Data from Vital and Health Statistics no. 136. DHHS pub. no. (PHS) 87–1250. Hyattsville, Md.: Public Health Service.

National Center for Health Statistics, Moss, A. J., and Parsons, V. L. 1986. Current estimates from the National Health Interview Survey, U.S., 195. *Vital and Health Statistics*, series 10, no. 160. DHHS pub. no. (PHS) 86–1588. Washington, D.C.: U.S. Government Printing Office.

NIH Consensus Panel. 1992. Diagnosis and treatment of depression in late life. *Journal of the American Medical Association* 268:1018–24.

Older Women's League. 1988. The picture of health for mid-life and older women in America. *Women and Health* 14:53–74.

Pinsky, J. L., Leaverton, P. W., and Stokes, J., III. 1987. Predictors of good function: the Framingham Study. *Journal of Chronic Disease* 40:159S–167S.

Rabin, D. L., and Stockton, P. 1987. *Long-term Care for the Elderly*. New York: Oxford University Press.

Simonsick, E. M., et al. 1993. Risk due to inactivity in physically capable older adults. *American Journal of Public Health* 83:1443–50.

Smyke, P. 1991. *Women and Health*. Atlantic Highlands, N.J.: Zed Books, Ltd.

U.S. Preventive Services Task Force. 1989. *Guide to Clinical Preventive Services*. Report of the U.S. Preventive Services Task Force. Baltimore: Williams and Wilkins.

U.S. Senate Special Committee on Aging. 1991. *Aging in America: Trends and Projections.* U.S. DHHS pub. no. (FCoA) 91–28001.

Verbrugge, L. M. 1984. A health profile of older women with comparisons to older men. *Research on Aging* 6:291–322.

Verbrugge, L. M., Lepkowski, J. M., and Imanaka, Y. 1989. Comorbidity and its impact on disability. *The Milbank Quarterly* 67:3–4.

Wagner, E. H., and LaCroix, A. Z. 1992. Effects of physical activity on health status in older adults I: observational studies. *Annual Review of Public Health* 13:451–68.

Wells, K. B., et al. 1989. The functioning and well-being of depressed patients: results from the Medical Outcomes Study. *Journal of the American Medical Association* 262:914–19.

Wenger, N. K., Speroff, L., and Packard, B., eds. 1993. *Proceedings of an N.H.L.B.I. Conference: Cardiovascular Health and Disease in Women.* Greenwich, Conn.: LeJacq Communications, Inc.

Wingard, D. L. 1982. The sex differential in mortality rates: demographic and behavioral factors. *American Journal of Epidemiology* 155:205–16.

Zook, C. J., and Moore, F. D. 1980. High cost utilizers of medical care. *New England Journal of Medicine* 302:996–1002.

III

Behavioral Well-Being

8

Depression and Self-esteem among Women

Mary Clare Lennon, Ph.D., M.S.

For the past several decades, a large body of literature has documented and attempted to explain the greater psychological distress and depression found among women than among men. In studies conducted in the general community, women have substantially higher rates of symptoms of psychological distress and depressive disorders than men (McGrath et al. 1990; Robins and Regier 1991; Kessler et al. 1994). This is found for measures of anxiety, depressed mood, and psychophysiological complaints—what Dohrenwend and colleagues (1980) called demoralization (see Dohrenwend and Dohrenwend 1976 and McGrath et al. 1990 for reviews). Similarly, this differential exists for measures designed to yield a psychiatric diagnosis of major depressive disorder and dysthymia according to criteria set forth by the *Diagnostic and Statistical Manual* of the American Psychiatric Association (Robins and Regier 1991; Kessler et al. 1994). While rates of disorders vary widely according to how they are defined, on average women have about twice as many depressive disorders as men (Weissman and Klerman 1977; McGrath et al. 1990; Paykel 1991). In contrast, men tend to have higher rates than women of acting-out disorders, such as antisocial behavior and drug and alcohol abuse (Lennon 1987; Robins and Regier 1991; Kessler et al. 1994).

The central question with respect to gender differences in mental health was put succinctly two decades ago by Bruce and Barbara Dohrenwend (1976), who asked: "What is there in the endowments and experiences of men and women that pushes them in these different deviant directions?" To date, most of the literature addressing this question has focused on explaining the excess of psychological distress and depression in women. Various risk factors for this excess have been examined, ranging from biological to psychological to social. While many reviewers conclude that women's risk for depressive disorders must be understood in a biopsychosocial context (e.g., McGrath et al. 1990), most empirical research does not examine biological, psychological, and social risks simultaneously (for an exception, see Kendler et al. 1993).

Research indicates that, to a large extent, psychological and sociological aspects of women's lives are related to their increased risk for depressive disorders (Jack 1991; Paykel 1991; Kendler et al. 1993). In contrast, biological factors, such as hormonal changes and genetic predisposition, appear to be less powerful contributors to gender differences in depressive disorders (Weissman and Klerman 1977; Merikangas, Weissman, and Pauls 1985). However, questions of etiology remain unanswered and pose a challenge for future researchers.

This chapter reviews some of the literature on sociological explanations for women's higher rates of psychological distress and depressive disorders and, using data from The Commonwealth Fund survey, examines empirically some social factors that may account for variations among women in symptoms of psychological distress. These include factors related to family, employment, and parenting, as well as poverty, social support, and health.

This chapter focuses primarily on depressed mood because depression is one of the most prevalent and debilitating mental disorders (McGrath et al. 1990). Correlates of women's self-esteem, an important component of depression, are also examined. Consideration of social factors, such as the nature of work, structure of family life, and poverty status—which may contribute to depressed mood or low self-esteem—is crucial for the development of appropriate intervention strategies and social policies.

THE COMMONWEALTH FUND SURVEY

Two aspects of well-being were included in The Commonwealth Fund survey: depressive symptoms and self-esteem. Studies generally find that there is a fairly high correlation between measures of these dimensions of well-being (Dohrenwend et al. 1980), and feeling worthless, an aspect of low self-esteem, is an important symptom of major depression (American Psychiatric Association 1987). However, there is some evidence that self-esteem may be a distinct component of well-being, in some cases independent of depression. For example, while the evidence of more depression among women is strong, comparisons of women and men on self-esteem often have failed to find differences (Hoelter 1983; Mackie 1983). While gender differences in self-esteem cannot be explored here because self-esteem is assessed only for women, these two aspects of well-being may be examined separately among women. Measurement of these variables is described below. Measurement of social and demographic variables is described throughout the chapter, in conjunction with the presentation of results.

METHODS OF DATA ANALYSIS

Data are analyzed using multiple regression procedures. These techniques allow for statistical adjustment of variables that potentially confound the associations of interest (i.e., between aspects of women's lives and their psychological well-being). The control variables are: age, education, income, race, Hispanic ethnicity, employment status, and marital status.[1] Multiple regression also permits testing for interaction effects to evaluate whether associations are constant across all women or are contingent on other factors, such as race, age, marital status, and parental status. Given the large number of analyses conducted and the large number of cases in the survey, a p level of 0.01 is used as the standard for statistical significance. The conventional p level of 0.05 is taken as an indicator of a trend of marginal statistical significance.

The prevalence of depressive symptoms is assessed with six items taken from the Center for Epidemiological Studies Depression (CES-D) Scale (Radloff 1977). These inquire into whether respondents experienced symptoms never, rarely, some of the time, or most of the time during the previous week. The six items are: I felt depressed; my sleep was restless; I enjoy life (scoring reversed); I had crying spells; I felt sad; I felt that people disliked me. Responses (ranging from 0 to 3) are summed to provide a scale of depressive symptoms, with resultant scale scores ranging from 0 to 18. The average depression score for the sample is 4.5 (SD = 3.3). While these items do not permit an assessment of the severity of depression, they do provide a reliable scale of depressive symptoms (Cronbach's alpha is 0.74 for women and 0.69 for men).

Self-esteem is assessed with ten items developed by Morris Rosenberg (1965). The scale inquires into aspects of self-acceptance with items such as: I feel that I have a number of good qualities; on the whole, I am satisfied with myself; I certainly feel useless at times (reverse scoring); I take a positive attitude toward myself. Response categories ranged from strongly agree (coded "3") to strongly disagree (coded "0"). In The Commonwealth Fund survey, self-esteem was assessed for women but not men. The average self-esteem score is 25.33 (SD = 4.77) and the reliability coefficient of the scale is 0.79 (Cronbach's alpha).[2]

RESULTS OF ANALYSES

Gender and Well-Being

As anticipated from the review of the literature above, women in the survey reported significantly more symptoms of depression than men, with a mean score of 4.82, compared with a mean of 3.75 for men (tab. 8.1). However, given different social and demographic characteristics of the women and men in the survey, gender differences in symptoms may turn out to be an artifact. For example, marriage is less prevalent among women (58.1%) than among men (65.9%), and more women

Table 8.1. Mean Depressive Symptoms, by Gender

	Women	Men	t-statistic
Mean depressive symptoms			
Unadjusted	4.82	3.75	8.63[b]
Adjusted[a]	4.77	3.74	7.72[b]
Adjusted mean depressive symptoms by marital status[a]			
Married	4.51	3.61	5.72[b]
Never married	4.69	3.23	5.13[b]
Widowed	4.61	4.60	0.02
Separated/divorced	5.41	4.39	2.41[c]

Source: Analysis of The Commonwealth Fund survey on women's health, 1993.

Note: Unweighted N = 2,515 women and 919 men.

[a] Adjusted for age, education, income, race, ethnicity, employment status, and marital status.

[b] $p < 0.001$.

[c] $p < 0.05$.

than men are separated or divorced (13.5% versus 8.2%) or widowed (13.4% versus 3%). In addition, 57.7 percent of women and 72.8 percent of men are employed. Because being married and being employed may enhance psychological well-being, it is possible that men's fewer depressive symptoms may be due to their greater likelihood of being married and employed. However, when we control for these statistically (along with age, education, income, race, and ethnicity), we find that women still exceed men in symptoms of depression. The mean depression scores, adjusted for these covariates (tab. 8.1), are quite similar to the unadjusted scores.

One of the contested issues in the study of gender and depression is whether differences between women and men are found primarily among married individuals and not among nonmarried persons. Gove and colleagues (Gove and Tudor 1973; Gove and Geerken 1977) contended that being married is especially detrimental to women's sense of well-being. Others (Fox 1980; Lowe and Smith 198 7) asserted that gender differences are no more pronounced among married persons than among individuals in other marital statuses. The survey data generally support the importance of gender, regardless of marital status. When respondents are categorized by marital status, significant gender differences are found for married and never-married individuals (tab. 8.1). The difference between separated or divorced women and men is of marginal significance, with women showing somewhat more symptoms than men. Widowed women and men exhibit similar levels of symptoms.[3]

Thus, this survey shows, as do many other studies of gender and depression, that more women than men report symptoms. To better understand the greater risk for depressive symptoms found among women, we next look more closely at the women in the sample in terms of some of the explanatory systems that have been offered in the literature.

Demographic Variables and Psychological Well-Being

We examined the association between demographic variables and psychological well-being for the sample of women as a whole. Depressive symptoms are negatively correlated with education and income. The literature suggests that the association of age with symptoms may be nonlinear (Newmann, Engel, and Jensen 1991; Kessler et al. 1992). This hypothesis was tested by regressing depressive symptoms and self-esteem on age and age squared. In the case of depressive symptoms, only the linear effect was significant (tab. 8.2). In the case of self-esteem, age has a curvilinear association, discussed below. As indicated by the mean depression scores, younger women have the highest level of symptoms and older women have the lowest. White women have lower symptoms than black/African American women, who have lower symptoms than women of other races. Finally, Hispanic women exceed non-Hispanic women in symptoms.

The results for self-esteem are somewhat different than those for depressive symptoms. Education and income are positively associated with self-esteem. As noted above, age shows a nonlinear association, with lower self-esteem reported by younger and older women than by

Table 8.2. Depressive symptoms and Self-esteem by Demographic Characteristics of the Sample of Women

Variable	Depressive Symptoms	Self-esteem
Education (correlation)	−0.12[a]	0.28[a]
Income (correlation)	−0.18[a]	0.25[a]
Age (mean):		
Younger than 35	5.29	25.37
35–54	4.72	25.77
55+	4.38	24.77
t-statistic (age)	−5.76[a]	−0.27
t-statistic (age squared)	−0.92	−5.26[a]
Race (mean):		
Black/African American	5.54	25.08
White	4.60	25.44
Other race	8.27	23.30
F-statistic	32.19[a]	4.38[b]
Ethnicity (mean):		
Hispanic	5.87	24.42
Non-Hispanic	4.70	25.49
t-statistic	4.67[a]	−2.98[b]

Source: Analysis of The Commonwealth Fund survey on women's health, 1993.

Note: Unweighted $N = 2,525$.

[a] $p < 0.001$.

[b] $p < 0.01$.

midlife women.[4] These results contrast with those for depressive symptoms, where older women show the lowest levels of symptoms. We also find that the relationship of self-esteem and race is statistically significant, with a tendency for white and black and African American women to report greater self-esteem than women of other races. Finally, Hispanic women reported significantly lower self-esteem than non-Hispanic women.

Social Role Theory

In the 1970s Gove and colleagues shaped the inquiry into the relationship of gender to psychological well-being with their social role perspective on gender differences (Gove and Tudor 1973, 1977; Gove and Geerken 1977; Gove, Hughes, and Style 1983). In their view, married women have higher rates of so-called mental illness than married men because their major social roles are frustrating and unrewarding. Gove and Tudor (1973) argued that, unlike men, who have two sources of gratification—work and family—many women have only their family roles as a major source of fulfillment and identification. Because many of the tasks of child care and housework are unskilled, repetitive, and isolating, they can be psychologically stressful. In addition, Gove and Tudor speculated that even if married women are employed, they have higher rates of psychological distress because their jobs tend to be low-level and unchallenging.

A number of studies dispute the evidence brought to bear on this question by Gove and Tudor. Prominent among these are Dohrenwend and Dohrenwend (1976, 1977), who observed that rates of mental disorder by gender have changed over time largely because the methodology used to assess disorder in community settings has changed. Moreover, Dohrenwend and Dohrenwend (1976) pointed out that Gove and Tudor relied heavily on data from hospitals and other mental health facilities. For many reasons, women are more likely than men to seek treatment for mental health problems (Greenley and Mechanic 1976; Horwitz 1977; Kessler, Brown, and Broman 1981). Biases in diagnostic and treatment practices may also affect the gender composition of psychiatric patients (Rosenfield 1982; Loring and Powell 1988; Potts, Burman, and Wells 1991). Nevertheless, studies conducted among general populations—like The Commonwealth Fund survey—support Gove and Tudor's contention that women have more mental health problems than men, but only with regard to particular types of problems—depression, anxiety, and demoralization (Lennon 1987; Robins and Regier 1991; Kessler et al. 1994).

Predictors of Psychological Well-Being among Women

During the past two decades, social role theory has informed a large number of studies of women's mental health. Many of these have focused on the importance of what until recently was considered the traditional female gender role: wife, mother, and homemaker. Empirical support for the hypothesis that women's traditional social roles are associated with distress is found in the significantly higher rates of depression and demoralization among married women than married men (Radloff 1975; Gove and Geerken 1977), among mothers of young children than mothers of older children or nonmothers (Radloff 1975, 1980; Gore and Mangione 1983; McLanahan and Adams 1987), and among housewives than employed women and men (Radloff 1975; Rosenfield 1980; Horwitz 1982).

Other studies have not supported aspects of social role theory, however. For example, as mentioned above, the contention that married women will be especially disadvantaged relative to women of other marital status has generally not been supported. And while results of comparisons of employed wives and homemakers have often been consistent with social role theory, many recent studies found no difference between homemakers and employed wives (see Thoits 1987 for a review). Similarly, many investigators have found support for role theory in the higher rates of distress exhibited by mothers of young children, but this finding is not consistently supported by others (Umberson and Gove 1989).

It is unclear at this stage whether the failure to find differences predicted by role theory is due to low levels of statistical power; to social, demographic, and economic changes in women's and men's lives since the 1960s; or to the failure to measure relevant aspects of women's lives. It is likely that each of these considerations plays a role. To study the relevance of women's social roles, many investigators have examined interaction effects—for example, between gender and marital status (Gore and Mangione 1983). The reduction in statistical power from such subgroup comparisons may explain the failure to detect effects, especially given the difficulty of assessing statistical interactions in survey research (McClelland and Judd 1993). Given the large number of women in The Commonwealth Fund survey

(N = 2,525), however, levels of statistical power are more than adequate for a number of important comparisons between subgroups.

In addition to statistical problems in the study of women's social roles, recent social changes in employment and family life have important implications for the study of psychological well-being in women and men. An important change has been the increased participation in the labor force by married women and mothers of young children. In studying the relation of wives' employment to their psychological well-being, Rosenfield (1992) found that the effect of employment has changed over time. She examined samples of married couples drawn from the same community 20 years apart, and found that while employed women had fewer symptoms of psychological distress than did homemakers in the 1960s, no differences in symptoms were apparent between these groups by the 1980s. She suggested that changing social norms and behaviors with respect to the increase in women's participation in the labor force mean that employment for women is less beneficial today than in the past.[5] While the issue of change over time cannot be addressed using the cross-sectional Commonwealth Fund survey, the survey does permit a timely examination of aspects of work and family life among a large sample of contemporary American women.

The third problem with the literature on social roles and psychological distress is that many studies report the simple comparison of women and men on the basis of social role occupancy, such as comparing married women to married men, housewives to employed women, on the basis of the number and/or configuration of social roles occupied (Thoits 1983, 1986; Froberg, Gjerdingen, and Preston 1986; Menaghan 1989). Building on results from these studies, more recent investigators considered factors that vary within social roles. For example, in studies of married individuals, researchers examined the quality of social roles, husbands' attitudes toward wives' employment, and the division of responsibility for housework and child care in the family (Lennon, Wasserman, and Allen 1991; Robinson and Spitze 1992; Ross, Mirowsky, and Huber 1993). These dimensions of family roles generally moderate the effects of employment for women. Thus, employed wives who have primary responsibility for family work or whose husbands object to their employment have more symptoms of psychological distress than do employed wives with more supportive husbands. The Commonwealth Fund survey contains indicators of such aspects of family life as well.

Employment, Marriage, Parenting, and Psychological Well-Being

Employment, marriage, and parenting for a subsample of women aged sixty-five or younger were examined (tab. 8.3). Older women are excluded because they are unlikely to be engaged actively in jobs and child care. The first column of the table shows the average depression scores adjusted for age, education, income, race, and ethnicity, and marital, employment, and parental status. The second column shows average self-esteem scores, adjusted for the same covariates. Looking at depressive symptoms first, we find that separated or divorced women have the highest depressive symptoms of all women. The effect of marital status is of marginal statistical significance. Employment and children are not associated with depressive symptoms. Results for self-esteem are generally similar, with no significant associations between marital, employment, and parenting status and self-esteem.

Thus, broad comparisons of women by marital, employment, and

Table 8.3. Adjusted Mean Depressive Symptoms and Self-esteem, by Marital, Employment, and Parental Status: Women Ages Sixty-five Years and Younger (unweighted $N = 1,856$)

	Depressive Symptoms	Self-esteem
Marital status		
Married	4.75	25.86
Never married	4.73	25.97
Widowed	4.85	26.17
Separated/divorced	5.51	25.39
F-statistic	4.01[a]	1.12
Employment status		
Employed	4.89	26.07
Not employed	5.03	25.63
t-statistic	−0.82	1.89
Parental status		
Children at home	4.86	25.65
No children at home	5.06	26.05
t-statistic	−1.15	−1.72

Source: Analysis of The Commonwealth Fund survey on women's health, 1993.

Note: Adjusted for age, education, income, race, ethnicity, marital status, employment status, and parental status.

[a] $p < 0.05$.

parenting status show no striking difference in depressive symptoms or self-esteem. However, these analyses are incomplete because they do not take role combinations into account. A more complex analysis is required to examine predictions from social role theory, such as the hypothesis that women in so-called traditional roles demonstrate lower well-being than other women. Such an evaluation entails testing for interactions among marital, employment, and parental status. For self-esteem, but not depressive symptoms, the three-way interaction is significant ($F = 8.82$, $p < 0.01$; $F = 4.14$, $p < 0.05$, respectively). For depressive symptoms, the two-way interaction of marital and employment status is significant ($F = 15.41$, $p < 0.001$). The adjusted mean scores for women categorized by various role constellations are presented (tab. 8.4). For clarity of presentation, women are classified as married or not, as employed or not, and as having children at home or not. Inspection of the results reveals that, as expected from tests of interaction effects, the effects are somewhat different for depressive symptoms and self-esteem.

Looking first at depressive symptoms, we find the highest symptoms among unemployed, unmarried women. As indicated by the absence of a three-way interaction effect, among unmarried, unemployed women, the difference in symptoms between those with and without children is not statistically significant. However, as a group, unemployed, unmarried women have significantly more depressive symptoms than other women. In addition, we find—contrary to social role theory—that women in so-called traditional roles (married, unemployed parents) have lower levels of symptoms than married, employed parents.

The results for self-esteem differ from those for depressive symptoms in that low self-esteem is found primarily among unmarried, unemployed mothers. This group differs significantly from each of the other groups. By way of contrast with the depression results, unmarried, unemployed women without children do not differ from other women in terms of self-esteem. Contrary to the predictions of role theory, there is no difference in self-esteem between women in traditional roles and other married women.

Responsibility for Housework and Child Care and Psychological Well-Being

In seeking to understand the lack of support for social role theory, it is important to recall the literature reviewed earlier that suggests that responsibility for housework and child care may moderate the benefi-

Table 8.4. Adjusted Mean Depressive Symptoms and Self-esteem, by the Interaction of Marital, Employment, and Parental Status: Women Ages Sixty-five Years and Younger (unweighted $N = 1,856$)

	Depressive Symptoms[a]	Self-esteem[b]
Marital status: married		
Employment status: employed		
Parental status:		
Children at home (unweighted $N = 524$)	4.71	25.77
No children at home (unweighted $N = 385$)	4.89	26.20
Employment status: not employed		
Parental status:		
Children at home (unweighted $N = 226$)	4.27	25.84
No children at home (unweighted $N = 178$)	4.69	25.87
Marital status: not married		
Employment status: employed		
Parental status:		
Children at home (unweighted $N = 144$)	4.42	26.14
No children at home (unweighted $N = 398$)	4.94	26.28
Employment status: not employed		
Parental status:		
Children at home (unweighted $N = 60$)	6.22	23.05
No children at home (unweighted $N = 140$)	5.80	25.87

Source: Analysis of The Commonwealth Fund survey on women's health, 1993.

Note: Adjusted for age, education, income, race, ethnicity, marital status, employment status, and parental status.

[a] Two-way interaction of employment status by marital status significant ($F = 15.41$; $p < 0.001$).

[b] Three-way interaction of employment status by marital status by parental status significant ($F = 8.82$; $p < 0.01$).

cial effects of employment for married women. The Commonwealth Fund survey inquired whether husbands/partners "take or share responsibility for housework or not." Response categories were Yes and No. The majority of women (75.8%) responded affirmatively. A similar question was asked of women with children at home about husbands' participation in child care. Ninety-three percent of women reported that their husbands take or share child care responsibility; only 7 percent said that their husbands do not share responsibility.

To examine these aspects of family life, analyses were restricted to married women, aged sixty-five or younger, and two-way interactions were tested for between employment and housework and between employment and child care (tab. 8.5). Husbands' involvement in housework does not interact with employment status but has a marginally significant main effect for depressive symptoms ($t = -1.91$, $p < 0.05$) and a significant main effect for self-esteem ($t = -3.26$, $p < 0.01$). Married women whose husbands are involved in housework show fewer depressive symptoms and higher self-esteem than women whose husbands do not share.

Child care shows similar significant relationships to depressive symptoms and self-esteem. Fewer symptoms and higher self-esteem are found among women whose husbands share child care. Given the high degree of relationship between sharing child care and housework (96% of husbands who share housework also share child care), it is difficult to separate the effects of involvement in housework from involvement in child care. Nevertheless, these results are consistent with

Table 8.5. Adjusted Mean Depressive Symptoms and Self-esteem, by Husbands' Participation in Housework and Child Care: Married Women Ages Sixty-five Years and Younger (unweighted $N = 1,182$ for housework analysis; unweighted $N = 683$ for child care analysis)

	Depressive Symptoms	Self-esteem
Housework		
Husbands share housework	4.48	25.90
Husbands do not share housework	5.27	24.84
t-statistic	-1.91^a	3.34^b
Child care		
Husbands share child care	4.51	26.05
Husbands do not share child care	5.52	24.30
t-statistic	-2.70^b	2.58^c

Source: Analysis of The Commonwealth Fund survey on women's health, 1993.

Note: Adjusted for age, education, income, race, ethnicity, employment status, and parental status.

[a] $p < 0.05$.

[b] $p < 0.001$.

[c] $p < 0.01$.

those of other investigators who show that husbands' involvement in child care is important for women's psychological well-being.

The Interaction of Work and Family and Psychological Well-Being

Studies of women's psychological well-being suggest that it is fruitful to examine the interaction of work and family roles for women. For example, Lowe and Northcott (1988) found higher symptoms of distress among female postal workers if they are married and their jobs offer little variety or challenge. Lennon and Rosenfield (1992) showed that the number of young children at home is associated with higher levels of distress among employed mothers with little job autonomy; among employed mothers with high job autonomy, children are not associated with distress (see also Hibbard and Pope 1987; Repetti 1988; Barnett and Marshall 1989). This research indicates the importance of examining the interaction of work and family conditions in relation to women's psychological well-being.

While The Commonwealth Fund survey did not include information about job stressors, it did inquire into difficulties that employed women experience in balancing work and family life. Women were asked the following question: "How difficult is it for you to balance your work and family responsibilities?" Responses were: very difficult (12.8%); somewhat difficult (32.1%); not very difficult (21.5%); and not difficult at all (33.5%). This variable was used as a continuous variable in the regression analysis to test the association of difficulty and well-being.

Depressive symptoms ($t = 11.15$, $p < 0.001$) and self-esteem ($t = -9.30$, $p < 0.001$) are associated with difficulties in balancing work and family life. The association between difficulties and psychological well-being is clearly linear, with increased levels of difficulty associated with more depressive symptoms and lower self-esteem (data not shown). Interactions between perceptions of difficulty and parental and marital statuses were tested for, but no evidence was found that parents differ from nonparents or that married women differ from nonmarried women on the association of difficulties balancing work and family life with either measure of well-being. However, it is important to note that women with children reported more difficulties balancing work and family life than women without children. Sixty-five percent of women with children reported that balancing work and family responsibility is somewhat or very difficult, compared with 29 percent of women without children. Thus, the increased depressive symptoms and decreased self-esteem experienced by women who find balancing work and family life difficult generally affect employed mothers.

Unemployment and Psychological Well-Being

As seen earlier, unemployment is associated with higher depressive symptoms for unmarried but not married women and with lower self-esteem for unmarried mothers. To examine possible mechanisms for these different associations, separate analyses were conducted for unemployed women aged sixty-five or younger. Of the unemployed, 63.5 percent are married and 36.5 percent are not. Respondents were asked whether they prefer being unemployed. More than half (57.8%) of married women and four of five (81.9%) unmarried women reported that they would prefer to have jobs. Given that unemployed, unmarried women reported higher depressive symptoms than other women, an analysis was undertaken to examine whether this could be accounted for by their desire for employment. An interaction between work preferences and marital status was tested as well. This turned out to be significant for depressive symptoms, but not for self-esteem.

Preferences for employment are associated with levels of depressive symptoms primarily among married persons (tab. 8.6). Married women who would prefer to work reported levels of symptoms as high as those reported by unmarried, unemployed women (regardless of their preference). The lowest level of symptoms is found among married, unemployed women who prefer being unemployed. With regard to self-esteem, work preference is an important factor, with women who would prefer to be employed averaging lower self-esteem than those who prefer being unemployed (tab. 8.6).

The Commonwealth Fund survey inquired further into the most important reason why unemployed women would prefer to work. Responses were classified as financial (need the money, need health insurance coverage), personal gratification (enjoy working, want to do something useful, gives me self-respect), and other reasons (am bored, friends work, to keep active/busy, other). The large majority of women gave financial reasons (65.2%), 18.9 percent were seeking personal gratification, and the rest (15.9%) cited other reasons. Whether reasons for preferring to work are associated with levels of psychological well-being was examined, and it was found that average levels of depressive

Table 8.6. Adjusted Mean Depressive Symptoms and Self-esteem, by Preference for Employment and Marital Status: Unemployed Women Ages Sixty-five Years and Younger (unweighted $N = 485$)

	Depressive Symptoms	Self-esteem
Marital status: Married		
Prefer to work	5.16	24.71
Prefer not to work	3.62	26.22
Marital status: Not married		
Prefer to work	5.83	24.09
Prefer not to work	5.16	26.27
F-statistic[a]	7.99[b]	0.37[c]

Source: Analysis of The Commonwealth Fund survey on women's health, 1993.

Note: Adjusted for age, education, income, race, ethnicity, and parental status.

[a] F-statistic is for the interaction of marital status and work preference.

[b] $p < 0.01$.

[c] Interaction of marital status and work preference not significant, but main effect of work preference significant at $p < 0.001$ ($t = -3.44$).

symptoms and self-esteem did not differ significantly by reason (not shown).

Unemployed women who would prefer to be working for pay were also asked, "If a suitable job were available in your area, would you be able to work or would it be not possible for you to work?" The majority (60.8%) believed that it would be possible for them to work if a job were available. However, the perceived availability of suitable work does not contribute to psychological well-being. Thus, regardless of perceived job availability, and regardless of the reason paid work is preferred, unemployed women who would like to be employed experience greater depressive symptoms and lower self-esteem than other women.

Other Predictors of Women's Psychological Well-Being

In seeking to understand interactions between jobs and family life, Lennon and Rosenfield (1992) suggested that the challenges and demands of both realms may influence an individual's sense of mastery over his or her life. Numerous investigations have demonstrated that the sense of personal control or mastery is crucial to an individual's feelings of well-being (Wheaton 1983; Mirowsky and Ross 1984; Rosenfield 1989). According to Rosenfield (1989), excessive demands can undermine feelings of mastery, whereas the ability to control situations can reinforce feelings of mastery. Low levels of mastery are also associated with higher rates of psychological distress and depressive disorders (Wheaton 1983; Rosenfield 1989; Link, Lennon, and Dohrenwend 1993).

Thus, some of the gender difference in rates of psychological distress and depression may be accounted for by characteristics of women's lives that decrease their sense of mastery and personal control. In addition to family demands and job stressors, women's sense of mastery may be compromised by their lower earnings and status at work and their higher rates of poverty, sexual abuse, discrimination, and victimization. Poor physical health status may affect perceptions of mastery as well. The relationship of some of these factors to well-being is considered below. In considering these factors, the entire sample of women is examined (unweighted $N = 2,525$).

Poverty and Psychological Well-Being

Poverty rates for women exceed those of men. Based on a rough indicator of poverty (categorizing as poor those women who receive at least one of the following: food stamps, AFDC, SSI, or public assistance/welfare), 11 percent of women in the sample are poor in contrast to 5.5 percent of men. When levels of well-being for women are classified by poverty status, rates of depressive symptoms are significantly higher among poor women ($t = 5.93$, $p < 0.001$). There is a trend, as well, for levels of self-esteem to be lower among poor women ($t = -2.01$, $p < 0.05$). As with other analyses, these are subject to a full set of statistical controls, indicating that the effects of poverty cannot be accounted for by age, education, income, employment, parenting, marriage, race, or ethnicity.

The effect of poverty status is not contingent on parental or employment status; when interactions between these variables are tested, none obtained statistical significance. However, it is important to point out that unmarried women are more likely to experience poverty than married women (17.2% versus 6.8%). And rates are far higher among unmarried parents than among unmarried nonparents (33.7% versus

13.3%). The fact that poverty status is operationalized in part as receipt of AFDC may confound this comparison, since nonparents are not eligible for this form of assistance. When levels of income are examined, however, the same pattern is found. The lowest levels of income are reported by single mothers. Thus, as seen earlier, this group is at an especially increased risk for experiencing poor psychological well-being, and some of the risk may be due to being poor.

Health Status and Psychological Well-Being

The Commonwealth Fund survey assessed perceived health status with one question: "Would you say your health, in general, is excellent, very good, good, fair, or poor?" The respective responses were: excellent (21.3%), very good (35.1%), good (28.8%), fair (11.2%), and poor (3.5%). Women who see their health as fair or poor reported very high depressive symptoms and very low self-esteem, compared with women with better health reports (tab. 8.7).[6] The average depressive

Table 8.7. Adjusted Mean Depressive Symptoms and Self-esteem, by Health Status (unweighted $N = 2,197$)

	Depressive Symptoms	Self-esteem
Perceived health		
Excellent	3.60	27.04
Very good	4.30	26.45
Good	5.07	25.32
Fair	6.66	23.53
Poor	7.36	22.30
t-statistic	14.14[a]	−12.33[a]
Disability status		
Has disability	6.12	24.13
No disability	4.44	26.14
t-statistic	8.81[a]	−7.65[a]

Source: Analysis of The Commonwealth Fund survey on women's health, 1993.

Note: Unweighted $N = 2,197$. Means adjusted for age, education, income, race, ethnicity, employment status, marital status, and parental status.

[a] $p < 0.001$.

symptoms score is twice as high among those in "poor" health as among those in "excellent" health. In interpreting this association, it is important to note that health perceptions are likely to reflect feelings of psychological distress and tendency to somatize distress (Barsky, Cleary, and Klerman 1992; Rodin and McAvay 1992).

Women were also asked whether "a disability, handicap, or chronic disease keeps you from participating fully in school, work, housework, or other activities." Sixteen percent responded affirmatively, and these women reported more symptoms of depression and lower self-esteem than other women (tab. 8.7). Of course, the chronic disease that limits activities may be a depressive disorder. Thus, like the association with perceived health, levels of depression may account for the correlation between disability and psychological well-being. Nevertheless, it is important to bear in mind that reports of perceived poor health and disability are quite high among women, with one in seven reporting that she cannot participate in activities fully or that her health is fair or poor; these women reported especially poor psychological well-being.

Social Support and Psychological Well-Being

In considering the ways in which women may be disadvantaged, it is also important to note that many women have social and psychological resources that may enhance their psychological well-being. Chief among these are their social relationships. A number of investigators have argued that women gain gratification and a sense of identity from their social ties (Gilligan 1982; Jack 1991). Social connectedness may also enhance feelings of psychological well-being (but for an argument about the constraints of social ties, see Kessler and McLeod 1984).

The availability of social support was assessed by the following question: "Is there someone in your life who's available to call on for help when you have a problem, or not?" The majority of women gave an affirmative response (94.6%). Women with negative responses reported far higher levels of depressive symptoms and lower self-esteem than women who receive support (tab. 8.8).

Respondents were also asked to characterize their relationship to the person(s) from whom support is available. The majority of women named a relative (58.7%), sibling, parent, spouse, or child. Fewer (19.2%) named nonrelatives such as friends, co-workers, neighbors, and clergy. Because multiple responses were possible, these data may

Table 8.8. Adjusted Mean Depressive Symptoms and Self-esteem, by Availability of Support (unweighted $N = 2,195$)

	Depressive Symptoms	Self-esteem
Support available		
Yes	4.59	26.00
No	6.86	22.67
t-statistic	-7.27^a	7.80^a
Number of supporters (b coefficient)	0.01	0.48
t-statistic	0.04	1.90^b

Source: Analysis of The Commonwealth Fund survey on women's health, 1993.

Note: Unweighted $N = 2,197$. Means adjusted for age, education, income, race, ethnicity, marital status, employment status, and parental status.

[a] $p < 0.001$.

[b] $p < 0.05$.

be used to assess the number of individuals available for support. Approximately 6 percent (5.8%) of women named more than one supporter. When the number of available supporters is added to the equation, along with the availability of support, there is a marginally significant increase in self-esteem ($t = 1.90$, $p < 0.05$), but no change in depressive symptoms. This suggests that the availability of a supporter is what matters for depressive symptoms, while the availability and, to a lesser extent, number of supporters affect self-esteem. Again, the direction of causality is ambiguous. It is likely that women with high self-esteem name more individuals as available for support. And depressed women may be less likely to recognize the availability of support that they may have access to, accounting for the association between the availability of support and both measures of psychological well-being.

SUMMARY OF FINDINGS

In this investigation, women reported more symptoms of depression than men, and this fact cannot be explained by differences in marital status or employment. Marriage, parenting, and employment all contribute to psychological well-being in specific combinations. Among women younger than sixty-five, paid employment appears beneficial for the unmarried but does not reduce symptoms among the married. Unemployment is associated with increased symptoms and lower self-esteem among wives who would prefer to be working for pay. For married women, regardless of employment status, having full responsibility for housework and child care is associated with more depressive symptoms and lower self-esteem. Among the unmarried, unemployed women with children at home show quite low psychological well-being, in terms of both high depressive symptoms and low self-esteem. Finally, among employed women, regardless of marital status, the perceived difficulty in balancing work and family responsibilities is related to increased symptoms and lower self-esteem. Other correlates of depressive symptoms and self-esteem are poverty, victimization, poor health, and the absence of social support.

These findings must be interpreted in the light of the cross-sectional nature of The Commonwealth Fund survey, which makes inferences about the direction of causality difficult. Thus, factors such as perceptions of difficulty in combining work and family life, evaluations of husbands' involvement in child care, poverty, and employment status each may have an origin in women's feelings of depression or in their low self-esteem. For example, among depressed individuals, evaluations of the difficulty of combining work and family responsibilities may be colored by feelings of depression. However, given the greater difficulty reported by mothers, it appears that reports of difficulty have some objective basis. Nevertheless, only prospective research can resolve issues of causal direction.

Another limitation of this study is the restricted range of outcome measures considered. As mentioned earlier, relative to men, women suffer more from depression and problems of low self-esteem. The exclusive focus on these disorders may overstate the problems that women experience. In addition, the reliance on a six-item scale to assess depressive disorder means that transient mood changes and severe depressive illness cannot be differentiated in this study. Future research should incorporate both a broader range of outcome measures and assessments of severity.

IMPLICATIONS FOR POLICY

The high rates of depressive symptoms among women and their association with aspects of women's lives suggest that health policy and treatment efforts must be sensitive to women's experiences. The relationship of psychological well-being to poverty, responsibility for housework and child care, unemployment, sexual abuse, difficulties balancing work and family life, and poor health suggest several avenues for intervention that may reduce the prevalence of depression among women, and possibly among men as well.

The factors that correlate with poor psychological well-being cannot be understood outside of the context in which they arise. The major social changes that have occurred in the United States in work and family life have meant that increasing numbers of women have gotten jobs, have been divorced, or have become single parents. The entry of mothers into the labor force has been dramatic. In 30 years, the rate of participation in the labor force by women with preschool children increased threefold: from one in five in 1960 to three in five today (Gibson 1993). The proportion of families headed by women doubled, from 9 percent to 20 percent, during that same time period.

And yet the pace of social change has not been even: women's participation in the labor force has not been accompanied by significant changes in household responsibility. Child care remains largely the mother's responsibility and household chores remain in the hands of women. Although there has been some reduction in the wage gap between women and men, gender disparities in earnings remain (Dabelko and Sheak 1992). Partly as a consequence of lower earnings and partly as a consequence of the increase in divorce and single parenting, rates of poverty have grown among women. Some of the consequences of such increasing social and economic stressors are reflected in the high rates of depression found among women.

Policies designed to reduce mental health problems in women, then, must be directed at reducing poverty, increasing access to child care, ensuring adequate wages, and encouraging men's involvement in family life. Because problems with managing and paying for child care have been shown to be associated with increased depressive symptoms among women (Lennon, Wasserman, and Allen 1991; Ross and Mirowsky 1988), policies geared to providing child care services could serve as primary prevention for women's mental health problems. The availability of child care, in turn, could alleviate some of the problems that make employment difficult for women who wish to be employed. As seen earlier, not working for pay when doing so would be preferred is associated with increased psychological distress.

The role of poverty in women's mental health needs to be addressed directly as well. The indicator of poverty status used in this research is a crude one, based on participation in social welfare programs. As a result, it underestimates poverty rates in the U.S. population (Lewis 1994). And rates of poverty are especially high among some groups of women, especially older women, African American women, and single mothers (Wilson-Ford 1990; Smock 1993; Lewis 1994). Thus, efforts designed to reduce poverty among women would also constitute primary prevention for women at risk.

IMPLICATIONS FOR RESEARCH

In addition to recommending that future research be prospective in design, I suggest that such future research be directed at situations that may increase women's risk for mental health problems. Among these are poverty—and its association with single parenthood, race, and age. In fact, research on women's mental health has not been sufficiently attentive to the diversity of women's experiences. The analyses conducted for this chapter examined the data for interactions with race, age, marital status, and parental status to ensure that findings could be generalized across these groups. While not many interactions were found, the problems of statistical power mentioned earlier made it difficult to closely examine some subgroups. I recommended, therefore, that future research obtain sufficient samples of subgroups at risk to understand similarities and differences among groups of women.

It is also important that other dimensions of work and family life be studied. In terms of family life, future research is required to specify the conditions under which the presence of children is positive or negative for well-being, for men and women. For example, the availability, quality, and cost of child care are pressing issues for many employed parents. More detailed information is required about the impact of various child care arrangements on parents'—and children's—well-being.

Other aspects of family life also require more detailed study. For example, some characteristics of household tasks, such as their routine, time pressure, and limited complexity, are associated with increased psychological distress (Schooler et al. 1983; Bird and Ross 1993; Lennon 1994), while others, such as autonomy, are associated with increased satisfaction (Lennon and Rosenfield 1993). The stresses and satisfactions that derive from domestic labor require more complete study in relation to women's and men's psychological well-being.

In addition to differentiating further the dimensions of family life, it is important to examine how characteristics of jobs interact with family life. For example, women in typically female jobs are likely to have low wages and little flexibility (Glass 1990), making combining work and family life more difficult and demanding. Moreover, women's continued responsibility for domestic work, in conjunction with job responsibilities, subjects them to greater pressures and demands, which may reduce mastery and psychological well-being. Further study is required to understand the conditions under which combining jobs and family life is particularly stressful.

Moreover, there is increasing evidence that the characteristics of women's jobs are related to their psychological well-being. For example, several studies show that low job control—for example, little decision-making authority—is associated with poor health in both women and men (Karasek, Gardell, and Windell 1987; Braun and Hollander 1988; Pugliesi 1988). Others find that job complexity is associated with physical and mental health in women and men (Adelmann 1987; Lennon 1987). The work of Kohn and colleagues suggests that occupational self-direction is related to women's psychological functioning in the same way it is to men's (Miller et al. 1979; Kohn and Schooler 1983; Schooler et al. 1983). Research in this area has only begun to uncover the ways in which jobs may directly enhance or diminish women's psychological well-being. While such efforts have been fruitful, studies have been cross-sectional in design, leaving unresolved crucial questions about causal direction. It is essential to the formation of sound social policy that large-scale prospective studies be undertaken to investigate issues of the relation of work and family life to the mental health of women.

Finally, it is important to consider broader social conditions that may reduce gender differences in depressive symptoms. These include access to economic and social resources that varies by gender, as well as differential socialization of boys and girls. Moreover, it is important to recall the other side of the epidemiological coin: the tendency for men to engage in antisocial and acting-out behaviors. These behaviors may be expressions of psychological difficulties experienced by men. They also affect the well-being of those close to them, such as parents, children, and partners. Women's mental health cannot be understood apart from the broad social context that shapes the health and well-being of men, as well as women.

NOTES

1. Women who described themselves as married but who were not living with their spouse ($N = 50$) were classified as separated.

2. The two well-being scales are negatively correlated in women ($r = -0.51$). This is a fairly high correlation, given the fact that unreliability of measurement attenuates correlations. In fact, correcting the correlation for attenuation results in an association of -0.67. In other words, if the scales had no measurement error, they would correlate at a fairly high level. Nevertheless, as we will see, there is some evidence for treating these as distinct aspects of well-being, because they are associated differently with some social variables.

3. When I tested for a two-way interaction between gender and marital status, I found that it did not add to the explained variance in symptoms. Thus, the apparent similarity of formerly married men and women (widows, separated/divorced) is not statistically reliable. In other words, the effects of gender are not conditioned on marital status, and women exceed men in depressive symptoms, regardless of marital status.

4. When sociodemographic characteristics are introduced into a multiple regression equation, the effect of age becomes linear for self-esteem. Thus, all subsequent analyses control for only the linear age effect.

5. As another example, in a study of changes in the rates of psychological distress over time, Kessler and McRae (1981) found that the gender difference in psychological distress has narrowed, largely due to the increase in distress experienced by men (see also Murphy 1985). It is important to note, however, that even with these trends, as a group, women still suffer significantly more from depressive disorders and general psychological distress than men.

6. Although the results are presented for each category of perceived health, in the regression equation perceived health was treated as a continuous independent variable and its effect tested using a *t*-test.

REFERENCES

Adelmann, P. K. 1987. Occupational complexity, control, and personal income: their relation to psychological well-being in men and women. *Journal of Applied Psychology* 72:529–37.

American Psychiatric Association. 1987. *Diagnostic and Statistical Manual of Mental Disorders*. 3rd ed., rev. Washington, D.C.: American Psychiatric Association.

Barnett, R. C., and Marshall, N. L. 1989. Multiple roles, spillover effects, and psychological distress. Working Paper no. 200, Wellesley College Center for Research on Women.

Barsky, A. J., Cleary, P. D., and Klerman, G. 1992. Determinants of perceived health status of medical outpatients. *Social Science and Medicine* 34:1147–54.

Bird, C. E., and Ross, C. E. 1993. Houseworkers and paid workers: qualities of the work and effects on personal control. *Journal of Marriage and the Family* 55:913–25.

Braun, S., and Hollander, R. B. 1988. Work and depression among women in the Federal Republic of Germany. *Women and Health* 14:3–26.

Brown, G. W., and Harris, T. 1978. *The Social Origins of Depression.* New York: Free Press.

Calhoun, L. G., Cheney, T., and Dawes, A. S. 1974. Locus of control, self-reported depression, and perceived causes of depression. *Journal of Consulting Psychology* 42:736–45.

Costello, E. J. 1982. Locus of control and depression in students and psychiatric outpatients. *Journal of Clinical Psychology* 36:661–67.

Dabelko, D. D., and Sheak, R. J. 1992. Employment, subemployment and the feminization of poverty. *Sociological Viewpoints* 8:31–66.

Dohrenwend, B. P., and Dohrenwend, B. S. 1977. Reply to Gove and Tudor's comment on sex differences and psychiatric disorders. *American Journal of Sociology* 82:1336–45.

———. 1976. Sex differences and psychiatric disorders. *American Journal of Sociology* 81:1447–54.

Dohrenwend, B. P., Shrout, P. E., Egri, G., and Mendelsohn, F. S. 1980. Measures of nonspecific psychological distress and other dimensions of psychopathology. *Archives of General Psychiatry* 37:1229–36.

Evans, R. 1981. The relationship of two measures of perceived control to depression. *Journal of Personality Assessment* 45:66–70.

Fox, J. W. 1980. Gove's specific sex-role theory of mental illness: a research note. *Journal of Health and Social Behavior* 21:260–67.

Froberg, D., Gjerdingen, D., and Preston, M. 1986. Multiple roles and women's mental and physical health: what have we learned? *Women and Health* 11:76–96.

Gibson, C. 1993. The four baby booms. *American Demographics* 15:36–40.

Gilligan, C. 1982. *In a Different Voice: Psychological Theory and Women's Development.* Cambridge, Mass.: Harvard University Press.

Glass, J. 1990. The impact of occupational segregation on working conditions. *Social Forces* 68:779–96.

Gore, S., and Mangione, T. W. 1983. Social roles and psychological distress: additive and interactive models of sex differences. *Journal of Health and Social Behavior* 24:300–312.

Gove, W. R., and Geerken, M. R. 1977. The effect of children and employment on the mental health of married men and women. *Social Forces* 56:66–79.

Gove, W. R., Hughes, M., and Style, C. B. 1983. Does marriage have positive effects on the psychological well-being of the individual? *Journal of Health and Social Behavior* 24:122–31.

Gove, W., and Tudor, J. 1977. Sex differences in mental illness: a comment on Dohrenwend and Dohrenwend. *American Journal of Sociology* 82:1327–36.

———. 1973. Adult sex roles and mental illness. *American Journal of Sociology* 78:812–35.

Greenley, J. R., and Mechanic, D. 1976. Social selection in seeking help for psychological problems. *Journal of Health and Social Behavior* 17:249–62.

Hibbard, J. H., and Pope, C. R. 1987. Employment characteristics and health status among men and women. *Women and Health* 12:85–103.

Hoelter, J. W. 1983. Factorial invariance and self-esteem: reassessing race and sex differences. *Social Forces* 61:834–46.

Horwitz, A. V. 1982. Sex role expectations, power and psychological distress. *Sex Roles* 8:607–23.

———. 1977. The pathways into psychiatric treatment: some differences between women and men. *Journal of Health and Social Behavior* 18:169–78.

Jack, D. C. 1991. *Silencing the Self: Women and Depression.* Cambridge, Mass.: Harvard University Press.

Kandel, D. B., Davies, M., and Raveis, V. 1985. The stressfulness of daily social roles for women: marital, occupational and household roles. *Journal of Health and Social Behavior* 26:64–78.

Karasek, R., Gardell B., and Windell, J. 1987. Work and nonwork correlates of illness and behavior in male and female Swedish white-collar workers. *Journal of Occupational Behavior* 8:87–207.

Kendler, K. S., et al. 1993. The prediction of major depression in women: toward an integrated etiologic model. *American Journal of Psychiatry* 150:1139–48.

Kessler, R. C., and McLeod, J. 1984. Sex differences in vulnerability to undesirable life events. *American Sociological Review* 48:620–31.

Kessler, R. C., and McRae, J. A. 1982. The effects of wives' employment on the mental health of married men and women. *American Sociological Review* 47:216–27.

Kessler, R. C., Brown, R. L., and Broman, C. L. 1981. Sex differences in psychiatric help-seeking: evidence from four large scale surveys. *Journal of Health and Social Behavior* 22:49–64.

Kessler, R. C., et al. 1992. The relationship between age and depressive symptoms in two national surveys. *Psychology of Aging* 7:119–26.

Kessler, R. C., et al. 1994. Lifetime and 12-month prevalence of DSM-III-R psychiatric disorders in the United States. *Archives of General Psychiatry* 51:8–19.

Kessler, R. C., and McRae, J. A. 1981. Trends in the relationship between sex and psychological distress, 1957–1976. *American Sociological Review* 47:216–227.

Kohn, M. L. 1972. Class, family, and schizophrenia. *Social Forces* 50:295–302.

Kohn, M. L., and Schooler, C. L., eds. 1983. *Work and Personality.* Norwood, N.J.: Ablex.

Krause, N., and Markides, K. A. 1985. Employment and well-being in Mexican American women. *Journal of Health and Social Behavior* 26:15–26.

Leggett, J., and Archer, R. P. 1979. Locus of control and depression among psychiatric inpatients. *Psychological Reports* 45:835–38.

Lennon, M. C. 1987. Sex differences in distress: the impact of gender and work roles. *Journal of Health and Social Behavior* 28:290–305.

———. 1994. Women, work, and well-being: the importance of work conditions. *Journal of Health and Social Behavior* 35:235–47.

Lennon, M. C., and Rosenfield, S. 1992. Women and distress: the contribution of job and family conditions. *Journal of Health and Social Behavior* 33:316–27.

———. 1993. Women and Mental Health: New Directions for Research. Paper presented at the American Sociological Association, Pittsburgh, Pa.

Lennon, M. C., Wasserman, G. A., and Allen, R. 1991. Husbands' involvement in child care and depressive symptoms among mothers of infants. *Women and Health* 17:1–23.

Lewis, R. 1994. These are not the best of times. *AARP Bulletin* 7:1044–1123.

Link, B. G., Lennon, M. C., and Dohrenwend, B. P. 1993. Socioeconomic status and depression: the role of occupations involving direction, control and planning. *American Journal of Sociology* 98:1351–87.

Loring, M., and Powell, B. 1988. Gender, race, and DSM-III: a study of the objectivity of psychiatric diagnostic behavior. *Journal of Health and Social Behavior* 29:1–22.

Lowe, G. S., and Northcott, H. C. 1988. The impact of working conditions, social roles, and personal characteristics on gender differences in distress. *Work and Occupations* 15:55–77.

Lowe, G. D., and Smith, R. R. 1987. Gender, marital status, and mental well-being: a retest of Bernard's his and her marriages. *Sociological Spectrum* 7:301–7.

Mackie, M. 1983. The domestication of self: gender comparisons of self-imagery and self-esteem. *Social Psychology Quarterly* 46:343–50.

McClelland, G. H., and Judd, C. M. 1993. Statistical difficulties of detecting interactions and moderator effects. *Psychological Bulletin* 114:376–90.

McGrath, E., et al., eds. 1990. *Women and Depression: Risk Factors and Treatment Issues.* Section I, pp. 1–14. Washington, D.C.: American Psychological Association.

McLanahan, S. S., and Adams, J. 1987. Parenthood and psychological well-being. *Annual Review of Sociology* 13:237–57.

Menaghan, E. G. 1989. Role changes and psychological well-being: variations in effects by gender and role repertoire. *Social Forces* 67:693–714.

Merikangas, K. R., Weissman, M. M., and Pauls, D. L. 1985. Genetic factors in the sex ratio of major depression. *Psychological Medicine* 15:63–69.

Miller, J., et al. 1979. Women and work: the psychological effects of occupational conditions. *American Journal of Sociology* 85:66–94.

Mirowsky, J., and Ross, C. E. 1984. Mexican culture and its emotional contradictions. *Journal of Health and Social Behavior* 25:2–13.

Murphy, J. M. 1985. Trends in depression and anxiety: men and women. *Acta Psychiatrica Scandinavica* 73:113–27.

Newmann, J. P., Engel, R. J., and Jensen, J. E. 1991. Age differences in depressive symptom experiences. *Journal of Gerontology* 46:224–35.

Paykel, E. S. 1991. Depression in women. *British Journal of Psychiatry* 158:22–29.

Pearlin, L. I. 1975. Sex roles and depression. In N. Datan and L. H. Ginsberg, eds., *Life-Span Developmental Psychology: Normative Life Crises.* New York: Academic Press.

Pearlin, L. I., et al. 1981. The stress process. *Journal of Health and Social Behavior* 22:337–56.

Potts, M. K., Burman, M. A., and Wells, K. B. 1991. Gender differences in depression detection: a comparison of clinician diagnosis and standardized assessment. *Psychological Assessment* 3:609–15.

Pugliesi, K. 1988. Employment characteristics, social support and the well being of women. *Women and Health* 14:35–58.

Radloff, L. S. 1980. Depression and the empty nest. *Sex Roles* 6:775–81.

———. 1977. The CES-D scale: a self-report depression scale for research in the general population. *Applied Psychological Measurement* 1:385–401.

———. 1975. Sex differences in depression: the effects of occupation and marital status. *Sex Roles* 1:243–65.

Repetti, R. L. 1988. Family and occupational roles and women's mental health. In R. M. Schwartz, ed., *Women at Work*. Los Angeles: Institute of Industrial Relations Publications, University of California.

Robins, L. N., and Regier, D. A. 1991. *Psychiatric Disorders in America: The Epidemiologic Catchment Area Study*. New York: Free Press.

Robinson, J., and Spitze, G. 1992. Whistle while you work?: the effect of household task performance on women's and men's well-being. *Social Science Quarterly* 73:844–61.

Rodin, J., and McAvay, G. 1992. Determinants of change in perceived health in a longitudinal study of older adults. *Journal of Gerontology* 47:373–84.

Rosenberg, M. 1965. *Society and the Adolescent Self-Image*. Princeton: Princeton University Press.

Rosenfield, S. L. 1992. The costs of sharing: wives' employment and husbands' mental health. *Journal of Health and Social Behavior* 33:213–25.

———. 1989. The effects of women's employment: personal control and sex differences in mental health. *Journal of Health and Social Behavior* 30:77–91.

———. 1982. Sex roles and societal reactions to mental illness: the labeling of deviant deviance. *Journal of Health and Social Behavior* 23:1824.

———. 1980. Sex differences in depression: do women always have higher rates? *Journal of Health and Social Behavior* 21:33–42.

Ross, C. E., and Mirowsky, J. 1988. Child care and emotional adjustment to wives' employment. *Journal of Health and Social Behavior* 29:127–38.

Ross, C. E., Mirowsky, J., and Huber, J. 1983. Dividing work, sharing work, and in-between: marriage patterns and depression. *American Sociological Review* 48:809–23.

Rotter, J. B. 1966. Generalized expectancies for internal vs. external control of reinforcement. *Psychological Monographs* 80:1–28.

Schooler, C., et al. 1983. Housework as work. In M. L. Kohn and C. Schooler, eds., *Work and Personality*. Norwood, N.Y.: Ablex.

Smock, P. J. 1993. The economic costs of marital disruption for young women over the past two decades. *Demography* 30:353–71.

Thoits, P. A. 1987. Negotiating roles. In F. Crosby, ed., *Spouse, Parent, Worker: On Gender and Multiple Roles*. New Haven: Yale University Press.

———. 1986. Multiple identities: examining gender and marital status differences in distress. *American Sociological Review* 51:259–72.

———. 1983. Multiple identities and psychological well-being: a reformulation and test of the social isolation hypothesis. *American Sociological Review* 48:174–87.

Umberson, D., and Gove, W. R. 1989. Parenthood and psychological well-being: theory, measurement, and stage in the family life course. *Journal of Family Issues* 10:440–62.

Weissman, M. M., and Klerman, G. L. 1987. Gender and depression. In R. Formanek and A. Gurian, eds., *Women and Depression: A Lifespan Perspective*. New York: Springer.

———. 1977. Sex differences in the epidemiology of depression. *Archives of General Psychiatry* 34:98–111.

Wheaton, B. 1983. Stress, personal coping resources, and psychiatric symptoms: an investigation of interactive models. *Journal of Health and Social Behavior* 24:208–29.

———. 1980. The sociogenesis of psychological disorder: an attributional theory. *Journal of Health and Social Behavior* 21:100–124.

Wilson-Ford, V. 1990. Poverty among black elderly women. *Journal of Women and Aging* 2:5–20.

9

Violence and Abuse
Implications for Women's Health

Stacey B. Plichta, Sc.D.

Women and girls in the United States face an uncomfortably high risk of being harmed by violence. An estimated 21 percent of adult women have been sexually abused as children (Leventhal 1990), 20 percent to 25 percent have been raped in adulthood (Kilpatrick, Veronen, and Best 1985; Koss 1987; Wyatt and Newcomb 1990), and 30 percent to 50 percent of married women have been physically assaulted by their spouses at least once (Council on Scientific and Ethical Affairs 1992). With the exception of spouse abuse, there are no nationally representative studies of the prevalence of these acts of violence against women and children.

Despite the high estimates of prevalence for experiencing violence, no comprehensive study of the effect of violence on physical and mental health (and subsequent use of health services) of women has been undertaken. Current research in this area suffers from several sampling and methodological flaws that limit its applicability. With the exception of a New Zealand study (Mullen et al. 1988), there are no large, demographically diverse studies. All prior studies of the health impact of violence use samples of women recruited at a single health service site, at a college, or through newspaper advertisements. These studies are also narrow in scope, usually focusing on only one or two potential effects of abuse (such as depression or chronic pain), rather than on a range of possible health outcomes.

Another major flaw of existing studies is their use of nonrandom samples that tend to be more urban and low-income and to have less education than the general U.S. population. Women with lower socioeconomic status are at higher risk of mental and physical health problems than other women (Bruce, Takeuchi, and Leaf 1991). While these studies reported that physical abuse is associated with poorer health status, it is not clear that the impact of physical abuse would be the same in the general population.

This chapter provides an analysis of data from The Commonwealth Fund survey. This survey is the first nationally representative survey to ask questions about child abuse and rape, and is one of the few national surveys to ask questions about violent crime and spouse abuse. More important, it provides information necessary to explore the relationship of experiencing violence to health status and to the use of health services. Finally, it examines the quality of physician-patient communication among women who have experienced violence.

STUDY METHODS

The Demographic Group of Interest

This chapter examines the prevalence of experiencing violence among all women ages eighteen to sixty-four. Elderly women (age sixty-five or older) are excluded from the analyses for several reasons. First, other studies indicate that exposure to violence, particularly the types of exposure measured in The Commonwealth Fund survey, is a much more salient issue for younger women. National data show that older women are at a much lower risk for exposure to rape (Maguire, Pastore, and Flanagan 1993) and spouse abuse (Hotaling and Finkelhor 1988); comparisons of studies from 1950 and 1980 indicate that they may also be much less likely to have been exposed to child abuse than younger women (Leventhal 1988). Second, a preliminary examination of the data from this survey confirms the hypothesis that older women report fewer experiences of violence. No women age sixty-five or older reported being raped in the past 5 years, and only one elderly woman reported experiencing spouse abuse in the past year; also, significantly fewer elderly women reported experiencing child abuse and/or other violent crimes. Third, older women are more likely to have health problems than younger women. Because older women are also less likely to experience violence, real differences in the health status of women experiencing violence and those not could be masked if older women were included in the analyses.

Measurement and Statistical Issues

Respondents answered a series of questions about child abuse, rape, violent crime other than rape, and spouse abuse, and their answers were coded according to specific rules (fig. 9.1). This survey over-sampled African American and Latina women to ensure that they would be well represented. The analyses presented in this chapter use sample weights that balance the data by age, race, education, insurance status, and Census region, so the results are representative of the 78.5 million women under age sixty-five residing in the United States (U.S. Bureau of the Census 1992).

Statistical tests of differences between women experiencing violence and those not are performed using the chi-square test when the variables are categorical (i.e., nominal or ordinal) and one-way analysis of variance (ANOVA) when one variable (such as the number of physician visits) is continuous and the other is categorical. Those tests of difference with a p-value of 0.01 or less are referred to as statistically significant. A more stringent p-value than the so-called traditional $p \leq 0.05$ is used because the large sample size makes it more likely that small, clinically inconsequential differences will attain a p-value of 0.05 (Selvin 1991).

Caveats

The major limitation of this study is that as a cross-sectional survey it depends on retrospective reporting by the participants. Its cross-sectional nature—that is, the asking of questions at only one point in time—makes it impossible to ascribe causality to statistical relationships. For example, this study can determine if a relationship exists between depressive symptoms and exposure to violence, but it cannot determine whether the violence is an underlying cause of the depressive symptoms. In addition, only bivariate statistical analyses are presented, which do not adjust for other factors, such as sociodemographic characteristics, which might moderate or mask the relationship of exposure to violence to the outcome variables of interest.

Another caveat is that the statistics do not fully document the extent of violence against women. Because this survey uses self-reported data, it depends on the participants' ability and willingness to remember and report events from their past. It is likely that traumatic events, such as child sexual abuse, are underreported because of either recall

Fig. 9.1. Measures of Violent Experiences
Source: The Commonwealth Fund Survey, 1993.

Child Abuse

Physical: "Do you feel that you were physically abused while you were growing up?"

Sexual: "Do you feel that you were sexually abused while you were growing up?"

Coding Rule: Those women responding yes to only the physical abuse question are coded as having experienced child physical abuse. Those women responding yes to the sexual abuse question are coded as having experienced child sexual abuse whether or not they report experiencing child physical abuse. Those women coded as "none" have not reported any child abuse, but they may or may not have reported violent crime and/or spouse abuse.

Violent Crime

Rape: "In the past five years, have you been a victim of rape or sexual assault?"

Other: "In the past five years, have you been a victim of a (1) mugging, robbery, or assault or (2) some other kind of physical crime?"

Coding Rule: Those reporting rape or sexual assault are coded as having been raped (whether or not they were exposed to other violent crimes), while those reporting a violent crime other than rape are coded as having experienced other violent crime (labeled "other" in the tables). Those women coded as "none" report no experiences of any violent crime in the past five years, but may or may not have reported child abuse and/or spouse abuse.

Spouse Abuse

Preamble: "No matter how well a couple gets along, there are just times when they disagree, get annoyed with the other person, or just have spats or fights because they're in a bad mood, or tired, or for some other reason. They also may use many different ways of trying to settle their differences. I'm going to read some things that you and your partner might do when you have an argument. I would like you to tell me whether, in the past five years, your spouse/partner ever: (1) pushed, grabbed, shoved, or slapped you, (2) kicked, bit, or hit you with a fist or some other object, (3) beat you up, (4) choked you, (5) threatened you with a knife or gun, (6) used a knife or gun on you."

Coding Rule: Spouse abuse is only measured for those women currently living with or married to a man (both are referred to as her spouse). These questions are from the Conflict Tactics Scale (CTS), a widely used instrument with good reliability and validity. A woman is coded as having experienced spouse abuse if she answered yes to any of these questions. Those women coded as not experiencing spouse abuse may or may not have reported child abuse and/or violent crime.

bias (these events may be too painful to remember) or social desirability bias (these events may be too shameful or painful to disclose). The measures of experiencing violence used in this survey may also lead to underestimating the prevalence of violence. The survey asks one question for child physical abuse and another for child sexual abuse. Asking only one question for each type of abuse has been shown to result in conservative estimates of child abuse (Leventhal 1990). Nor does this study measure the lifetime prevalence of spouse abuse, rape, or nonsexual violent crime. Thus, it is not possible to examine the impact of lifetime exposure to violence on health.

RESULTS OF SURVEY ANALYSES

The Prevalence of Child Abuse among U.S. Women

The risk of experiencing violence starts in childhood (tab. 9.1). Of all women responding to The Commonwealth Fund survey, 18.3 percent reported being either physically or sexually abused as a child; 6.8 percent reported physical abuse only; 11.5 percent reported sexual abuse (with or without physical abuse). When these percentages are projected to the U.S. population of 1991, one can estimate that 5.3 million women were physically abused as children (but not sexually abused) and that 9.0 million women were sexually abused as children (with or without physical abuse). In addition, sexual and physical abuse are strongly related; almost half of women who experienced child sexual abuse also experienced child physical abuse.

No other national data exist that indicate the prevalence of adult women who experienced child abuse. However, several studies of single metropolitan areas (and one state) have randomly selected, demographically representative samples. One study, of Texas residents, reported a lifetime prevalence rate of child physical abuse among adults to be 7.6 percent (Sapp and Carter 1978). Other studies of clinical and college populations reported rates of childhood physical abuse of 4 percent to 21 percent (Drossman et al. 1990; DiTomaso and Routh 1993). These variations largely result from differences in the measurement and definition of child physical abuse.

Previously reported prevalence rates of adult women experiencing child sexual abuse range from 7 percent to 60 percent (Wyatt 1985; Siegel et al. 1987; Saunders et al. 1992). This wide variation is again mainly due to differences in measurement and definition. When sexu-

Table 9.1. Prevalence of Exposure to Violence in U.S. Women
(weighted N = 2,052)

	Percentage Exposed	Estimated Number Exposed (in millions)[a]
Exposed to child abuse[b]	18.3	14.4
Physical abuse only	6.8	5.3
Sexual abuse	11.5	9.0
Exposed to a violent crime in the past 5 years[c]	12.0	9.4
Nonsexual violent crimes only	9.1	7.1
Rape or sexual assault	2.9	2.3
Exposed to spouse abuse in the past year[d]	8.4	4.4
Severely abused	3.2	1.7

Source: Analysis of The Commonwealth Fund survey on women's health, 1993.

[a] This survey uses a representative sample of U.S. women. When sample weights are used, the results can be projected to the population and estimates of the number of U.S. women exposed to violence can be made. In 1991 there were 78.5 million women from the ages of eighteen to sixty-four living in the United States; 52.483 million of these women were married to or cohabiting with a male (U.S. Bureau of the Census 1992). The estimates of the number of women exposed to violence presented here are based on these Census data.

[b] Child physical abuse and child sexual abuse are mutually exclusive categories. Respondents reporting child physical abuse, but not child sexual abuse, are coded as physically abused. Respondents reporting child sexual abuse are coded as sexually abused whether or not they also report physical abuse.

[c] Nonsexual violent crime and rape are mutually exclusive categories. Respondents are counted as exposed to a nonsexual violent crime if they report that they were the victim of a mugging, robbery, nonsexual assault, or some other kind of physical crime in the past 5 years and did not report exposure to rape. Respondents are counted as exposed to rape or sexual assault whether or not they also report exposure to a nonsexual violent crime.

[d] Only those respondents who are currently married or living with someone are asked the spouse abuse questions (N = 1,324). Spouse abuse is measured using the Conflict Tactics Scale. Respondents coded as severely abused reported being punched, kicked, beaten up, or threatened with or injured by a weapon (Gelles and Straus 1988).

al abuse is defined as sexual contact with a child age sixteen or under by a perpetrator at least 5 years older, the range narrows somewhat, to 7 percent to 40 percent (Leventhal 1990). Applying this definition to most community-based surveys published by 1989, Leventhal (1990) estimated that 21 percent of all adult women in the United States and Canada were sexually abused as children.

The Commonwealth Fund survey provides a more conservative estimate of women experiencing child sexual abuse (11.5%) than previous estimates and the synthetic rate (21%) calculated by Leventhal (1990). This is partly due to differences in methodology (telephone survey with only one question for each type of child abuse). Studies using a similar methodology reported comparable estimates of abuse from 7 percent to 11 percent (Sapp and Carter 1978; Siegel et al. 1987; Mullen et al. 1988). Other surveys, which ascertained child abuse with multiple questions and/or used a face-to-face interview or self-answered questionnaire, typically reported a much higher prevalence (Leventhal 1990).

The Prevalence of Rape and Other Violent Crime

During the past 5 years, 12 percent of women participating in this survey experienced a violent crime, 9.1 percent a nonsexual crime, and 2.9 percent a rape or sexual assault (tab. 9.1). Projected to the U.S. population, one can estimate that 7.1 million women have experienced a violent crime in the past 5 years and 2.3 million women have been raped or sexually assaulted.

The National Crime Victimization Survey (NCVS) reported a one-year incidence rate of experiencing violent crime in 1991 of 2.3 percent. The NCVS is a nationally representative survey of approximately 42,000 randomly selected households each year (Maguire, Pastore, and Flanagan 1993). It asks respondents if they have experienced specific crimes other than rape. The only study to examine lifetime exposure to violent crime in women reported a prevalence rate of 14.9 percent (Koss, Koss, and Woodruff 1991).

No randomly selected, nationally representative study of one-year incidence rates or the lifetime prevalence of rape has ever been done to allow direct comparison with The Commonwealth Fund findings of 2.9 percent of women experiencing a rape or a sexual assault in the past 5 years. The NCVS reported that 0.1 percent of women are raped each year. This estimate is likely to be low because the NCVS does not ask directly about rape, but reports the responses of women who volunteer that they have been raped. Other studies reported the lifetime prevalence of rape to be 20 percent to 25 percent (Kilpatrick, Vernonen, and Best 1985; Koss 1987; Wyatt and Newcomb 1990). These studies have randomly selected, representative samples from single metropolitan areas; one is a nationally representative study of college students (Koss 1987).

The Prevalence of Spouse Abuse

More than 8 percent of the women in The Commonwealth Fund survey who are married or cohabitating ($N = 1,324$) reported suffering physical abuse from their partner in the past year; 3.2 percent reported being severely abused (defined as being kicked, punched, beaten up, hit with an object, or threatened with or hurt by a weapon) (tab. 9.1). Projected to the U.S. population in 1991, one can estimate that 4.4 million women were physically abused by a partner, and 1.7 million of these women experienced severe abuse.

Spouse abuse is the only form of violence against women for which there are data from other large, nationally representative studies, as well as from two statewide surveys. Their findings are similar to this study—that 8.3 percent to 11.3 percent of all women married to or living with a man are physically abused by that man each year and 3 percent are severely abused (Schulman 1979; Teske and Parker 1983; Straus and Gelles 1986). Other studies indicated that spouse abuse incidents rarely occur only once; they are usually part of a continuing and escalating pattern of physical and emotional abuse against the woman (Teske and Parker 1983; Bowker and Maurer 1987; Walker 1989).

Violence and Demographic Characteristics

The Commonwealth Fund survey confirms what previous studies have indicated: no woman, regardless of age, racial/ethnic group, marital status, education, or income, is immune to experiencing violence; however, some groups of women are at especially high risk for certain types of violence. While few measures of socioeconomic status (SES) are significantly related to experiencing child abuse, there are significant relationships between almost all the measures of SES and experiencing violence as an adult (tab. 9.2).

Overall, lower SES is related to higher levels of experiencing violence; women receiving welfare payments (a proxy measure for poverty status) are much more likely to report child abuse, violent crime, and spouse abuse. Less-educated women, especially those who did not graduate from high school, are also significantly more likely to report exposure to rape and spouse abuse; however, college-educated women are more likely than other women to report violent crimes other than rape.

Prior studies have found few differences in SES other than age and marital status to be related to being abused as a child (Wyatt 1985; Leventhal 1990); however, a number of socioeconomic factors have been found to put women at higher risk for experiencing violence as an

Table 9.2. Socioeconomic Characteristics and Exposure to Violence

	Percentage of Women in Each Demographic Category Exposed to				
	Child Abuse		Violent Crime		Spouse Abuse
	Physical	Sexual	Other	Rape	Any Physical
Age					
18–44	7.4	12.6	10.8	4.1	9.8
45–64	6.1	8.8[a]	5.5	0.3[b]	5.9
Race					
African American	4.5	12.3	8.3	1.7	16.0
Latina	5.3	12.8	11.5	3.6	10.3
White/Other	7.6	11.1	9.0	3.0	7.5[a]
Education					
Below high school	3.7	12.1	7.6	3.4	16.3
High school	9.0	10.9	8.2	3.2	8.2
College	6.6	11.5	12.2	1.7[a]	4.3[b]
Welfare[c]					
No	6.8	10.2	8.4	2.3	6.8
Yes	8.0	18.6[b]	13.8	6.7[b]	24.0[b]
Marital status					
Single	6.7	7.9	11.2	7.7	N/A
Divorced	8.0	17.1	13.3	4.8	N/A
Live together	10.9	12.2	11.9	2.9	13.7
Married	6.4	10.5[b]	6.9	0.9[b]	7.9[b]
Geographic location[d]					
Central city	6.4	10.9	12.6	3.2	12.9
Suburbs	7.0	12.5	8.9	3.8	4.3
Rural	9.8	10.6	6.0	0.9	9.7
Very rural	5.1	8.9	2.1	0.8[b]	12.7[b]

Source: Data from The Commonwealth Fund survey on women's health, 1993.

[a] Significant at $p \leq 0.01$.

[b] Significant at $p \leq 0.001$.

[c] Respondents are coded as on welfare if they receive food stamps, Aid to Families with Dependent Children, Supplemental Security Income, public assistance or welfare payments from the state or local welfare office.

[d] These terms are identical to measures used by the Bureau of the Census (1992). *Central city* is a metropolitan statistical area (MSA); *suburb* is a remainder MSA; *rural* is a county outside an MSA with at least one town with more than 2,500 residents; *very rural* is a county outside an MSA with fewer than 2,500 residents in the largest town.

adult. Younger urban women have been found to be at higher risk for spouse abuse (Telch and Linquist 1984; Follingstad et al. 1988; Hotaling and Finkelhor 1988), rape, and other violent crime (Maguire, Pastore, and Flanagan 1993). Unmarried (single or divorced) women are also at high risk for rape and other violent crime (Maguire, Pastore, and Flanagan 1993). The findings on economic status are mixed: several studies reported no relationship between economic status and exposure to violence (Schulman 1979; Lockhart 1987), while others reported that lower economic status is related to higher levels of violent experiences (Rath, Jarratt, and Leonardson 1989; Amaro et al. 1990; Maguire, Pastore, and Flanagan 1993). Overall, race has not been shown to be consistently related to any type of violence among women (Hotaling and Finkelhor 1988; Leventhal 1990; Maguire, Pastore, and Flanagan 1993).

THE RELATIONSHIP OF EXPERIENCES OF VIOLENCE TO HEALTH STATUS

Physical Health and Violence

A strong relationship exists between experiencing violence and poor health status (tab. 9.3). This study found that women who experienced child abuse or spouse abuse are almost twice as likely as nonabused women to rate their own health as fair or poor. An increased reporting of poorer health, as measured by self-report or the GHQ (general health questionnaire), was reported in previous studies of child abuse (Mullen et al. 1988; Rosenberg and Krugman 1991), rape (Golding et al. 1988; Mullen et al. 1988; Waigandt et al. 1990), and spouse abuse (Jaffe et al. 1986; Mullen et al. 1988). Clinical studies also reported that women exposed to violence have more somatic symptoms (such as headaches, chronic back pain, and gastrointestinal distress), which may indicate that they have poorer general health (Golding et al. 1988; Drossman et al. 1990; Felitti 1991).

Women who were abused as a child or raped as an adult are also much more likely to have a disability that prevents them from participating fully in school, housework, paid employment, or other activities. This survey found that almost 33 percent of women who were raped, and more than 20 percent of women who experienced child abuse, reported such a disability (compared with just over 14% of all

Table 9.3. Exposure to Violence and Physical Health

	Child Abuse			Violent Crime			Spouse Abuse	
	None	Physical	Sex	None	Other	Rape	No	Yes
% Rates own health fair/poor	11.8	16.1	21.1[a]	12.7	15.5	20.0	10.7	20.5[b]
% Disabled[c]	13.9	21.6	24.0[a]	14.8	18.6	32.2[a]	14.2	12.7
% Gyn diagnosis[d]	15.2	22.0	36.2[a]	16.6	27.4	30.2[a]	16.0	45.9[a]
% UTI in past 5 years[d]	6.7	13.9	27.0[a]	16.5	22.0	41.8[a]	16.4	26.6
% STD in past 5 years[f]	1.5	9.8	7.2[a]	1.8	6.7	15.6[a]	1.0	6.4[a]

Source: Data from The Commonwealth Fund survey on women's health, 1993.

Note: Numbers cited are percentages.

[a] Significant at $p \leq 0.001$ by the chi-square test.

[b] Significant at $p \leq 0.01$ by the chi-square test.

[c] Respondent says she has a disability that keeps her from participating fully in school, work, housework, or other activities.

[d] In the past 5 years, respondent has been told by a doctor that she had severe menstrual problems, endometriosis, or reproductive problems (like infertility).

[e] In the past 5 years, respondent has been told by a doctor that she had a urinary tract infection.

[f] In the past 5 years, respondent has been told by a doctor that she had a sexually transmitted disease.

women reporting neither type of violence). An earlier study, which examines disability in adults exposed to child abuse, reported that 32 percent have a permanent disfigurement or disability (Martin and Elmer 1992). In a review of child abuse studies, Rosenberg and Krugman (1991) suggested that disabilities in adults exposed to child abuse may result from scars, untreated injuries, or untreated sexually transmitted diseases. Rape has also been found to result in permanent disabilities, usually related to sexual functioning (Becker, Skinner, and Abel 1986; Gise and Paddison 1988; Chapman 1989).

This study found that the relationship between violence and poor gynecological health is fairly strong (tab. 9.3). Women who experience violence are much more likely to report a gynecological diagnosis by a physician during the past 5 years than nonabused women (this includes diagnoses of severe menstrual problems, endometriosis, and infertility).[1] Of women under age fifty, 22 percent of those physically abused as children, 36 percent of those sexually abused as children, 27 percent of those who experienced a violent crime other than rape, 30 percent of those who were raped, and 45 percent of women physically abused by a spouse reported a gynecological diagnosis. This compares with approximately 16 percent not exposed to these types of violence. Women abused as children, raped, or victimized by a violent crime also reported much higher rates of diagnosed urinary tract infections (UTIs) than nonexposed women.

While no other study directly examines the relationship of violence to menstrual disorders and UTIs, a number look at the relationship between pelvic pain, which is often related to menstrual and UTI problems (Howard 1993), and exposure to violence. In general, these studies (usually small, clinical, retrospective case-control design) reported that experiencing child abuse (Domino and Haber 1987; Mullen et al. 1988), rape (Chapman 1989; Reiter and Gambone 1990; Peters et al. 1991), or spouse abuse (Haber 1985; Chapman 1989; Schei 1990) is strongly associated with chronic pelvic pain.

Sexually transmitted diseases (STDs) are also a potential outcome of experiencing sexual violence. Women who were raped in the past 5 years reported the highest rate (15.1%) of STD diagnosis (tab. 9.3). Other studies, of clinical populations, also reported a high prevalence of STDs among women who were raped, and attributed at least some portion of this prevalence to the rape (Jenny et al. 1990; Glaser et al. 1991; Davies and Clay 1992). Women who experienced child abuse (physical and sexual), violent crime, or spouse abuse also reported higher STD rates than other women. Rosenberg and Krugman (1991) suggested that adult women who were sexually abused as children may have untreated STDs resulting from this abuse. The high rate of STDs among women who reported that they were only physically abused as children is, however, intriguing and its meaning unclear. Women who were abused by their spouses in the past year may have sex partners (e.g., the abusive male) who are less likely to be sexually monogamous and thus put them at higher risk for STD acquisition. Related to this point, women in this study who reported experiencing spouse abuse were much more likely than other women who are married or living with a male to say that a sex partner had refused to wear a condom in the past year.

Although the rate of injury immediately following a violent incident is not measured in this survey, other studies indicated that violence is a primary cause of acute injury for women. Rates of physical injury among women who reported experiencing rape range from 40 percent to 71 percent (Everett and Jimerson 1977; Cartwright 1987; Geist 1988). Research on spouse abuse indicates that almost half of all incidents may lead to injury (Berk et al. 1983; Klaus and Rand 1984), and that half of these injuries require immediate medical attention (Schulman 1979; Teske and Parker 1983). In addition, several surveys found that between 7 percent and 33 percent of women presenting to emergency rooms are there because of a spouse abuse incident (Goldberg and Tomlanovich 1984; Flaherty and Kurz 1985; McLeer et al. 1989).

Mental Health and Violence

This study found significant differences in the prevalence of emotional problems, with women who experienced violence reporting more problems (tab. 9.4). Women exposed to child abuse and/or to spouse abuse are much more likely to have low self-esteem than other women. Other studies reported lower self-esteem in women who were abused as children (National Research Council 1993), were raped (Carmen, Riecker, and Mills 1984; Kilpatrick, Veronen, and Best 1985; Murphy et al. 1988), or experienced spouse abuse (Walker 1989).

Table 9.4. Exposure to Violence and Mental Health

	Child Abuse			Violent Crime			Spouse Abuse	
	None	Physical	Sexual	None	Other	Rape	No	Yes
Low self-esteem[a]	19.9	23.9	26.6[b]	20.9	19.0	28.9	18.1	37.3[c]
Depression/anxiety diagnosis[d]	12.7	26.7	32.7[c]	14.1	24.4	45.6[c]	14.0	31.9[c]
Depressive symptoms[d]	38.6	52.1	55.7[c]	40.0	49.7	62.9[c]	34.2	74.0[c]
Suicide ideation[e]	4.4	10.7	23.1[c]	5.3	17.1	26.7[c]	4.9	14.4[c]

Source: Data from The Commonwealth Fund survey on women's health, 1993.

Note: Numbers cited are percentages of women in each abuse category with the health outcome.

[a] Self-esteem is measured by the Rosenberg's Self-Esteem Scale (Rosenberg 1965). A low score is assigned to any woman who did not, on average, "strongly agree" with any positive self-esteem statement (a score of 20 or less).

[b] Significant at $p \leq 0.01$ by the chi-square test.

[c] Significant at $p \leq 0.001$ by the chi-square test.

[d] In the past 5 years, the respondent was told by a physician that she had a depression or anxiety disorder.

[e] Respondent scored high on a scale of depressive symptoms, a subset of six items from the CES-D scale (Radloff 1977).

[f] Respondent says she has thought about ending her life in the past year.

Women who have experienced violence are also much more likely to report receiving a diagnosis of a depressive or anxiety disorder from a physician in the past 5 years (tab. 9.4). These diagnoses are especially high among women who were raped (45.6%). Women who experienced violence are also more likely to have a high level of current depressive symptoms; this is especially true for women who were physically abused by their spouses in the past year (74% compared to 34.2% of nonabused women).

Depression has been one of the most studied outcomes of experiencing violence, with reports of high rates of depression in women who experienced child abuse (Felitti 1991; Pribor and Dinwiddie 1992; Saunders et al. 1992), rape (Ellis, Atkenson, and Calhoun 1981; Frank and Stewart 1984; Mackey et al. 1992), and spouse abuse (Shields and Haneke 1983; Jaffe et al. 1986; Amaro et al. 1990). Many of these authors noted that the depression persists years after the violent event. Higher levels of anxiety disorders (both panic and phobia types) are also apparent in women who were abused as children (Burnam et al. 1988; Mullen et al. 1988; Pribor and Dinwiddie 1992; Saunders et al. 1992), raped (Kilpatrick et al. 1981; Calhoun, Atkenson and Resnick, 1982), or abused by their spouses (Stewart and deBlois 1981; Jaffe et al. 1986).

Suicide ideation, which has been linked to depression, is much higher in the surveyed women who have experienced violence (tab. 9.4), especially in women abused as children (23.1% versus 4.4%) or raped (26.7% versus 5.3%). High levels of suicide ideation and suicide attempts have been previously documented in women who experienced child abuse (Felitti 1991; Saunders et al. 1992), rape (Burgess and Holmstrom 1979; Ellis et al. 1981), or spouse abuse (Carmen, Riecker, and Mills 1984; Amaro et al. 1990; Bergman and Brismar 1991). Stark and colleagues (1979) examined the temporal relationship between suicide attempts and violence, finding no difference in suicide attempts before the first recorded incident of spouse abuse but a strong difference after the first assault (26% versus 3%).

Behavioral Responses

The two behavioral responses commonly associated with experiencing violence are substance abuse and the intergenerational transmission of violence. This study finds that women who were abused as children or who experienced violent crime are more likely to use tobacco and alcohol than other women (tab. 9.5); spouse abuse, however, is not signifi-

Table 9.5. Exposure to Violence and Substance Use

	Child Abuse			Violent Crime			Spouse Abuse	
	None	Physical	Sexual	None	Other	Rape	No	Yes
Uses tobacco currently	25.0	36.3	34.9[a]	25.5	36.4	38.0[a]	23.3	32.0
Used alcohol in the past month	51.6	60.5	58.3[a]	51.4	66.2	60.7[a]	51.2	58.4
Used tranquilizers in the past year	7.1	6.6	11.7	6.9	10.9	19.9[a]	7.8	6.7
Ever used illicit drugs[b]	22.0	45.3	42.3[a]	23.2	46.1	45.8[a]	24.0	40.0[a]
Used illicit drugs in the past month	1.1	7.8	5.5[a]	1.4	8.2	2.2[a]	1.1	6.9[a]
Counseled by a doctor about substance use[c]	13.2	23.1	22.2[a]	14.6	17.4	16.5	12.0	23.2[a]

Source: Data from The Commonwealth Fund survey on women's health, 1993.

Note: Numbers cited are percentages of women in each abuse category who use substances.

[a] Significant at $p \leq 0.001$ by the chi-square test.

[b] Illicit drugs include marijuana, cocaine, crack cocaine, heroin, amphetamines, and depressants.

[c] Counseled by a doctor in the past year about smoking, drinking, or drug use.

cantly related to greater use of alcohol (tab. 9.5). Also of note is that there were no differences in the level of drinking (neither in the number of drinks consumed in the past 2 weeks nor in the level of heavy drinking, defined as drinking an average of three drinks per day). However, women who experienced violence are almost twice as likely to have ever used illicit drugs, to use illicit drugs currently, or to have been counseled by a physician for tobacco, drug, or alcohol use in the past year than other women.

The results of this study seem to differ somewhat from the results of previous studies of alcohol and drug abuse among women who experienced violence. Those studies found higher rates of alcoholism and drug addiction among women who experienced child abuse (Burnam et al. 1988; Bushnell, Wells, and Oakley-Brown 1992; Pribor and Dinwiddie 1992), rape (Frank et al. 1981), or spouse abuse (Jaffe et al. 1986; Miller, Downs, and Gondoh 1989; Amaro et al. 1990). Miller, Downs, and Gondoh (1989) reported that spousal violence scores are among the strongest predictors of alcoholism in women, even after controlling for income, violence in family of origin, and having an alcoholic husband.

While this study reported higher rates of use of illicit drugs by women who experienced violence and higher rates of use of alcohol by women exposed to child abuse and rape, it does not agree with previous studies of alcoholism and spouse abuse. This may be due to several factors. First, this study examines only the use of, not abuse of or addiction to, alcohol. Second, very few study participants (whether exposed to violence or not) reported heavy use of alcohol; most of the previous studies of alcoholism and spouse abuse used clinical samples of alcoholic women. The rarity of heavy drinking in this sample makes it impossible to examine such drinking as an outcome. Third, there really may be no connection between the use of alcohol and experiencing spouse abuse; the findings of previous studies may be suspect due to their small, nonrepresentative samples.

Another behavioral problem of interest is the intergenerational transmission of child abuse. While this survey did not ask any questions regarding the perpetration of child abuse by the respondents, other studies examined this issue. In general, they estimated that approximately 30 percent of women abused as children will in turn abuse their own children (National Research Council 1993; Oliver 1993).

Cognitive Responses to Violence

A number of other studies have examined differences in cognitive functioning related to exposure to violence. The prevalence of multiple personality disorder, and less extreme levels of disassociative symptoms (such as spontaneous self-hypnosis, self-anesthesia, feelings of being "disconnected" and of being "out of one's body") are reported to be much higher in women exposed to child abuse than in other women (DiTomasso and Routh 1993; Hendricks-Matthews 1993; National Research Council 1993). One review of child abuse studies (Beitchman et al. 1992), however, maintained that there is insufficient evidence to support a strong link between multiple personality disorder and child sex abuse. The presence of visual hallucinations and flashbacks in women exposed to child abuse (Terr 1991; Hendricks-Matthews 1993) or rape (Sorenson et al. 1991) has also been reported. However, no link has been established between schizophrenia and experiencing violence (Burnam et al. 1988; Pribor and Dinwiddie 1992).

Interpersonal Responses Related to Violence

This survey found that experiencing physical or sexual abuse as a child is significantly related to experiencing future violence as an adult (tab. 9.6). The impact of experiencing child sexual abuse is especially striking; 8 percent of women sexually abused as children reported that they were raped in the past 5 years (compared with 2.1% of women not abused as children), and 17.9 percent of women abused as children reported they were abused by a spouse in the past year (compared with 7.1% of those not abused as children).

Other studies also reported that past violence is a factor for future risk. Several reported a significant relationship between child abuse and experiencing any violence as an adult (National Research Council 1993), especially rape (Browne and Finkelhor 1986; Russell 1986; Coons et al. 1989; Terr 1991) or spouse abuse (Hotaling and Finkelhor 1988; Coons et al. 1989). Only one study found no relationship between child sexual abuse and experiencing violence as an adult (Atkeson, Calhoun, and Morris 1989). Also, being raped as an adult may be a risk factor for future rape (Coons et al. 1989; Sorenson et al. 1991; Scott, Lefley, and Hicks 1993).

Several reasons may underlie the increased risk of adult violence suffered by those who experienced child abuse. Women abused as children may have low self-esteem and view themselves as deserving of physical abuse or as incapable of stopping the abuse (Walker 1989). They may also believe that physical abuse is a normal part of a relationship. Finally, women exposed to child abuse may have dissociative

Table 9.6. Child Abuse and Adult Exposure to Violence

Child Abuse	Violent Crime			Spouse Abuse	
	None	Other	Rape	No	Yes
None	89.1	8.8	2.1	92.9	7.1
Physical abuse only	68.8	26.9	4.3	90.0	10.0
Sexual abuse, with or without physical abuse	65.4	26.6	8.0[a]	82.1	17.9[a]

Source: Data from The Commonwealth Fund survey on women's health, 1993.

Note: Numbers cited are percentages.

[a] Significant at $p \leq 0.001$ by the chi-square test.

symptoms that may make the abuse seem unreal or that make it difficult for them to recognize a potentially violent situation (Coons et al.
1989).

Violence and the Use of Health Services

Not surprisingly, given their increased level of health problems, this
study found that women who experienced violent crime and child
abuse reported significantly more use of health care than other women
(tab. 9.7). Women who experienced violent crime, rape, or child abuse
see more physicians and make more physician visits than other wom-
en. Despite much higher levels of use of services, women who were
raped or who experienced violent crime or child abuse are still significantly more likely than other women to say that they needed, but did
not receive, medical care in the past year.

Other studies also reported a similar increase in the use of services
among women who were abused as children (Drossman et al. 1990;
Felitti 1991), were raped (Golding et al. 1988; Koss, Koss, and Woodruff
1991), or experienced violent crimes other than rape (Koss, Koss, and
Woodruff 1991). This increased use can be both immediate and long-
term; in a large study of female HMO patients, the severity of victimization is the strongest predictor of medical visits over the next year
(Koss, Koss, and Woodruff 1991).

Table 9.7. Violence and the Use of Health Services

	Child Abuse			Violent Crime			Spouse Abuse	
	None	Physical	Sexual	None	Other	Rape	No	Yes
Mean number of doctors	1.98	2.22	2.44[a]	2.01	1.95	3.63[a]	2.04	2.09
Mean number of visits	4.90	7.63	7.17[a]	5.18	6.71	9.88[a]	5.38	6.51
Percentage needed and did not get medical care in the past year	12.9	22.2	29.0[b]	13.9	23.1	38.1[b]	12.2	37.6[b]

Source: Data from The Commonwealth Fund survey on women's health, 1993.
[a] Significant at $p \leq 0.01$ by the ANOVA F-test.
[b] Significant at $p \leq 0.001$ by the chi-square test.

This survey found significant unmet need in obtaining medical services among women abused by their spouses (tab. 9.7). While there is no significant difference in the number of physicians seen or the number of physician visits physically abused women are significantly more likely than other women to say that they needed and did not get care in the past year. Although previous research indicates that women who experience spouse abuse use more mental health care (Stark, Flitcraft, and Frazier 1979) and may use more primary care (Rath, Jarratt, and Leonardson 1989), anecdotal evidence suggests that abusive men may prevent their spouses from getting medical care, especially when these men are the cause of the injury (Walker 1989; Plichta et al. 1993).

Survey respondents who experienced spouse abuse are also more likely than other women to name the emergency room as their primary source of health care. Previous studies have shown that 7 percent to 33 percent of emergency room visits by women are due to spouse abuse (Flaherty and Kurz 1985; Golding et al. 1988; McLeer et al. 1989).

One possible explanation for the finding that women who experienced violence have unmet need for medical care may be differential access to care. This, however, is only partly supported by the survey data. Women experiencing violence are just as likely as other women to have a usual source of care and to see an obstetrician-gynecologist. Further, women experiencing child abuse and violent crime are just as likely to have health insurance as other women, but those exposed to spouse abuse are less likely to have insurance.

Physician-Patient Communication Patterns

One explanation for the difference in the unmet need for care may be a lack of communication between women and their physicians. Because exposure to violence often cannot be detected except by the woman disclosing the information to her physician, it is especially important that the quality of communication be examined. This survey measured the ease of communication with the physician, the perceived ability of the physician to listen, the perceived seriousness with which the physician treats the respondent, and any inappropriate sexual behavior by the physician.

Women who experienced violence reported consistently poorer quality communication with their physicians than other women (tab. 9.8), specifically reporting that it is much more difficult to talk to their

Table 9.8. Exposure to Violence and Physician–Patient Communication

Response	Child Abuse			Violent Crime			Spouse Abuse	
	None	Physical	Sexual	None	Other	Rape	No	Yes
Difficult to talk to physician	15.1	14.0	16.8	16.0	20.8	17.5[a]	15.5	34.2[b]
Physician does not listen well	5.4	8.8	11.0[b]	5.9	5.1	9.8	5.4	17.1[b]
Physician talked down to them	25.2	42.2	44.7[b]	27.1	36.7	50.0[b]	29.2	35.7
Physician told them a medical problem was "all in their head"	15.0	35.0	39.5[b]	17.7	20.7	28.5[b]	20.3	28.3[b]
Sexually harassed by a physician	4.6	8.7	15.7[b]	5.5	11.4	9.6	6.2	12.7[b]

Source: Data from The Commonwealth Fund survey on women's health, 1993.

Note: Numbers cited are percentages in each abuse category that said they had the communication problem.

[a] Significant at $p \leq 0.01$ by the chi-square test.

[b] Significant at $p \leq 0.001$ by the chi-square test.

physician and that their physician does not listen well. They are more likely than women who did not experience violence to say that their physician does not take them seriously; a higher percentage also reported that a physician talked down to them and told them a medical problem was "all in their head." Of great concern is the high level of sexually inappropriate behavior by physicians reported by women exposed to child abuse, rape, and other violent crime.

It is not surprising that women who are exposed to violence report communication problems with their physicians and thus often fail to disclose abuse. This survey reveals that only 9.1 percent of women who were abused by their spouses and 26.4 percent of women who were sexually abused as children had ever discussed the abuse with a physician. In fact, the majority of women abused by their spouses (61%), and a substantial minority of women who were sexually abused (32.2%), did not discuss the abuse with anyone. Other studies found similar or lower levels of disclosure (Hamberger, Saunders, and Hovey 1992; Pribor and Dinwiddie 1992; Saunders et al. 1992).

IMPLICATIONS FOR POLICY

As this study has demonstrated, violence against women is an endemic problem in the United States; the findings indicate that literally millions of adult women have been physically or sexually abused in childhood, raped, physically abused by their spouses, or have been victims of another type of violent crime. Clearly, a national, multitiered policy of preventing child abuse, rape, and spouse abuse is needed, and health care providers should be among the leaders in devising and implementing this effort. Violence, as this study demonstrates, has a significant negative effect on physical and mental health, it increases the use of health services, and it interferes with open communication between women and their physicians.

A policy agenda that seeks to reduce women's exposure to violence and the harm it causes must address the legal, social, and instrumental components (i.e., food, clothing, shelter) as well as those that are related to health. Although the needs of women who are at risk or who have been exposed to violence cannot be met solely by the health care system, these women most often turn to health care providers for help (Bowker and Maurer 1987). The health care system, therefore, must be able to respond to these women effectively. A number of health professional organizations, including the American Medical Association (Council on Scientific and Ethical Affairs 1992), the American Academy of Nursing (1993), the American College of Obstetricians and Gynecologists (1988), and the American Public Health Association (personal communication, APHA 1992), all have recently begun to discuss the prevention of violence and the best way to offer assistance to women who have already been exposed to violence. However, none of these organizations has yet proposed a set of policies that provide for a coordinated and cohesive response on the part of the health care system.

Any cohesive response to violence against women by the health care system should address the primary and secondary prevention of violence. Prevention entails: (1) education for the providers and consumers of health care, (2) assessment of women for their risk of victimization, (3) the detection and documentation of past exposure, and (4) the treatment of any negative health impact stemming from the violent experience. Furthermore, a mechanism is necessary to coordinate the efforts of health care providers with those of the legal system, the social welfare system, and community-based organizations that seek to provide instrumental needs (such as battered women's shelters and rape crisis centers).

Professional Education

Before health providers can engage in the primary and secondary prevention of child abuse, rape, and spouse abuse, they must learn the risk factors, indicators, estimated prevalence, and sequelae of abuse (Council on Scientific and Ethical Affairs 1992). Currently, less than half of all U.S. medical schools offer training in issues related to domestic violence, and there is little reason to believe that instruction about child abuse or rape is any more common (Holtz, Hames, and Safran 1989). Numerous studies and panels have recommended educating health care providers, and several professional organizations have provided educational materials in the form of pamphlets, special journal issues, and technical bulletins (American College of Obstetricians and Gynecologists 1988; Braham, Furniss, and Holtz 1992; Council on Scientific and Ethical Affairs 1992). These works provide a good starting point for individual health care providers to begin to learn about the impact of violence on women.

Health care systems should actively encourage health care providers to become knowledgeable about violence and its sequelae through the promotion of professional education. Clinics and hospitals can offer in-service education focusing on the health aspects of violence, including identification, treatment, and referral of women exposed to violence. Schools training health professionals can incorporate training about violence into their curricula, and the agencies that accredit health professionals could include questions about violence in their professional boards and exams. Professional societies can provide incentives for health practitioners to educate themselves about violence by offering courses on the subject for continuing education credit.

Primary Prevention of Violence

The primary prevention of violence involves creating policies to assist women in avoiding violent events and to prevent violent people (usually male) from perpetrating child abuse, rape, spouse abuse, and other violent crimes. While preventing perpetrators from committing crime is primarily the responsibility of the legal system, health care providers can participate in public awareness efforts to decrease the social acceptability of child and spouse abuse. However, the main role of providers should be to educate their patients about how to minimize their personal risk of a violent event occurring.

Health care institutions need to implement protocols that screen women for their risk. These protocols should include providing information to women on their personal risk of experiencing rape or spouse abuse and some anticipatory guidance on how to minimize that risk. All women must be assessed for this risk; while this study found that several sociodemographic factors increase the risk of spouse abuse and rape, all women are at some risk of these events occurring. Because the one event that clearly put all woman at risk for future violence (either rape or spouse abuse) is having been physically or sexually abused as a child, any screening instrument for the risk of future violence should include exposure to child abuse as one of its questions.

One place where this screening and education process could be integrated is with routine gynecological care. This study, as well as earlier work, found that women who were raped or physically abused by a spouse are at higher risk than other women for sexually transmitted diseases and gynecological problems. This finding suggests that spouse abuse and rape prevention strategies (especially date rape) could be discussed most naturally in the context of good sexual health practices.

Prevention strategies aimed at child abuse can be undertaken by health care professionals either in the pediatrician's office or in the school. Pediatricians may want to provide anticipatory guidance to parents regarding the risk factors for child abuse and the safety precautions that can help minimize a child's risk of being abused. In addition to teaching parents about avoiding child abuse, children can be reached directly through the public school system. Much of the public health education children receive is in elementary and secondary schools. Many schools currently offer courses in personal health, family life, and living skills. School nurses and health educators could incorporate information and skills development around violence prevention (especially of child abuse and dating violence) into existing health curricula (Vanderschmidt et al. 1993).

Many authors have noted that the level of sexual, physical, and mental battering of women in a society is directly related to the degree that societal values support aggressive, domineering, and hierarchical behavior by men and silence on the part of women (Stark, Flitcraft, and

Frazier 1979; Tifft 1993). In addition to providing educational interventions at the patient level, health care providers and their professional organizations can become involved in activities to increase societal awareness about violence against women. One such public health activity, which began in June 1994, is a national media campaign to break the silence surrounding spouse abuse, to change societal values regarding male violence, and to provide individuals with concrete actions they can take to reduce the level of violence in their own community. This public awareness campaign, "There's No Excuse" (for domestic violence), was commissioned by the Family Violence Prevention Fund and is being sponsored by the Ad Council. This campaign was designed with the involvement of professional medical organizations and will be run for at least 5 years. As part of this campaign, community action kits will be made available to anyone who calls a toll-free number; these kits will help individuals organize locally against domestic violence. Health care providers may want to use the information available in these kits to take a leadership role in their own communities (Family Violence Prevention Fund, personal communication).

Secondary Prevention of Violence

Secondary prevention of violence involves the provision of care to women who have already experienced a violent event; the goal is to treat problems stemming from the violence and to prevent future incidents from occurring. The results of this and other studies indicate that there is a great need for the secondary prevention of violence. More than 4 million women are abused by their spouses each year; over 9 million women experience a violent crime over a 5-year period (for 2.2 million of these women, the crime is rape or sexual assault); and over 14 million women were abused as children (as noted earlier, experiencing child abuse puts a woman at a higher risk for experiencing violence as an adult). It is important for health care providers to detect and document these incidents so that they can treat any health damage related to the violence, refer those who require nonmedical assistance to other sources of help, and help their patients reduce their risk of future incidents.

Detection of exposure to violence will probably not occur without action on the part of health care providers. Several studies, including this one, found that the vast majority of women do not disclose their experiences of violence to physicians. In fact, this study found that physician-patient communication is significantly poorer for women who have experienced violence than for other women. Available information suggests that physicians may not be sensitive to issues of violence or may hold attitudes that prevent them from addressing woman abuse. These include: "Family matters are private"; "Violence against women is not a health issue"; and "Working with victims of violence is a hopeless cause" (Burge 1989:364–65). The findings related to lack of disclosure and poor communications indicate that health care institutions must take the lead in adopting institution-wide policies that encourage open communication about violence issues. Health care institutions should screen for experiences of child abuse, rape, violent crime, and spouse abuse as a part of standard intake procedures.

In addition to screening for exposure to violence, it is important that health care facilities adopt protocols that require documentation of any physical injury related to the violent incident(s). Documentation is especially important for women as they begin to work with the legal system to prevent future incidents of violence (e.g., to obtain protection from or prosecution of the perpetrator). Several groups have already designed, tested, and validated such protocols for child and spouse abuse (Council on Scientific and Ethical Affairs, 1992; Taylor and Campbell 1992; Campbell and Humphreys 1993), as well as for recording physical evidence from rape (Dunn and Gilchrist 1993).

The Health Care Provider as a Connector to Other Services

The effective prevention of violence requires a coordinated response of medical and psychological services as well as legal services, contact with a social worker, safe housing, and other nonmedical resources. Because health care providers are often the first place women turn for help, providers need to be able to connect with nonmedical resources for these women. The creation of a referral list of services is a fairly low-cost way for health care providers to begin to help women coordinate the various services they need (Berk et al. 1983; Tilden 1989; Stenchever and Stenchever 1991).

A referral list is not enough, however. Health care providers should be prepared to offer direct assistance, because they may be the only available source of help. This is especially true in those situations where the violence is recent (such as a woman coming in to be treated for injuries due to rape) or when there is an immediate danger of the violence recurring (such as with spouse abuse). In the case of rape, health care providers should have access to a rape crisis team. In the case of spouse abuse, health care providers must address the immediate safety of the patient herself and her children; this may involve developing an exit plan with the woman, assessing her other health risks (such as the likelihood of her committing suicide or the presence of a gun in the house), and assessing any risks to her children (such as the likelihood of their being hit or sexually abused) (Campbell and Humphreys 1993).

Developing a Community-Wide Response to Violence

Ultimately, the effective prevention of violence requires participation by and coordination from many community groups that normally do not interact. Because the outcomes of violence are most often related to health, local public health agencies may want to take the lead in establishing a multidisciplinary community board to develop a realistic community response to violence. Board members should be drawn from local groups that are concerned about violence, including public health clinics, community health centers, hospitals, law enforcement, courts, community residents, child and family services, therapists, academics, battered women's shelters, and rape crisis centers (Elliot 1993).

There are several practical reasons for different agencies to be interested in participating in such a board. One is that a change in policy by one group (such as a community health center) may result in an increased demand for the services of another agency; if all involved know of these changes in advance, they will be better prepared to handle the increased client flow. A more important reason is to enable the community to establish an integrated response to the prevention of violence that is appropriate to individual community circumstances.

IMPLICATIONS FOR RESEARCH

Policies regarding the prevention of violence need a solid underpinning of accurate, comprehensive information. However, much work remains to be done. First, it is essential that definitions of child abuse and rape acceptable to most researchers be developed; there currently are no commonly accepted definitions of child abuse (National Research Council 1993) or rape (Russell 1983). Without this, it will be difficult to compare directly and synthesize the results of different studies. Second, basic epidemiological studies are needed to establish the risk factors for violence and to document and monitor the one-year and lifetime prevalence rates of child abuse, rape, and spouse abuse. Economic analyses of the direct and indirect costs to society of child abuse, rape, and spouse abuse are especially important. Currently there are no useful estimates of the total medical, legal, or social services used, or of the total losses to the women exposed to violence (such as days of work lost). Finally, there is pressing need to design, evaluate, and refine effective interventions for the primary and secondary prevention of violence.

The epidemiology of child abuse, spouse abuse, and rape is not well understood; in fact, the yearly incidence of rape and child abuse, and the lifetime prevalence rates of rape, nonsexual violent crime, and spouse abuse have never been accurately measured in the United States. Although the U.S. Department of Justice conducts the National Crime Victimization Survey (NCVS) each year, it does not ask any direct questions about spouse abuse or rape (women are counted as having been raped if they volunteer this information to the interviewer) (Maguire, Pastore, and Flanagan 1993). A low-cost way to accurately measure and monitor the one-year incidence of experiencing rape and spouse abuse would be for the NCVS to include items that measure these events in their questionnaire. Another U.S. survey that could include measures of child abuse, spouse abuse, and rape is the Health Interview Survey; the advantage of monitoring violence in a health survey is that it would give researchers the ability to examine the relationship among violence, health status, and the use of health services over time. Continual monitoring of one-year prevalence rates of child abuse, spouse abuse, and rape would be crucial for providing information on the level of need for prevention and medical services and for providing an indication of the effectiveness of any interventions.

The medical costs to society of violence against women are unknown. The one study that attempted to estimate the direct medical costs of spouse abuse used data from the 1980 National Crime Victimization Survey, which underestimates spouse abuse by a factor of at least 10 (McLeer et al. 1989). An estimate of the direct medical cost of rape or child abuse would assist policy makers in determining the allocation of resources for violence prevention. To estimate this cost, the following information is needed: (1) the differences in the type and quantity of medical and mental health services used by women experiencing and not experiencing violence in the United States, (2) the number of temporary and permanent injuries suffered as a result of experiencing violence, and (3) the number of days of productive functioning lost (either paid work or housework) as a result of the violence. However, no studies currently exist that would provide even rough estimates of this information. A detailed, nationally representative survey with an explicit focus on violence and the use of health services could focus these issues.

Finally, research is essential to develop effective primary and secondary prevention strategies for women exposed to violence and for the perpetrators of violence. A screening protocol for a woman's exposure to and risk of future violence that is short, inexpensive, effective, and useful in a variety of settings is a priority for development and testing. A better understanding of the factors that put a woman at increased risk for violence (especially the role of child abuse) would give us a better understanding of how to develop interventions. Program development must be directed toward crafting preventive interventions for violent men. If one woman resolves a violent situation by leaving an abusive male (often the only feasible alternative), that male may still victimize other women and children. To date, treatment programs for child molesters, wife abusers, and rapists have not enjoyed much success and have high drop-out and recidivism rates (Ceasar and Hamberger 1989).

Effective interventions for women who have been abused as children, raped, or physically abused by their spouses need to be developed. Interventions, where they exist, are often highly fragmented and may involve an uncoordinated combination of crisis centers, battered women shelters, 12-step programs, and medical/mental health visits by professionals with no training in violence issues. While curriculum development for educating health care professionals about violence is needed, health care professionals alone cannot prevent violent events from occurring. As noted before, much of the care that women who are at risk or who have experienced violence require (such as legal services) is outside the realm of health care providers. A "team approach" to women exposed to violence, similar to that taken with children who have been abused, is essential.

NOTE

1. Gynecological diagnoses are asked of only women under age fifty.

REFERENCES

American Academy of Nursing. 1993. Violence as a nursing priority: policy implications. *Nursing Outlook* March–April:83–92.

American College of Obstetricians and Gynecologists. 1989. *The Battered Woman.* ACOG Technical Bulletin 124. Washington, D.C.: ACOG.

Amaro, H., Fried, L., Cabral, H., and Zuckerman, B. 1990. Violence during pregnancy and substance use. *American Journal of Public Health* 80:575–79.

Atkeson, B. M., Calhoun, K. S., and Morris, K. T. 1989. Victim resistance to rape: the relationship of previous victimization, demographics and situational variables. *Archives of Sexual Behavior* 18:497–507.

Becker, J. V., Skinner, L. J., and Abel, G. G. 1986. Level of post-assault functioning in rape and incest victims. *Archives of Sexual Behavior* 15:37–49.

Beitchman, J. H., Zucker, K. J., Hood, J. E., and DaCosta, G. A. 1992. A review of the long-term effects of child sexual abuse. *Child Abuse and Neglect* 16:101–18.

Bergman, B., and Brismar, B. 1991. Suicide attempts by battered wives. *Acta Psychiatrica Scandinavia* 83:380–84.

Berk, B. A., Berk, S. F., Loseke, D. R., and Rauma, D. 1983. Mutual combat and other family violence myths. In D. Finkelhor, ed., *The Dark Side of Family Violence.* Beverly Hills: Sage Publications.

Bowker, L., and Maurer, L. 1987. The medical treatment of battered wives. *Women's Health* 12:25–27.

Braham, R., Furniss, K. K., and Holtz, H. 1992. Nursing protocol on domestic violence. *Nurse-Practitioner* November:24–31.

Browne, A., and Finkelhor, D. 1986. Impact of child sexual abuse: a review of the research. *Psychological Bulletin* 92:66–77.

Bruce, M. L., Takeuchi, D. T., and Leaf, P. J. 1991. Poverty and psychiatric status. Longitudinal evidence from the New Haven epidemiologic catchment area study. *Archives of General Psychiatry* 48:470–74.

Burge, S. K. 1989. Violence against women as a health care issue. *Family Medicine* 21:368–73.

Burgess, A. W., and Holmstrom, L. L. 1979. Adaptive strategies and recovering from rape. *American Journal of Psychiatry* 136:1278–82.

Burnam, M. A., Stein, J. A., Golding, M., Siegal, J. M., Sorenson, S. B., and Forsythe, A. B. 1988. Sexual assault and mental disorders in a community population. *Journal of Consulting and Clinical Psychology* 56:843–50.

Bushnell, J. A., Wells, J. E., and Oakley-Browne, M. A. 1992. Long-term effects of intrafamilial sexual abuse in childhood. *Acta Psychiatrica Scandinavia* 85:136–42.

Campbell, J., and Humphreys, J. 1993. *Nursing Care of Survivors of Family Violence.* St. Louis: Mosby.

Calhoun, K. S., Atkenson, B. M., and Resnick, P. A. 1982. A longitudinal evaluation of fear reactions in victims of rape. *Journal of Counseling Psychology* 29:655–61.

Carmen, E., Riecker, P., and Mills, T. 1984. Victims of violence and psychiatric illness. *American Journal of Psychiatry* 141:378–83.

Cartwright, P. S. 1987. Factors that correlate with injury sustained by survivors of rape. *Obstetrics and Gynecology* 70:44–46.

Ceasar, P. L., and Hamberger. 1989. *Treating Men Who Batter: Theory, Practice and Programs.* New York: Springer.

Chapman, J. D. 1989. A longitudinal study of sexuality and gynecologic health in abused women. *Journal of the American Osteopath Society* 89:619–24.

Coons, P. M., Bowman, E. S., Pellow, T. A., and Schneider, P. 1989. Posttraumatic aspects of the treatment of victims of sexual abuse and incest. *Psychiatric Clinics of North America* 12:325–35.

Council on Scientific and Ethical Affairs. 1992. Violence against women. *Journal of the American Medical Association* 1267:3184–89.

Davies, A. G., and Clay, J. C. 1992. Prevalence of sexually transmitted disease infection in women alleging rape. *Sexually Transmitted Diseases* September–October:298–300.

DiTomasso, M. J., and Routh, D. K. 1993. Recall of abuse in childhood and three measures of disassociation. *Child Abuse and Neglect* 17:477–85.

Domino, J. V., and Haber, J. D. 1987. Prior physical and sexual abuse in women with chronic headache and clinical correlates. *Headache* 27:310–14.

Drossman, D. A., et al. 1990. Sexual and physical abuse in women with functional or organic gastrointestinal disorders. *Annals of Internal Medicine* 113:828–33.

Dunn, S. F. M., and Gilchrist, V. J. 1993. Sexual assault. *Primary Care* 20:359–73.

Elliot, B. A. 1993. Community responses to violence. *Primary Care* 20:495–502.

Ellis, E. M., Atkenson, B. M., and Calhoun, K. S. 1981. An assessment of long-term reactions to rape. *Journal of Abnormal Psychology* 90:263–66.

Ellis, E. M., Calhoun, K. S., and Atkenson, B. M. 1980. Sexual dysfunction in victims of rape. *Women and Health* 5:39–47.

Everett, R. B., and Jimerson, G. K. 1977. The rape victim: a review of 117 consecutive cases. *Journal of Abnormal Psychology* 50:88–90.

Felitti, V. J. 1991. Long-term medical consequences of incest, rape and molestation. *Southern Medical Journal* 84:328–31.

Flaherty, E. W., and Kurz, D. E. 1985. Battering victims: Identification in Emergency Rooms. Final Report, NIMH Grant #RO1.MH37180.

Follingstad, D. R., Rutledge, D. S., Polek, D. S., and McNeil-Hawkins, K. 1988. Factors associated with patterns of dating violence toward college women. *Journal of Family Violence* 3:169–82.

Frank, E., and Stewart, B. D. 1984. Depressive symptoms in rape victims: a revisit. *Journal of Affective Disorders* 7:77–85.

Frank, E., Turner, S. M., Stewart, B. D., Jacob, M., and West D. 1981. Psychiatric symptoms and the response to sexual assault. *Comprehensive Psychiatry* 22:479–87.

Geist, R. F. 1988. Sexually related trauma. *Emergency Medicine Clinics of North America* 6:439–66.

Gelles, R. J., and Straus, M. A. 1988. *Intimate Violence: The Causes and Consequences of Abuse in the American Family.* New York: Simon and Schuster.

Gise, L., and Paddison, P. 1988. Rape, sexual abuse and its victims. *Psychiatric Clinics of North America* 11:629–48.

Glaser, J. B., Schachter, J., Benes, S., Cummings, M., Frances, C. A., and McCormack, W. B. 1991. Sexually transmitted diseases in post pubertal female rape victims. *Journal of Infectious Diseases* 164:726–30.

Goldberg, W. G., and Tomlanovich, M. C. 1984. Domestic violence in the emergency department. *Journal of the American Medical Association* 251:3259–64.

Golding, J. M., et al. 1988. Sexual assault history and use of mental health services. *American Journal of Community Psychology* 16:625–44.

Haber, J. 1985. Abused women and chronic pain. *American Journal of Nursing* 85:1010–11.

Hamberger, L. K., Saunders, D. G., and Hovey, M. 1992. Prevalence of domestic violence in community practice and the role of physician inquiry. *Family Medicine* May-June:283–87.

Hendricks-Matthews, M. K. 1993. Survivors of abuse: health care issues. *Primary Care* 20:391–406.

Herman, J. L., Perry, J. C., and van der Kolk, B. A. 1989. Childhood traumas in borderline personality disorder. *American Journal of Psychiatry* 146:490–95.

Holtz, H., Hames, C., and Safran, M. 1989. Education about domestic violence in U.S. and Canadian medical schools, 1987–1988. *Morbidity and Mortality Weekly Report* 38:17–19.

Hotaling, G., and Finkelhor, D. 1988. *Family Abuse and Its Consequences: New Directions for Research*. Beverly Hills: Sage Publications.

Howard, F. M. 1993. The role of laparoscopy in chronic pelvic pain: promise and pitfalls. *Obstetrical and Gynecological Survey* 48:357–87.

Jaffe, P., Wolfe, D., Wilson, S., and Zak, L. 1986. Emotional and physical health problems of battered women. *Canadian Journal of Psychiatry* 31:625–28.

Jenny, C., et al. 1990. Sexually transmitted diseases in victims of rape. *New England Journal of Medicine* 322:713–16.

Kilpatrick, D. G., Resnick, P. A., and Veronen, L. J. 1981. Effects of a rape experience: a longitudinal study. *Journal of Social Issues* 37:105–22.

Kilpatrick, D. G., Veronen, L. J., and Best, C. L. 1985. Factors predicting psychological distress among rape victims. In C. R. Figley, ed., *Trauma and Its Wake: The Study and Treatment of Post-Traumatic Stress Disorder*. New York: Brunner/Mazel.

Klaus, P., and Rand, M. 1984. *Family Violence*. Bureau of Justice Statistics Special Report, U.S. Department of Justice. Washington, D.C.: U.S. Government Printing Office.

Koss, M. P. 1987. Rape Incidence and Prevalence: A Review and Assessment of the Data. Presented at the September 1987 National Institute of Mental Health conference: State of the Art in Sexual Assault Research, Charleston, S.C.

Koss, M. P., Koss, P. G., and Woodruff, W. J. 1991. Deleterious effects of criminal victimization on women's health and medical utilization. *Archives of Internal Medicine* 151:342–47.

Lazzaro, M. V., and McFarlane, J. 1991. Establishing a screening program for abused women. *Journal of Nursing Administration* October:24–29.

Leventhal, J. M. 1990. Epidemiology of child sexual abuse. In R. K. Oates, ed., *Understanding and Managing Child Sexual Abuse*. Sydney, Australia: W. B. Saunders.

Leventhal, J. M. 1988. Have there been changes in the epidemiology of sexual abuse of children during the 20th century? *Pediatrics* 82:766–73.

Lockhart, L. 1987. A re-examination of the effects of race and social class on the incidence of marital violence: a search for reliable differences. *Journal of Marriage and the Family* 49:603–10.

McCann, I. L., Sakheim, K. D., and Abrahamson, D. J. 1988. Trauma and victimization: a model of psychological adaptation. *Counseling Psychologist* 16:531–94.

Mackey, T., Sereika, S. M., Weissfeld, L. A., Hacker, S. S., Zender, J. F., and Heard, S. L. 1992. Factors associated with long-term depressive symptoms of sexual assault victims. *Archives of Psychiatric Nursing* February:10–25.

McLeer, S., Anwar, R., Herman, S., and Maquiling, K. 1989. Education is not enough: a system's failure in protecting battered women. *Annals of Emergency Medicine* 18:651–53.

Maguire, K., Pastore, A. L., and Flanagan, T. J., eds. 1993. *Sourcebook of Criminal Justice Statistics, 1992*. U.S. Department of Justice, Bureau of Justice Statistics. Washington, D.C.: U.S. Government Printing Office.

Martin, J. A., and Elmer, E. 1992. Battered children grown up: a follow-up study of individuals severely maltreated as children. *Child Abuse and Neglect* 16:75–87.

Miller, B. A., Downs, W. R., and Gondoh, D. M. 1989. Spousal violence among alcoholic women as compared to a random household sample of women. *Journal of Studies on Alcohol* 50:533–40.

Miller, J., et al. 1978. Recidivism among sexual assault victims. *American Journal of Psychiatry* 135:1103–4.

Mullen, P. E., Romans-Clarkson, S. E., Walton V. A., and Herbison, G. P. 1988. Impact of sexual and physical abuse on women's mental health. *Lancet* 1:841–45.

Murphy, S. M., et al. 1988. Rape victims' self-esteem: a longitudinal analysis. *Journal of Interpersonal Violence* 3:355–70.

National Research Council. 1993. *Understanding Child Abuse and Neglect*. Washington, D.C.: National Academy Press.

Oliver, J. E. 1993. Intergenerational transmission of child abuse: rates, research, and clinical interpretations. *American Journal of Psychiatry* September:1315–19.

Peters, A. A. W., van Dorst, E., Jellis, B., van Zuuren, E., Hermans, J., and Trimbos, J. B. 1991. A randomized clinical trial to compare two different approaches in women with chronic pelvic pain. *Obstetrics and Gynecology* 77:740–44.

Plichta, S. B. 1992. The effects of woman abuse on health care utilization and health status: a literature review. *Women's Health Issues* 2:154–63.

Plichta, S. B., Hoppe, B. M., Hirsch, E., and Weisman, C. S. 1993. The Invisible Factor: Violence in the Lives of Patients. Presented at the 121th Annual Meeting of the American Public Health Association, San Francisco.

Pribor, E. F., and Dinwiddie, S. H. 1992. Psychiatric correlates of incest in childhood. *American Journal of Psychiatry* 149:52–56.

Radloff, L. S. 1977. Centers for Disease Control Depression Scale (CES-D). *Applied Psychological Measurement.*

Rath, G. D., Jarratt, L. G., and Leonardson, G. 1989. Rates of domestic violence against adult women by men partners. *Journal of American Board of Family Practice* 2:227–33.

Reiter, R. C., and Gambone, J. C. 1990. Demographic and historic variables in women with idiopathic chronic pelvic pain. *Obstetrics and Gynecology* 75:428–32.

Rosenberg, A. 1965. *Society and the Adolescent Self-Image.* Princeton, N.J.: Princeton University Press.

Rosenberg, D. A., and Krugman, R. D. 1991. Epidemiology and outcome of child abuse. *Annual Review of Medicine* 42:217–24.

Russell, D. E. 1983. The incidence and prevalence of intrafamilial and extrafamilial sexual abuse of female children. *Child Abuse and Neglect* 7:133–46.

———. 1986. *The Secret Trauma.* New York: Basic Books.

Sapp, A. D., and Carter, D. L. 1978. *Child Abuse in Texas.* Houston: Sam Houston State University, College of Criminal Justice.

Saunders, B. E., Villeporteaux, L. A., Lipovsky, J. A., Kilpatrick, D. G., and Veronen, D. J. 1992. Child sexual assault as a risk factor for mental health disorders among women: a community survey. *Journal of Interpersonal Violence* 7:189–204.

Schei, B. 1990. Psychosocial factors in pelvic pain. *Acta Obstetrica Gynecologia Scandenavia* 69:67–71.

Schulman, M. A. 1979. *Survey of Spousal Violence against Women in Kentucky.* Harris Study #792701. Conducted for the Kentucky Commission on the Status of Women. Washington, D.C.: U.S. Government Printing Office.

Scott, C. S., Lefley, H. P., and Hicks, D. 1993. Potential risk factors for rape in three ethnic groups. *Community Mental Health Journal* 29:133–41.

Selvin, S. 1991. *Statistical Analysis of Epidemiological Data.* New York: Oxford University Press.

Shields, N., and Haneke, C. 1983. Battered wives' reaction to marital rape. In D. Finkelhor, ed., *The Dark Side of Family Violence.* Beverly Hills: Sage Publications.

Siegel, J. M., Sorenson, S. B., Golding, J. M., Burnam, M. A., and Stein, J. A. 1987. The prevalence of childhood sexual assault. *American Journal of Epidemiology* 126:1141–53.

Sorenson, S. B., Siegel, J. M., Golding, J. M., and Stein, J. A. 1991. Repeated sexual victimizations. *Violence and Victims* Winter:299–308.

Stark, E., Flitcraft, A., and Frazier, W. 1979. Medicine and patriarchal violence: the social construction of a private event. *International Journal of Health Services* 98:461–93.

Stenchever, M. A., and Stenchever, D. H. 1991. Abuse of women: an overview. *Women's Health Issues* 1:187–92.

Stewart, M. A., and deBlois, C. S. 1981. Wife abuse among families attending a child psychiatry clinic. *Journal of the American Academy of Child Psychiatry* 20:845–62.

Straus, M. A., and Gelles, R. J. 1986. Societal change and change in family violence from 1975 to 1985. *Journal of Marriage and the Family* 48:465–79.

Taylor, W. K., and Campbell, J. C. 1992. Treatment protocols for battered women. *Response to the Victimization of Women and Children* 14:10–21.

Telch, C., and Lindquist, C. 1984. Violent vs. non-violent couples: a comparison of patterns. *Psychotherapy* 21:242–48.

Terr, L. C. 1991. Childhood traumas: an outline and overview. *American Journal of Psychiatry* 148:10–20.

Teske, R., and Parker, M. 1983. *Spouse Abuse in Texas: A Study of Women's Attitudes and Experiences*. Houston: Criminal Justice Center, Sam Houston State University.

Tifft, L. L. 1993. *The Battering of Women*. Boulder, Colo.: Westview Press.

Tilden, V. P. 1989. Response of the health care delivery system to battered women. *Issues in Mental Health Nursing* 10:309–20.

U.S. Bureau of the Census. 1992. *Statistical Abstract of the United States, 1991*. 112th ed. Washington, D.C.: U.S. Government Printing Office.

Vanderschmidt, H. F., Lang, J. M., Knightwilliams, V., and Vanderschmidt, G. F. 1993. Risks among inner-city young teens: the prevalence of sexual activity, violence, drugs and smoking. *Journal of Adolescent Health* June: 282–88.

Waigandt, A., Wallace, D. L., Phelps, L., and Miller, D. A. 1990. The impact of sexual assault on physical health status. *Journal of Traumatic Stress* 3:93–102.

Walker, L. 1989. *The Battered Woman*. New York: Harper and Row.

Wyatt, G. E. 1985. The sexual abuse of Afro-American and white-American women in childhood. *Child Abuse and Neglect* 9:507–19.

Wyatt, G. E., and Newcomb, M. 1990. Internal and external mediators of women's sexual abuse in childhood. *Journal of Consulting and Clinical Psychology* 58:758–67.

IV

Socioeconomic Circumstances

10

Poverty, Access to Health Care, and Medicaid's Critical Role for Women

Barbara Lyons, M.H.S.
Alina Salganicoff, Ph.D.
Diane Rowland, Sc.D.

Millions of American women live in poverty today, and millions more struggle on the edge of poverty. Despite stereotypes to the contrary, a close examination of the characteristics of these women reveals an astonishingly diverse population. While limited income serves as a common thread, women are poor for a range of reasons. Some were born into poverty and have been poor all their lives. Many have not had access to the education and resources needed to enable them to leave poverty. Others are poor because current caregiving responsibilities limit their ability to participate in the workforce. Still others must cope with chronic disease and disabilities that limit their employment opportunities.

Economic and social issues may eclipse the immediacy of health issues faced by low-income women. Thus, it is impossible to consider this population group's health needs in isolation because factors affecting their health extend beyond common health policy boundaries. Such concerns as welfare, housing, education, and employment all relate to how health issues affect low-income women. Given the complexity of issues that these women face, health insurance coverage and access to the health care system are vital.

Low-income women rely on a patchwork of public and private funding to meet their varying health care needs. Medicaid, the federal–state means-tested health program, is the leading financier of health care services for poor women and their families and provides essential coverage for a broad range of health services, including pregnancy-related, reproductive, and preventive health care. The critical role of Medicaid for low-income women has grown over the past decade, largely because of federal eligibility expansions to cover more pregnant women and children. Policy choices that affect how this program is structured and financed are enormously important to the health of low-income women and their families. Despite Medicaid's prominent role as an insurer of low-income women millions of poor and near-poor women remain uninsured.

Because few poor women have private employer-based insurance coverage, exclusion from Medicaid generally translates into being un-insured. For these low-income women, access to health care services can be severely compromised. Because they lack the resources to ob-tain health care from the private sector, many of these women rely on publicly funded providers or programs for their medical care. Public hospitals, community and migrant health centers, Title X-funded fami-ly planning clinics, and Title V-funded maternal and child health pro-grams are indispensable sources of care for economically disadvan-taged women. Problems in gaining access to health care can result in postponing preventive care or early treatment of health problems, as well as in going without needed care. This lack of care can have serious consequences for low-income women.

This chapter draws on national survey data to profile the socio-economic characteristics of nonelderly low-income women, describe their health needs and access to health care, and examine the role of insurance coverage. Drawing on this analysis, the policy and research implications related to health care delivery and financing are then discussed, with a particular emphasis on the key role of Medicaid for adult women under age sixty-five. A substantial number of women age sixty-five or older also have low incomes, and face many problems with insurance coverage to supplement Medicare and with access to health care; however, a discussion of the health care issues facing older wom-en is beyond the scope of this essay.

DATA SOURCES AND METHODS OF ANALYSIS

Findings are based on analysis of two national databases and are repre-sentative of noninstitutionalized civilian adult women ages eighteen to sixty-four. The demographic profile and estimates of health insurance coverage are based on the analysis of the Current Population Survey (CPS) of March 1993. Conducted annually by the U.S. Bureau of the Census, the CPS provides nationally representative estimates of the noninstitutionalized civilian population living in the United States.[1] The survey included a sample of 11,712 women age eighteen to sixty-four years in 1992.

The health profile is based on analysis of The Commonwealth Fund survey. This telephone survey of 2,525 women was conducted in February and March 1993 and provides information on health status, use of health care services, and barriers to care. Data were weighted by age, race, education, insurance status, and Census region, utilizing March 1992 CPS as nationally representative. The sampling design and survey methods are detailed elsewhere (Harris and Associates 1993).

Among the 2,065 women ages eighteen to sixty-four who completed the survey, 111 did not report information on family income and are excluded from this analysis. These women differed si ;nificantly from the women who did report their income. They were more likely to be racial and ethnic minorities, unemployed, poorly educated, and older than the other group. In addition, they were in considerably poorer health and used fewer health services than the group that reported income. For analytic purposes, the remaining 1,954 women were grouped by their total 1992 household income level into two categories, poor/near-poor and nonpoor. The poor/near-poor category included 705 women and reflects family income below 200 percent of poverty, adjusted for family size based on Census Bureau poverty thresholds for 1992. The nonpoor sample consisted of 1,249 women with incomes at or above 200 percent of the federal poverty threshold.

RESULTS OF SURVEY ANALYSIS

One out of three American women falls in the low-income category. Among the nearly 80 million adult women ages eighteen to sixty-four living in the United States in 1992, analysis of the March 1993 Current Population Survey reveals that about 25 million had incomes under 200 percent of the poverty level (Kaiser Commission on the Future of Medicaid 1994). Of these, 11 million women were living on an income below 100 percent of the federal poverty level. (The federal poverty level in 1992 was set at $7,299 for a single individual under age sixty-five and $11,186 for a family of three.[2]) Another 13.5 million women are near-poor and live on the edge of poverty, with incomes between 100 percent and 200 percent of poverty. Thus, nearly one-third of American women live on limited incomes and regularly confront difficult choices in purchasing necessities for themselves and their families, such as food, housing, utilities, and clothing, in addition to health care services.

Poor women make up one-third of the total U.S. population under age sixty-five living in poverty, with children accounting for 45 percent and adult men the remaining 22 percent. But this statistic underestimates the impact of poverty on women by ignoring family relationships. Almost all poor families include women, whose lives are influenced not only by programs and policies that serve them, but also by those that affect their children and other members of their families.

Poverty disproportionately affects women compared with men. Poverty rates among women are 1.5 times those of men, with 14 percent of women living in poverty compared with 10 percent of men. The percentages of women and men who make up the near-poor (100–199% poverty) are equivalent. Although increasing numbers of women have been participating in the workforce, the number of women living in poverty and the poverty rates among women have been rising steadily (U.S. Bureau of the Census 1993, 1991a, 1991b).

The higher poverty rates among women reflect many factors related primarily to employment and family responsibilities. Women provide more caregiving for children and elderly parents; these obligations disrupt and limit employment (Clancy and Massion 1993; Piacentini and Foley 1992). As a consequence, women are less likely to be employed. When they are in the labor force, women hold jobs that are more apt to be part-time and low-wage. In addition, women are more likely to face discrimination in the workplace, earning less than men who hold similar positions. These differences in employment result in women having less access to health insurance through the workplace, as well as lower income levels and fewer economic opportunities than men.

SOCIODEMOGRAPHIC PROFILE

Age, family structure, racial/ethnic background, education, and work status are closely associated with the risk of women living in poverty. Younger women are particularly at risk for poverty. Among women ages eighteen to twenty-nine, 20 percent are poor and an additional 20 percent are near-poor. These are the years when many women first enter the labor market and often hold low-wage jobs or are enrolled in educational programs. In addition, many of these women are starting families and therefore may not be able to participate fully in the workforce. As women age, their poverty rates fall until they reach the fifty-five to sixty-four age range, when rates begin to rise. The increase in the poverty rate among this older group reflects increasing limitations in the ability to work because of a higher incidence of health problems, as well as income reductions resulting from the loss of a spouse through death, separation, or divorce.

Although poverty disproportionately affects younger women, poor women span all ages. Forty percent of poor women are under age thirty; 36 percent are between thirty and forty-four years of age (tab. 10.1). For these women in their childbearing years, access to reproductive health care services is fundamental. About one-quarter of non-elderly poor women (24%) are age forty-five or older. Many of these women may be poor because they are unable to work as a result of health problems and chronic conditions. Despite a greater incidence of breast and cervical cancer among these women, a number of studies have found that older women are less likely to receive preventive screening tests than younger women who are at lower risk (Hayward et al. 1988; Norman et al. 1991; Calle et al. 1993). Thus, the health needs of poor women are diverse, and coverage of health care services for poor women must extend beyond reproductive health needs.

Low educational levels are associated with an increased risk of living in poverty. One-third (34%) of women who have less than a high school education are poor, compared with 12 percent of those who completed high school and 8 percent of those with some college education. A number of studies also confirmed that low educational attainment is associated with a decreased likelihood of receiving timely preventive services such as Pap smears, clinical breast exams, and mammography (Hayward et al. 1988; Norman et al. 1991; Calle et al. 1993; Howe and Bzduch 1987). Because 40 percent of poor women and 27 percent of near-poor women have not completed high school, special efforts may be required to help these women identify health care needs, gain access to the health care system, and understand treatment alternatives and plans.

Being a member of a racial or ethnic minority is also associated with a higher risk of poverty. More than half of all African American (54%)

and all Hispanic (56%) women live on incomes less than 200 percent of poverty, compared with 25 percent of white women. Almost half (49%) of all poor women are members of racial and ethnic minority groups, in contrast to 18 percent of the nonpoor. A woman's race and ethnicity have been found to figure prominently in her risk of not having had such preventive services as Pap smears and mammographies (Hayward et al. 1988; Norman et al. 1991; Calle et al. 1993; Howe and Bzduch 1987). This diversity means that translation services and cultural competency issues are critical to ensuring low-income women access to health services.

Reflecting the younger age distribution of all poor women, almost half (56%) of poor women have children in the household and more than one-third (35%) head single-parent families. These women not only must care for their own health needs but also are usually the sole caregivers for their children. This responsibility can affect the use of health care services, as well as employment and income. For example, if a small child is sick or needs health care, the mother must arrange for care and may need time off from work. This can translate into lower earnings. Alternatively, if the woman herself needs care, she must either take her children with her or arrange for child care. Thus, obtaining health care can place an additional financial burden on women beyond the cost of medical care itself by forcing women to forgo earnings or purchase additional enabling services.

Despite common misperceptions, more than half (53%) of poor women live in households where someone is employed. At higher income levels, the likelihood of living in a working household increases to 84 percent of near-poor and 95 percent of nonpoor women. However, poor women are much less likely to live in households where the worker is fully employed than higher-income women. Only 16 percent of poor women and 54 percent of near-poor women live in a household with a full-time, full-year worker, compared with 83 percent of nonpoor women. Part-time and part-year work in service or seasonal industries is much more common among poor persons. This pattern of employment means that health insurance is much less likely to be available through the workplace or to be affordable for low-income women.

This profile of poor women reveals a population that is predominately young, poorly educated, and disproportionately made up of racial and ethnic minorities. Many low-income women are balancing multiple responsibilities—raising families and working. As a result of differences in the risk of poverty, low-income women are strikingly

Table 10.1. Characteristics of Women Eighteen to Sixty-four Years, by Poverty Level, 1992

	Poor (<100% Poverty)	Near-Poor (100–199% Poverty)	Nonpoor (200%+ Poverty)	Total
Age	100.0%	100.0%	100.0%	100.0%
18–29 years	40.3%	33.3%	24.0%	27.8%
30–44 years	36.0%	38.1%	41.0%	39.8%
45–54 years	11.6%	14.3%	20.9%	18.5%
55–64 years	12.2%	14.3%	14.2%	13.9%
Family Structure	100.0%	100.0%	100.0%	100.0%
Two parents, no children	10.2%	19.3%	40.1%	32.4%
Two parents, children	21.3%	36.7%	36.4%	34.4%
Single, no children	33.6%	27.7%	19.3%	22.7%
One parent, children	34.9%	16.3%	4.2%	10.6%
Employment	100.0%	100.0%	100.0%	100.0%
Full-time, full-year	15.6%	53.8%	83.4%	68.9%
Part-time or part-year	36.9%	29.8%	11.7%	18.3%
Not working	47.5%	16.4%	4.9%	12.8%
Insurance	100.0%	100.0%	100.0%	100.0%
Medicaid	44.8%	13.6%	1.7%	9.7%
Employer	8.9%	40.2%	78.5%	62.3%
Individual	9.7%	11.4%	9.2%	9.6%
Other	3.0%	4.6%	1.8%	2.4%
Uninsured	33.6%	30.2%	8.9%	16.0%
Total respondents (in millions)	79.4	11.1	13.5	54.8

Source: Data from the March 1993 Current Population Survey.

different from higher-income women in their racial and ethnic composition, family characteristics, and education. Their characteristics often compound their difficulty in getting care and mean that they have special needs and vulnerabilities that should be considered in meeting their care needs beyond the basic issue of lacking financial resources.

HEALTH INSURANCE COVERAGE

Insurance matters for all Americans, but it is especially important for those who lack the financial resources to purchase health care services directly. Health insurance is critical for low-income women and their families because it reduces financial barriers to care. The importance of health insurance coverage in increasing access to care among low-income populations is well documented in research literature (Weissman and Epstein 1994).

Health insurance coverage differs markedly between lower- and higher-income women. Low-income women are more than three times as likely to be uninsured as nonpoor women. About one-third of poor (34%) and near-poor (30%) women are uninsured, compared to 9 percent of women with incomes of 200 percent of poverty or greater. Poor and near-poor populations who are without health insurance coverage are less likely to obtain health care services, including preventive and primary care, than those with higher incomes.

Medicaid plays a critical role for low-income women, particularly among the poor. Almost half (45%) of poor women and 14 percent of near-poor women are covered by Medicaid. Medicaid's restrictive categorical and income eligibility criteria, however, leave many of the poorest and most vulnerable women outside its safety net (Rowland et al. 1991). Medicaid coverage is usually available only to women receiving cash assistance through Aid to Families with Dependent Children (AFDC) or to low-income pregnant women. The eligibility thresholds for AFDC vary enormously across states, ranging from 16 percent of the federal poverty level in Alabama to 72 percent in Alaska. The national average for AFDC eligibility is 42 percent of poverty or $5,231 for a family of three. Currently, states are required to cover pregnant women up to 133 percent of poverty, and thirty-four states have extended coverage to pregnant women at higher income levels (National Governors' Association 1994). Although coverage of pregnancy-related services is critically important to the health of a woman and her baby, Medicaid coverage for the woman ceases shortly after childbirth unless she becomes eligible for AFDC. Women without children are generally ineligible for Medicaid, regardless of how poor they are, unless they are disabled.

A small number of women are eligible for Medicaid coverage because they are disabled and qualify for assistance under the federal Supplementary Security Income (SSI) program, which is also a means-tested categorical program. Because SSI is a federal program, there is little variability in the financial criteria used to determine eligibility across states. To qualify for SSI, nonelderly women must be blind or disabled, and only those with severe physical or mental impairments and who meet the financial criteria are eligible.

For poor women, employer-provided health insurance is a minor source of coverage. Only 9 percent of poor women have employer-based coverage. This is not surprising, given the lower levels of workforce attachment among the poor population. The role of employer coverage increases to 40 percent among near-poor women and 78 percent among nonpoor women, reflecting stronger family attachments to the workforce.

About 10 percent of poor and 11 percent of near-poor women purchase individual private health insurance. These policies are frequently expensive, are less comprehensive than group insurance, and may represent a economic hardship for low-income women. The poor women who are covered by these policies are often still at risk for many out-of-pocket expenses and higher financial burdens.

Thus, the health insurance picture for low-income women is quite mixed. Some have coverage through Medicaid, but eligibility is linked to receipt of welfare or pregnancy; and others have private health insurance. However, one-third of low-income women have no insurance coverage and are vulnerable to significant financial risk if a health care problem arises.

HEALTH PROFILE

Poverty has long been associated with greater incidence of health problems and greater need for health care services. Across a wide range of health measures, poor and near-poor women are sicker and more likely to have disabilities than their nonpoor counterparts. These health problems can adversely affect quality of life, limit employment opportunities, and severely strain the limited financial and social resources of low-income women and their families.

The Commonwealth Fund survey provides important information on how the health of economically disadvantaged women differs from that of their more affluent counterparts. Self-reported health status provides a generally accurate overall gauge of the many dimensions of health and well-being. Low-income women are more than twice as likely to rate their health as fair or poor as are higher-income women. Among the poor and near-poor, 19 percent of women reported fair or poor health, compared with 8 percent of the nonpoor (fig. 10.1). Self-reported poorer health status is associated with greater need for and use of health care services.

Poor and near-poor women are consistently more likely to experi-

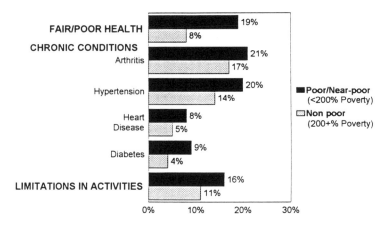

Fig. 10.1. Percentage of Women Ages Eighteen to Sixty-four Years Reporting Selected Health Problems, by Poverty Level, 1993
Source: Analysis of The Commonwealth Fund survey on women's health, 1993.

ence chronic health conditions than more affluent women. About one in five low-income women has arthritis or hypertension (fig. 10.1). Nearly one in ten reported heart disease or diabetes. Because many of these conditions require ongoing monitoring by health care providers and treatment with prescription drugs, low-income women need assistance to pay for medical care and prescription drugs.

Low-income women are also more likely than women with higher incomes to report that a disability, handicap, or chronic disease keeps them from participating fully in school, work, housework, or other activities. Sixteen percent of poor and near-poor women reported these limitations, compared with 11 percent of those who are nonpoor (fig. 10.1). Women with disabilities also require assistance to obtain home health care, medical supplies, and long-term care. It is worth noting that gender disparities in income are also found among the populations with disabilities. Women with disabilities have considerably lower mean earnings than their disabled male counterparts. In fact, men with work disabilities have higher mean annual incomes than able-bodied women (Hooley et al. 1992).

Given the financial and social difficulties and health problems low-income women face, it is not surprising to find a relationship between socioeconomic factors and mental health. Low-income women are disproportionately more likely to show evidence of mental health problems and distress. Eighteen percent of poor and near-poor women indicated that they had experienced anxiety or depression, compared with 14 percent of nonpoor women (fig. 10.2).[3]

Low self-esteem is also pervasive among low-income women. One-quarter of poor and near-poor women reported experiencing problems with low self-esteem, compared with 12 percent of nonpoor women.[4] Poor and near-poor women are also more likely to report that they have had suicidal thoughts during the past year and are twice as likely to report that they are not as satisfied as nonpoor women with their lives. These findings highlight the importance of mental health services to low-income women and are consistent with other research showing that women enduring economic and social difficulties are at higher risk for mental health problems (Belle 1990). This research shows that poor women have greater difficulty fulfilling social roles, have less control over life events and their environments, and experience severe constraints on coping strategies. The social problems faced by low-income women compound their health care needs.

ACCESS TO HEALTH CARE

Many of the disparities in access to health care between poor persons and those with higher incomes have diminished in recent years, largely because of Medicaid and other publicly funded health programs.

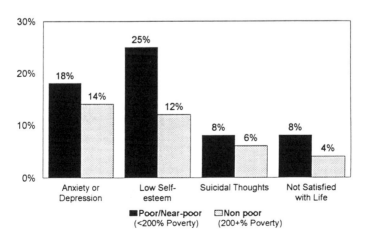

Fig. 10.2. Percentage of Women Ages Eighteen to Sixty-four Years with Selected Mental Health Concerns, by Poverty Level, 1993

Source: Analysis of The Commonwealth Fund survey on women's health, 1993.

However, nearly three decades after the start of the War on Poverty in the mid-1960s, income-related inequalities in access still persist. Access to health care is also influenced by a broad range of factors, including, but not limited to, the availability, affordability, and accessibility of health care services. Given the greater physical and mental health needs of the low-income population, poor and near-poor women should need more health care. Analysis of The Commonwealth Fund survey data, however, reveals that across a range of measures—such as the use of physician services and preventive care—low-income women still generally use less care and face considerably more barriers to care than those with greater financial resources.

The use of physician services is commonly viewed as a broad indicator of achieved access to care or, in other words, entry into the health care system. Despite greater health problems and need for care, low-income women are twice as likely as higher-income women to report that they made no visits to the physician during the past year (tab. 10.1). Twelve percent of poor and near-poor women made no physician visits in the past year, compared with 6 percent of higher-income women. Among the low-income population, the critical role of insurance coverage is evident. Women without insurance, particularly those who are poor or near-poor, are considerably more likely to go without medical care than their publicly and privately insured low-income counterparts. About 5 percent of low-income women on Medicaid and 10 percent of those with private insurance coverage made no physician visits during the past year, compared with 22 percent of uninsured low-income women.

Once they enter the health care system, low-income women appear to make slightly more physician visits than others. Among women with at least one physician visit, low-income women had 6.7 mean annual visits, compared with 6.2 annual visits for nonpoor women. It is difficult to gauge, however, the quality or appropriateness of the care they receive or whether their use is commensurate with their need for care.

The differences in the levels of use among the poor population again highlight the vital role of insurance, particularly among those with limited incomes. Uninsured low-income women use considerably less care, even after gaining entry into the system, than those with Medicaid or private insurance. Women with Medicaid coverage made 8.4 mean annual visits and privately insured women made an average of 6.4 visits, compared with 6.0 for uninsured women. The differences by type of insurance coverage are largely attributable to Medicaid policy with regard to eligibility and coverage. Recent modifications of Medicaid eligibility levels have increased coverage to large numbers of pregnant women, who tend to be high users of physician care. In addition, women who are medically needy or disabled—categorical Medicaid eligibility groups—are by definition high users of care. Medicaid also permits providers to charge only nominal amounts of co-payments. In contrast, many private insurance policies can have high deductible charges and co-payment levels that are financially burdensome to low-income women.

In addition to assessing the level of use of medical care, there are other ways of gauging access to the health system. A strong predictor of access to care has been the presence of a primary care provider or a usual source of care. Higher levels of provider–patient continuity, which can lead to better quality of care and higher levels of patient satisfaction, have been found to be associated with having a usual source of care (Starfield 1992). In 1993, 80 percent of nonpoor and 79 percent of low-income women reported that they have a usual source of care (tab. 10.1).

Although in aggregate there appear to be few differences by income in the percentage of women with a usual source of care, a closer examination reveals that within the low-income population, those who are uninsured face more barriers than those with Medicaid or private insurance. Low-income women who have Medicaid coverage are the most likely to have a usual source of care. Among poor and near-poor women, 85 percent of those with Medicaid reported a usual source of care, compared with 80 percent of those with private insurance and 69 percent of those who were uninsured (tab. 10.2).

Having a regular source of care is also associated with increased use of key preventive services. Preventive services like Pap smears and mammography are among the most important precautions women can take to prevent or reduce their chances of mortality from breast cancer or invasive cervical cancer. Guidelines issued by the American Cancer Society (1992) recommend that women begin to have regular Pap smears at age eighteen or when they become sexually active, whichever is earlier, and continue throughout adulthood. Mammography, along with clinical breast exams, improves breast cancer survival through the detection of malignant tumors at early stages.

Despite increases in the use of these preventive services in recent years, income-related gaps in use persist (Makuc et al. 1989). Low-

Table 10.2. Use of Health Care Services by Women Ages Eighteen to Sixty-four Years, by Poverty Level and Insurance, 1993

	Poor/Near-Poor (<200% of Poverty)				Nonpoor (200% + of Poverty)
	Private	Medicaid	Uninsured	Total	Total
No physician visits	9.9%	5.4%	21.7%	12.1%	6.4%
Usual source of care	79.8%	84.6%	68.9%	77.9%	79.5%
Pap smear in past year	66.8%	71.8%	46.7%	62.2%	74.4%
Clinical breast exam	64.0%	65.3%	43.3%	58.6%	74.8%
Mammography[a]	49.0%	54.2%	39.3%	47.0%	67.8%
Mean annual number of physician visits for users	6.4	8.4	6.0	6.7	6.2
Total respondents (unweighted)	1,617	214	228	705	1,249

Source: Data from The Commonwealth Fund survey on women's health, 1993.

Note: Percentages are calculated based on weighted sample to reflect national distribution.

[a] Women fifty to sixty-four years.

income women are less likely to have received a Pap smear, clinical breast exam, or mammogram during the past year than those with higher incomes (tab. 10.1). Approximately 62 percent of low-income women between ages eighteen and sixty-four years reported having a Pap smear during the past year and 59 percent reported having a clinical breast exam conducted by a health care provider in the past year. In contrast, 75 percent of nonpoor women reported receiving the same services. Among women fifty to sixty-four, for whom yearly mammograms are recommended (American Cancer Society 1992), only half (47%) of poor and near-poor women reported receiving the service in the past year, compared with two-thirds (68%) of nonpoor women. The use of preventive services is related to having a regular source of care, knowledge that services are available, and financial ability or insurance coverage to pay for services (Collins et al. 1994).

Lack of insurance coverage deters the use of preventive services for all women, but particularly for low-income women. Within the low-income population, women on Medicaid are most likely to have had clinical breast exams or Pap smears, with uninsured women lagging behind. Among poor and near-poor women, 65 percent of Medicaid beneficiaries and 64 percent of those with private insurance had a breast exam during the past year, compared with 43 percent of those without insurance. Similarly, 72 percent of those with Medicaid, 67 percent of those with private insurance, and 47 percent of those with no insurance reported having a Pap smear in the past year. The greater incidence of these preventive services among the Medicaid population could be due to the comprehensive coverage of health care services Medicaid affords to those whom it covers. In contrast, many private insurance plans do not extend coverage of preventive services to policy holders, forcing them to pay for services directly or to go without care.

In addition to examining the differences in the rates of access to the health care system, it is critical to assess the degree to which women are unable to obtain health care services that they believe they need. Low-income women generally are not only less likely to get care but also more likely to report that they postponed or delayed care that they feel was needed. Almost one-quarter (23%) of poor and near-poor women indicated that they did not get needed medical care during the past year, compared with 10 percent of nonpoor women. When asked why they did not get needed care, prohibitive cost was the leading reason given. Nearly two-thirds (61%) of low-income women who reported they went without needed medical care responded that the care costs too much, compared with 39 percent of higher-income women. One-quarter of low-income women reported that they did not get needed care because it was not covered by their insurance, a slightly lower rate than that of nonpoor women (30%). Poor women are less likely to have private health insurance; therefore, coverage issues are less relevant to them.

IMPLICATIONS FOR POLICY

The results of this analysis reveal that low-income women experience multiple and interrelated economic, health, and social vulnerabilities. In many cases these problems reflect limited education, lack of paid employment or work in low-paying jobs, difficulties in securing child care, and poor health status. Compounding these problems, insurance coverage is uneven, inadequate, or absent, and access to health care and the use of health services by low-income women lag behind that of higher-income women, despite their greater health needs. These gaps are serious, creating barriers to appropriate care and leading to adverse health consequences.

The Role of Medicaid for Low-Income Women

Because low-income women have limited access to employer-based insurance and cannot afford to purchase private individual policies, they are highly dependent on public coverage through Medicaid. Expanded to fill gaps in the private market, Medicaid is the predominant source of insurance coverage for poor women and is an important source for near-poor women.

Medicaid plays several important roles for low-income women. The program serves as a primary source of coverage for women receiving cash assistance through AFDC, as a predominant source of pregnancy-related coverage for poor and near-poor women, and as a safety net for women with disabilities covered by SSI.

Medicaid's coverage of women receiving AFDC has been enormously important. Today, millions of low-income women receive AFDC and, therefore, are eligible for Medicaid. This coverage provides a comprehensive set of health care services. It has been instrumental in ensuring that very poor women have access to health care services and that their health expenses do not consume income needed for their family's basic living expenses.

The role of Medicaid in pregnancy-related care has increased substantially during the past decade as a result of federal and state efforts to expand coverage to women whose incomes are above AFDC levels. One-third of all deliveries in this country are paid for by Medicaid, and 80 percent of pregnant women who are poor and one-third of those who are near-poor have Medicaid coverage (Holahan et al. 1995). Expanded eligibility, coupled with simplified enrollment and expanded outreach efforts, have served to improve coverage and access to prenatal care for pregnant women (U.S. General Accounting Office 1991; Piper, Mitchell, and Ray 1994).

For low-income nonelderly women with disabilities, Medicaid is an insurer of health care, covering basic medical services and long-term care. Medicaid provides this coverage for individuals eligible for SSI benefits, and it is particularly important for low-income women with AIDS, chronic mental health problems, and other severe disabilities. Many of these women have complex health and medical needs. Often they have fallen through the cracks in the private insurance system and have turned to Medicaid as a last resort.

Medicaid is important to low-income women, not only for their own coverage but also in its coverage of their children. Today, Medicaid covers

80 percent of poor children and one-quarter of near-poor children (Holahan et al. 1995). Its coverage of children is comprehensive, providing access to services for children and financial protection for the family.

For Medicaid-eligible women, a comprehensive set of services has been available with little or no cost sharing. Although problems persist related to provider participation in the program, Medicaid has greatly improved access to health care services for low-income women.

Despite Medicaid's accomplishments, the program is not without limitations. The combination of financial and categorical eligibility restrictions that have characterized Medicaid since its inception continue to place a stranglehold on the program's effectiveness. Despite significant federal and state expansions of eligibility for Medicaid over the past decade, eligibility policy is not always consistent with effective public health and policy objectives.

The focus of Medicaid coverage—pregnant or very poor women with families receiving welfare—leaves gaps in coverage and creates barriers to coordinated and comprehensive care. Women who fall outside Medicaid's eligibility categories or who have family incomes just above AFDC levels are typically excluded from Medicaid, regardless of health needs, and are at great risk for being uninsured. For example, a woman who is not pregnant and has no children is not eligible for Medicaid assistance, unless she is disabled. This policy creates difficulties for older low-income women, who have not yet reached age sixty-five when they automatically become eligible for Medicare. Many of these women may be developing chronic conditions and have health care needs that could benefit from medical care, but cannot afford private insurance premiums or direct payments for health care services.

In addition, Medicaid's coverage of low-income women continues to vary enormously by state and across eligibility categories. This stands in the way of simplifying eligibility and improving program participation. Moreover, these eligibility categories and income levels cause many women to move on and off Medicaid coverage over relatively short periods of time. This lack of continuous coverage creates tremendous obstacles for low-income women in obtaining comprehensive and coordinated care, and for their health care providers.

Loss of Medicaid coverage places women and their families at enormous financial risk for health expenses. This policy creates tremendous disincentives to poor women to increase earning levels above Medicaid eligibility thresholds and is inconsistent with efforts to reform the welfare system. An additional failure in the current system is that, among poor persons, those who are working run the greatest risk of not having insurance. Low-income women in working households are three times more likely to be uninsured than those at higher income levels.

Health Insurance Coverage of Low-Income Women

One in three low-income women is uninsured. Lack of insurance among low-income women is associated with diminished access to health care across a broad range of indicators, including having a regular source of care, access to physician and other medical services, and use of preventive care. These findings corroborate those of other studies, which found lower levels of use among the low-income population and that insurance plays a critical role in improving access to care, particularly for low-income populations (Institute of Medicine 1993).

Health insurance coverage is important because it reduces financial barriers to health care. Low-income women are likely to have fewer discretionary dollars to spend after providing basic necessities for themselves or their families. Thus, the cost of health care services is much more likely to affect women at lower income levels and can create serious access problems. The Commonwealth Fund survey found that financial factors are the foremost reason cited by low-income women for not getting needed care. While other factors, such as health-seeking behaviors, racism, the availability of providers, and patient health knowledge, may also influence access, health insurance is absolutely essential because low-income women do not have the financial means to pay for care directly.

Medicaid has been the primary vehicle used to expand coverage for low-income women. The program continues to be an essential source of financing, particularly for pregnant women and mothers. Budgetary pressures facing the program may, however, jeopardize the program's coverage of low-income women. In addition, many women remain outside the reach of Medicaid or private insurance. Private insurance is unaffordable to low-income women because of high premiums and the typical benefit package often does not meet the complex health needs of low-income women.

The Scope of Health Services for Low-Income Women

The greater incidence and prevalence of a wide range of health problems among low-income women highlight the importance of covering a broad range of health care services, including preventive services, medical care, and mental health services. Policy makers have increasingly recognized the value of covering preventive services and over the past decade there has been an increase in the coverage and use of services, such as Pap smears and mammograms. However, many low-income women still do not receive these services at recommended rates. Delaying or forgoing preventive care can have serious, adverse health consequences.

Although the importance of preventive care and other medical benefits, such as physician and hospital care, are recognized, other services are also critical to enable low-income women to gain access to care. Important enabling services typically include help with translation, transportation, and child care. Education and outreach efforts are necessary to inform low-income women about health care issues and to promote greater compliance with treatment plans. In addition, providers need to be culturally competent and aware of the multiple dimensions of the health problems facing low-income women.

An important finding of The Commonwealth Fund survey is the higher incidence of mental health problems among low-income women. Lack of economic resources places low-income women at risk for psychological difficulties. Problems such as low self-esteem, anxiety, depression, and suicidal thoughts can complicate health needs and create serious family, social, and employment issues. Access to mental health services is, therefore, an important component of comprehensive coverage for poor and near-poor women.

Also less readily appreciated are the needs of poor women with chronic health conditions and functional limitations. For these women, health needs extend far beyond mammographies and Pap smears. Case management and support with health and social needs are critical to improve the quality of life for these low-income women.

Uncovered services, whether medical or enabling, can be financially prohibitive for low-income women. For them, the comprehensiveness of the health insurance benefit package is crucial. These women do not have the financial resources to draw on to pay directly for care that is not covered.

In addition, particular care must be taken to ensure that cost-sharing levels are not excessive. Even nominal cost-sharing levels can create barriers to care or strain the ability of low-income women to meet other essential living expenses for themselves and their families.

The Implications of the Rapidly Evolving Health Care System for Low-Income Women

Given the greater health care needs and lack of income among poor and near-poor women, how health care is structured and delivered is of critical importance to low-income women. In the absence of reform at the federal level, states are aggressively seeking major restructuring of health care services for their low-income populations (Rosenbaum and Darnell 1995). Typically, these programs offer simplified and broadened eligibility to expand coverage for the uninsured population previously excluded from Medicaid. These expansions are financed in part through projected cost savings obtained by the increased use of managed care and payments by near-poor beneficiaries.

Depending on how these programs are structured and financed, the potential exists to improve longstanding gaps in insurance coverage and access to care. However, careful attention to how these changes affect low-income women previously eligible for Medicaid and newly eligible for coverage is needed. Careful evaluation of these demonstrations will be needed to assess whether coverage and access to care for low-income women is improved or diminished.

Facing enormous pressure to control spending, many state Medicaid programs are turning to managed care to expand access and control spending. The number of Medicaid beneficiaries enrolled in managed care doubled from 1993 to 1994, reaching nearly 8 million (Rowland et al. 1995). Because most of these enrollees are women and their children, these organizational changes in the delivery system have important implications for low-income women.

The increasing use of managed care for the Medicaid population has potential benefits as well as drawbacks. The concept of managed care holds the promise of improving access to care—if appropriately implemented, administered, and monitored. By ensuring that beneficiaries have a primary care provider responsible for coordinating care, we could improve access and quality. However, in some cases these changes may cause substantial disruption of traditional care patterns for both routine and specialty services, with positive or negative implications for access and the quality of care. The effect of these new constraints on health status is largely unknown. In addition, financial incentives offered to plans and providers should be monitored closely to ensure that they do not result in underservice to beneficiaries.

Of particular importance to low-income women is how reproductive, mental health, and specialty services are handled by managed care plans. Important questions include assessing whether providers are adequately trained in determining when these services are appropriate and whether low-income women who need these services are able to access them.

In sum, insurance coverage issues are vitally important to the health and economic well-being of low-income women and their families. Addressing the gaps in health coverage among low-income women is a policy priority. Expansions of eligibility for Medicaid over the past decade have expanded coverage to many low-income women and children and have undoubtedly slowed the growth in the number of Americans without insurance. Efforts to eliminate gaps in coverage and to provide a comprehensive benefit package for low-income women should continue. The important gains that have been made under Medicaid need to be safeguarded in an era of budget constraints.

ACKNOWLEDGMENTS

We would like to express appreciation to Li-Yu Huang, Lois Simon, and Marguerite Ro for their research assistance.

NOTES

1. A detailed description of the 1993 Current Population Survey is presented in U.S. Bureau of the Census (1993).

2. Poverty levels are updated every year to reflect changes in the Consumer Price Index. The poverty definition used by the Bureau of the Census is based on pretax money income only, excluding capital gains, and does not include the value of noncash benefits such as employer-provided health insurance, food stamps, or Medicaid.

3. Respondents were asked how often they experienced six symptoms of depression in the past week (felt depressed, had restless sleep, enjoyed life, had crying spells, felt sad, felt disliked). Each frequency level was assigned a numerical score ranging from 0 to 3 (0 = never; 1 = rarely, 2 = some of the time, 3 = most of the time). A total score was created by adding the frequency level for each item. Scores could range from 0 to 18. "Low" depressive symptoms is defined as scores 0–2; "low moderate" is defined as scores 3–5; "moderate" is defined as scores 6–11; "high or major" is defined as scores 12–18.

4. The Rosenberg Self-Esteem Scale, from *Measures of Psychological Attitudes, 1991*, was used. Respondents were read ten statements regarding self-esteem.

A 4-point ordinal scale of agreement/disagreement was used. Based on the score distribution, respondents with scores of 0–21 were assigned to the "low" category, 22–26 to the "moderate" category, and 27–30 to the "high" category.

REFERENCES

Aday, L. A., Andersen, R., and Fleming, G. 1980. *Health Care in the U.S.: Equitable for Whom?* Beverly Hills: Sage Publications.

American Cancer Society. 1992. *Cancer Facts and Figures, 1992.* Atlanta.

Belle, D. 1990. Poverty and women's health. *American Psychologist* 45:385–89.

Calle, E., Flanders, W., Thun, M., and Martin, L. 1993. Demographic predictors of mammogram and Pap smear screening in the U.S. *Journal of the American Public Health Association* 83:53–60.

Clancy, C. M., and Massion, C. T. 1993. American women's health care: a patchwork quilt with gaps. *Journal of the American Medical Association* 268:1918–20.

Collins, K. S., Rowland, D., Salganicoff, A., and Chait, E. 1994. Assessing and improving women's health. In C. Costello and A. J. Stone, eds., *The American Woman, 1994–1995: Where Do We Stand?* New York: W. W. Norton Co.

Harris, Louis, and Associates. 1993. *The Health of American Women.* Conducted for the Commonwealth Fund.

Hayward, R. A., et al. 1988. Who gets screened for cervical and breast cancer? *Archives of Internal Medicine* 148:1177–81.

Holahan, J., Winterbottom, C., and Rajan, S. 1995. The Changing Composition of Health Insurance Coverage in the United States. Background report prepared for the Kaiser Commission on the Future of Medicaid: Washington, D.C.

Hooley, J., Riley, T., and Hazard, E. 1992. *Familiar Faces: A Status of America's Vulnerable Populations: A Chartbook.* Portland, Maine: Center for Vulnerable Populations.

Howe, H. L., and Bzduch, H. 1987. Recency of Pap smear screening: a multivariate model. *Public Health Reports* 102:295–301.

Institute of Medicine. 1993. *Access to Health Care in America.* Washington, D.C.: National Academy Press.

Kaiser Commission on the Future of Medicaid. 1994. Unpublished analysis of the March 1993 Current Population Survey.

Makuc, D., et al. 1989. National trends in the use of preventive health care by women. *American Journal of Public Health* 79:21–29.

National Governors' Association. 1994. State coverage of pregnant women and children. *MCH Update.* Washington, D.C.: National Governors' Association.

Norman, S. A., et al. 1991. Demographics, psychosocial, and medical correlates of Pap testing: a literature review. *American Journal of Preventive Medicine* 7:219–26.

Piacentini, J., and Foley, J. 1992. *EBRI Databook on Employee Benefits*. 2nd ed. Washington, D.C.: Employee Benefits Research Institute.

Piper, J., Mitchell, E., and Ray, W. 1994. Presumptive eligibility for pregnant Medicaid enrollees: its effects on prenatal care and perinatal outcome. *American Journal of Public Health* 84:1626–30.

Rosenbaum, S., and Darnell, J. 1995. *Medicaid Section 1115 Demonstration Waivers: Approved and Proposed Activities as of July 1995*. Report prepared for the Kaiser Commission on the Future of Medicaid, Washington, D.C.

Rowland, D., Feder, J., Lyons, B., and Salganicoff, A. 1991. *Medicaid at the Crossroads*. A report of the Kaiser Commission on the Future of Medicaid, Baltimore, Md.

Rowland, D., Rosenbaum, S., Simon, L., and Chait, E. 1995. *Medicaid and Managed Care: Lessons from the Literature*. A report of the Kaiser Commission on the Future of Medicaid, Washington, D.C.

Starfield, B. 1992. *Primary Care: Concept, Evaluation and Policy*. New York: Oxford University Press.

U.S. Bureau of the Census, Current Population Reports. 1991a. *Poverty in the United States, 1988 and 1989*. Series P-171. Washington, D.C.: U.S. Government Printing Office.

———. 1991b. *Poverty in the United States, 1990*. Series P-175. Washington, D.C.: U.S. Government Printing Office.

———. 1993. *Poverty in the United States, 1992*. Series P-185. Washington, D.C.: U.S. Government Printing Office.

U.S. General Accounting Office. 1991. *Prenatal Care: Early Success in Enrolling Women Made Eligible by Medicaid Expansions*. Washington, D.C.: U.S. Government Printing Office.

Weissman, A., and Epstein. 1994. *Falling Through the Safety Net: Insurance Status and Access to Care*. Baltimore: Johns Hopkins University Press.

11

Employment and Women's Health

Heidi I. Hartmann, Ph.D.
Joan A. Kuriansky, J.D.
Christine L. Owens, J.D.

In the past several decades, more and more women in the United States have joined the labor force, raising many questions about the immediate and long-term consequences of employment in the lives of women. This chapter discusses the relationship between employment and the general health of women. This relationship has two dimensions. First is the role of employment in providing health insurance, which in turn governs access to health care. Because insurance is the focus of another chapter, here we look more closely at the second dimension—the question of whether working women are healthier women.

Thirty years ago, when women entered the workforce in rapidly increasing numbers, the impact of women's employment on their families began to draw the attention of researchers (Voydanoff 1987). More recently, the emphasis has shifted to the interplay between the health of the women themselves and a variety of factors, such as employment, marital status, and motherhood. The studies have consistently found that working women are healthier than nonworkers, reporting less chronic illness, fewer limitations on their activity, fewer doctor's visits, and better overall health status (Nathanson 1980; Waldron 1980; Verbrugge 1982). Conversely, women with higher incidences of health problems or who rate their health as poor are less likely to join the workforce, or, if employed, to remain in the workforce (Voydanoff 1987).

One of the most comprehensive studies of the relationship between women's health and each of three social roles (employment, marriage, and parenthood) was the National Health Interview Survey (NHIS) for the years 1964–65 and 1977–78 (Verbrugge and Madans 1985). For virtually every indicator of health status, employed women were healthier than nonworkers. Employed women had fewer restricted activity and disability days, experienced lower rates of long-term limitations, and assessed their own health status more favorably than nonworkers. While African American women had less favorable health profiles than white women, workers of both races were healthier than nonworkers in their race groups. The authors also examined the multiple roles of women as employees, wives, and mothers to determine which roles or combinations of roles correlate with good health. They concluded that for all women, the employment variable was most strongly and consistently tied to good health.

A subsequent analysis using more recent NHIS data reached the same conclusion (Anson and Anson 1987). In testing their hypothesis that transitions into and out of the workforce are associated with differences in health status, the authors found that: (1) respondents with the strongest and most continuous attachment to the labor force were the healthiest; (2) the next healthiest respondents were recent entrants into the workforce; (3) the health conditions of unemployed women and women voluntarily out of the workforce a year or more were comparable to each other, but both groups were less healthy than employed women; and (4) least healthy of all were women who had recently left the labor force. The authors concluded that transition into and out of the workforce is related to women's health status.

Other researchers have hypothesized that the relationship between employment and health is governed by specific job attributes, as well as workers' actual preferences to work (Verbrugge 1985; Voydanoff 1987). One such study measured the relationship between three indicators of health status and three job descriptor indexes (social support/integration from work, intrinsic qualities such as challenge and variety, and occupational status) (Hibbard and Pope 1987). For women, a positive correlation was found between occupational status and social support/integration and all three health indicators. In contrast, a study of older male and female workers and retirees found that job attributes were relatively unimportant in predicting the health of respondents (Herzog, House, and Nelson 1991). Another study found that midlife women who worked reported better health than full-time homemakers (Adelmann et al. 1989).

APPROACH TO ANALYSES

In general, the data analyses that follow paint a similar picture of the connection between employment status and health condition for women included in The Commonwealth Fund survey. Respondents were asked a host of questions about their health status and health insurance coverage, as well as their employment status. Nonworking respondents were asked whether they would prefer to work. When the overall health conditions of workers and nonworkers are compared, our analysis shows that, on the whole, employed women are healthier than nonworkers. (The term *nonworkers*, as used here, includes unemployed persons who wish to work but cannot find jobs, those who may prefer to work but have not been looking, and those who are not working by choice.) In general, this finding is consistent with other research studies.

Table 11.1. Characteristics of the Sample Population: Working and Nonworking Women (all ages)

		Working Women			Nonworking Women
	Total	All	Full-Time	Part-Time	
Age[a]					
18–29	23%	27%	27%	29%	17%
30–39	23	29	30	26	15
40–49	18	23	25	19	11
50–64	18	16	17	16	20
65+	18	4	2	10	38
Total	100%	100%	101%	100%	101%
Race/ethnicity[b]					
White	79%	78%	78%	78%	80%
African American	12	12	13	11	12
Latina	8	8	7	9	7
Asian and other	1	2	2	2	1
Total	100%	100%	100%	100%	100%
Marital status					
Single	18%	22%	22%	21%	13%
Divorced/separated	13	16	19	8	9
Married	55	57	55	63	53
Widowed	14	5	4	9	25
Total	100%	100%	100%	100%	100%

(*continued*)

Table 11.1. (*Continued*)

		Working Women			Nonworking Women
	Total	All	Full-Time	Part-Time	
Educational attainment[c]					
Less than high school	21%	12%	9%	19%	33%
High school	37	37	37	39	38
Some college	19	21	21	21	15
College+	23	30	33	22	14
Total	100%	100%	100%	100%	100%
Family income					
<$15,000	27%	17%	15%	22%	41%
$15,001–$50,000	45	54	56	47	34
$50,001+	19	25	26	22	11
Don't know	9	5	3	9	15
Total	100%	100%	100%	100%	101%
Health insurance coverage[d]					
With health insurance	88%	87%	88%	86%	88%
No health insurance	12	13	12	14	12
Total	100%	100%	100%	100%	100%
Sample size[e]	2,525	1,442	1,044	399	1,056
Percentage of total sample	100%	57%	41%	16%	42%

Source: Data from The Commonwealth Fund survey on women's health, 1993.

[a] Age: frequency missing = 14.

[b] Race/ethnicity: frequency missing = 15.

[c] Educational level: frequency missing = 6 (not sure/refused).

[d] Data for workers taken from self-assessment tables. Total number of workers = 1,442.

[e] Working/Nonworking status is unknown for 26 sample members.

The analyses of the survey data are presented in several parts. The first covers all female respondents and examines their demographic characteristics, employment behavior, and health insurance coverage. The next reports on their health conditions in relation to their employment status. The analysis then looks at the subgroup of nonworking respondents separately, comparing those who would prefer to work at paid employment with those who would prefer not to do so.

The final section presents recommendations suggested by this research for health and employment policy initiatives as well as several directions for further research that would likely prove fruitful. For example, if we seek to understand what about employment per se may make women healthier, or whether nonworking women are prevented from working because of ill health, the results of this survey would need to be augmented. The data currently available do not help answer the long-established question of whether only healthy people work or work makes people healthy.

THE DEMOGRAPHIC, EMPLOYMENT, AND HEALTH INSURANCE PROFILE OF THE SURVEY RESPONDENTS

Workers Compared to Nonworkers

The respondents' overall rate of participation in employment is similar to that of women in the United States as a whole. Nearly six of every ten (57%) respondents (who were eighteen years of age or older) are employed either full- or part-time, compared with approximately 56 percent in the national data (Bureau of Labor Statistics 1994a). Among nonworking respondents, slightly fewer than half say they would prefer to work. As table 11.1 shows, the nonworking group, compared with the working group, (1) is older (38% of the nonworkers are sixty-five years old or older, compared with only 4% of the working group), (2) is more likely to be widowed (25% compared with 5%), (3) is less likely to be single or divorced/separated (9% compared with 16%), (4) is less well educated (33% have not completed high school, compared with 12%), and (5) has lower family income (41% compared with 17% have annual family incomes of $15,000 or less). The nonworkers are slightly less likely to be women of color.

When only the working-age nonworkers (those ages eighteen to sixty-four) are compared with the same-age workers (data not shown), the same generalizations hold for this subpopulation as for the sample as a whole. The nonworkers are older (one-third are ages fifty to sixty-four, compared with one-sixth of the workers), more likely to be widowed rather than single or divorced/separated, less well educated (with nearly one-third not having completed high school), and with lower family income (41% have incomes of $15,000 or less). This group of working-age nonworkers is slightly more likely to be of color than the comparably aged working group.

As in the national population, significant differences exist among the respondents from the different race/ethnic groups. In general, the African American women who responded to the survey are younger than the white women, and the Hispanic women are the youngest of all, with fully one-third under thirty years of age. While 20 percent of the white respondents are sixty-five or older, only 8 percent of the Hispanic respondents and 13 percent of the African American respondents are. African American women are the most likely to be single and the least likely to be married. Hispanic women also have higher non-marriage rates than white women, but they are less likely to be widowed, probably because they are a much younger group. While all three race/ethnic groups have about the same proportion of women with some college education, the Hispanic and African American women have less education overall than the white women, since proportionately more women of color have not finished high school and proportionately fewer have graduated from college. As is the case among the national population, the African American and Hispanic survey respondents have lower family incomes. Women of Asian or Pacific American or Native American background (generally referred to as "other") are a small part of the sample population, approximately one percent. Thus, little can be said about them with statistical confidence, and they are generally dropped from the remainder of the analysis.

Factors Affecting Participation in Employment

Many factors are known to affect women's decisions to participate in paid employment. The labor market behavior of the survey sample population appears to be similar to the behavior of other populations of women that have been studied. These variations among women imply significant challenges in generalizing the employment–health connection for women.

Rates of participation in employment,[1] by age, for full-time and part-time workers as well as for the two together again mirror national patterns. Employment increases through middle age and then tapers off as workers near retirement. Approximately 13 percent of those over sixty-five in this sample work (the figure from federal data is 9%, Bureau of Labor Statistics 1994b), while 75 percent of women in their forties work (approximately the same proportion as in the federal data). If employed women are generally healthier, the decline in employment with age challenges us to consider the implications for good health in older women. One solution to maintaining the involvement of older women in work is part-time employment. Part-time work, which does not represent a large portion of employment for most women, is more common than full-time work among those sixty-five or older. In fact, women sixty-five or older are five times more likely to work part-time than full-time (tab. 11.1).

We examined employment participation rates by race and ethnicity for the survey sample. Rates of employment are about the same for non-Hispanic whites and African Americans across the life cycle. Hispanic women tend to work less during the earlier, childbearing years than either African Americans or whites, but they work more at age sixty-five or older.

Marital status and educational attainment levels (discussed below) may bear directly on women's health because they also affect participation in work as well as access to health insurance (Yoon et al. 1994). For all women, being single or divorced increases the likelihood of employment, yet participation in employment for married women is only a few percentage points below that for single women, across all age groups. Single women work more when young, whereas divorced women work more when older. Widowed women work less than any of these marital status groups.

Employment behavior, including full-time and part-time employment, varies by race and ethnicity among the marital status groups. White women work most when single or divorced, while African American women have the highest rate of employment when married, including a very high rate of full-time employment. Married-couple African American families, then, are likely to depend more on the wives' earnings than other married couples do.

For the sample, as for the female labor force as a whole, higher education levels correspond to greater participation in employment, and this is true across all racial/ethnic groups (fig. 11.1). Employment is low for those without high school education, and this is true among all age groups (not shown); among those with less education, Hispanic women work the most. At all educational levels, African American and Hispanic women work considerably more than white women. Thus, the apparent equality of participation among white and African American women, and the lower participation for Hispanic women, actually reflect the generally lower levels of education attained by women of color compared with white women. When white women and women

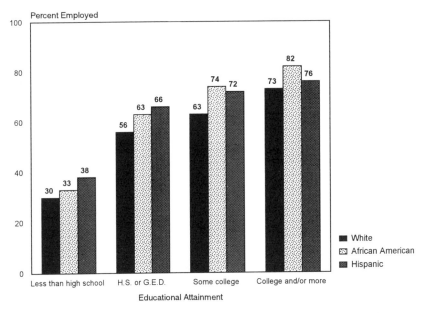

Fig. 11.1. Employment Participation, by Education and Race/Ethnicity (All Ages)
Source: Analysis of The Commonwealth Fund survey on women's health, 1993.

of color with the same educational levels are compared, women of color clearly work more.

Health Insurance Coverage for Workers and Nonworkers

Among all survey respondents, 88 percent reported having some type of health insurance, leaving only 12 percent without any—a figure similar to that reported in national data for the same time period.[2] Eighty-eight percent of those working full-time and 86 percent of those working part-time indicated they have insurance (tab. 11.1). On average, 87 percent of all working women reported having health insurance, leaving 13 percent without any, virtually identical to the sample as a whole.

Among nonworking women, as with the survey population as a whole, relatively few overall (12%) lack health insurance coverage entirely. Among nonworking Hispanic and African American women, the proportions without health insurance are higher: 28 percent and 18 percent, respectively (data not shown). Among marital categories, nonworking single women are the least likely to have health insurance,

with 23 percent reporting that they do not have any coverage. However, nearly two-fifths (38%) of the nonworking women are sixty-five
years of age or older and are likely being covered through Medicare.
However, excluding this retired portion of nonworkers leaves a relatively high proportion lacking insurance (data not shown): 19 percent
(compared with 20% as reported in the March 1993 Current Population
Survey).

Of all those who reported having no insurance,[3] 58 percent are
working and 39 percent are nonworkers of working age (the small
remaining group are nonworkers sixty-five or older) (tab. 11.2). Well
over half of all survey respondents without health insurance are in the
paid labor force. Of the 58 percent of the uninsured who are working,
about one-third work part-time and two-thirds work full-time.

Summary Profile of Respondents

Participation in employment by survey respondents parallels national
labor force participation rates for all women and for women within the

Table 11.2. Distribution of Women without Health
Insurance

	Women without Health Insurance	
	Number	Percentage
Sample population		
All ages	314	100
Under age 65	303	96
Workers (all ages)[a]	181	58
Full-time	126	40
Part-time	55	18
Under age 65	179	57
Nonworkers (all ages)[a]	131	42
Work preferrers[b]	96	31
Voluntary nonworkers[b]	33	11
Under age 65	124	39

Source: Data from The Commonwealth Fund survey on wom-
en's health, 1993.

[a] Work status: frequency missing = 26.

[b] Work preference: frequency missing = 47.

three race/ethnic groups studied. The higher the level of education, the more likely a woman is to work full-time. At all educational levels, women of color are much more likely than white women to be employed. More single and divorced women work full-time than do married or widowed women. Among all married women, by far, more African Americans work than whites or Hispanics, and the great majority of those women work full-time. For all women, employment participation peaks between the ages of forty and forty-nine; after age fifty part-time work increases as a proportion of all employment among women.

A large majority of survey respondents carry health insurance, with about 88 percent of both workers and nonworkers receiving some type of health insurance (tab. 11.1). Nearly as high a percentage of part-timers as full-timers reported having some type of insurance, and as many nonworkers are covered as full-time workers. Among all non-working Hispanic and African American women, the portion of those lacking health insurance is higher than for white nonworkers. Non-working single women were the most likely to lack insurance (data not shown).

In general, working women are younger than nonworking women. They tend to be better educated, be single or divorced rather than widowed, and have higher family incomes. Of the nonworking women, nearly two-fifths are sixty-five years of age or older.

EMPLOYMENT STATUS AND HEALTH OUTCOMES

The survey data were scrutinized for information regarding a possible relationship between being employed and being healthy using four conventional measures of health status: (1) incidences of four specific health conditions (hypertension, heart disease, arthritis/bursitis, and anxiety/depression); (2) use of sick leave by full- and part-time employees; (3) incidence of disability; and (4) respondents' self-assessment of health status. For each measure, analyses were conducted for all female respondents by employment status (full-time workers, part-time workers, and nonworkers); for all white, African American, and Hispanic women; and for respondents across age groups. We also investigated whether having health insurance was related to how women in these different employment and demographic categories reported their health status.

Specific Health Conditions

Among all respondents, rates of hypertension, heart disease, arthritis/bursitis, and depression/anxiety are higher for nonworkers than for workers (tab. 11.3). The differences are especially pronounced for heart disease and hypertension, with nonworkers reporting more than 2.5 times as much heart disease (12% versus 5%) and hypertension (with nonworkers reporting an incidence of 34% compared with only 13% for workers). Among workers, full- and part-time workers reported about the same incidence of these two specific health conditions and of anxiety/depression. Arthritis/bursitis is significantly more common among part-time than among full-time workers, and even more common among nonworkers.

To some extent these findings result from the age difference between the working and nonworking populations; the nonworkers are older on average. Excluding those sixty-five or over from the comparison shows the same direction of difference between workers and nonworkers, with nonworkers generally reporting more of each specific health condition, but the differences are somewhat smaller (tab. 11.3). For example, for arthritis/bursitis, only 25 percent of women nonworkers under age sixty-five reported this diagnosis, compared with 36 percent of nonworkers regardless of age. In comparison, workers under age sixty-five still reported substantially less (16%). Hypertension is also substantially less prevalent among nonworking women

Table 11.3. Incidence of Specifically Diagnosed Health Conditions for All Women, by Employment Status (all ages)

	Hypertension	Heart Disease	Arthritis or Bursitis	Anxiety or Depression
All women	22%	8%	26%	15%
Under age 65	15	6	19	16
All workers	13	4	18	14
Full-time	13	4	16	14
Part-time	11	5	23	13
Under age 65	11	4	16	14
Nonworkers	34	12	36	16
Under age 65	24	10	25	20

Source: Data from The Commonwealth Fund survey on women's health, 1993.

under sixty-five than among those of all ages (24% versus 34%), while the incidence of heart disease and anxiety/depression shows less difference between the under sixty-five and all-age groups.

The percentages of respondents reporting each of these four specific health diagnoses for workers and nonworkers were compared for those with and without health insurance (fig. 11.2). Among working women, those without health insurance generally reported slightly higher incidences of specific health conditions, especially arthritis/bursitis and anxiety/depression; it may be somewhat more difficult for working women with these conditions to get access to health insurance through employment.

Among nonworking women, those with health insurance reported higher incidences of hypertension, heart disease, and arthritis/bursitis than those without insurance, while the reverse is true of anxiety/depression. Because under the U.S. health care system, nonworkers must often purchase health insurance at substantial cost, it may be that

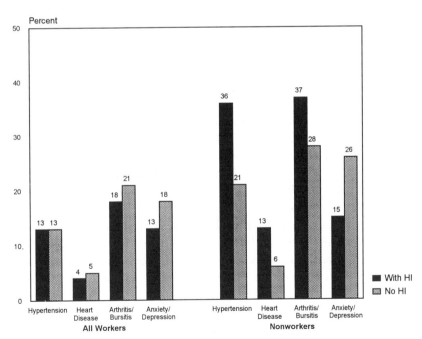

Fig. 11.2. Specifically Diagnosed Health Conditions Reported by Working and Nonworking Women, by Health Insurance Coverage (All Ages)

Source: Analysis of The Commonwealth Fund survey on women's health, 1993.

those who are less healthy are more likely to purchase insurance because they know they need it more. On the other hand, those who are healthier are more likely to take their chances and avoid the cost of obtaining insurance. Because most health policies offer less coverage for mental health needs than for physical health needs, we do not see any self-selection regarding health insurance purchase and anxiety/ depression. As noted, many of the nonworking women are sixty-five or older and have Medicare, as well as a higher incidence of many of these conditions.

When the racial/ethnic groups are compared, some differences in the incidences of the four health conditions reported by respondents are found. Nonworkers in each race/ethnic group reported higher incidences of all four health conditions than workers (often reporting two to three times the incidence among workers).

For most of these specific conditions, African Americans, workers and nonworkers, reported higher rates than whites; depression/ anxiety is an exception, with African Americans reporting less than whites. Among working women, African Americans and whites reported the same rate of heart disease (5%); among nonworkers, African Americans indicated they have more heart disease (15% versus 11% for whites). This racial difference is especially pronounced for hypertension, with African American working women experiencing nearly three times (28%) the rate of hypertension of whites (10%).

The incidence rates vary more for Hispanics. Hispanic nonworking women reported having hypertension (27%) less often than African Americans (40%) and whites (34%); working Hispanic women still reported hypertension (13%) less often than working African American women (28%), but more often than working white women (10%). For heart disease, Hispanic and white women show identical rates, while African American nonworking women have more. The data on Hispanic women indicate they have the lowest rate of diagnosed arthritis/bursitis. This may be because Hispanic women in the sample are younger, and they may also have less access to health care and therefore obtain fewer diagnoses. For depression/anxiety, Hispanic working women report less than whites but more than African Americans, while Hispanic nonworking women reported more than both white and African American women.

Most but not all specific health conditions increase with age, for both workers and nonworkers. In general, as above, the nonworkers reported having more specific diagnosed health conditions than workers in all age groups (except for arthritis/bursitis in the sixty-five-plus age group). Reported hypertension and heart disease increase substantially with age; differences among workers and nonworkers are greatest for midlife respondents. Arthritis/bursitis shows the most rapid increase with age; smaller differences between workers and nonworkers are reported than with the other physical health conditions. One condition, anxiety/depression, decreases with age; older women, workers and nonworkers, suffer less than middle-aged women (ages thirty to sixty-four years) from these mental health conditions.

Use of Sick Leave

Average use of sick leave was analyzed by employment status (full- or part-time) for all women and by race and age. The average number of days of sick leave for all workers is 4.3 days (data not shown). Overall, full-time workers have a higher mean number of days of sick leave used (4.8 days) than part-time workers (2.8 days), most likely because they worked more days over the course of the year.

Average use of sick leave differs among the race/ethnic groups, with African Americans using the most (7.2 days) and Hispanics the least (3.0 days); white women workers use, on average, 4.0 days of sick leave. Because African Americans generally reported more specific health conditions than whites, their greater use of sick leave is to be expected. Hispanic women's low use of sick leave is surprising, given that they, too, generally reported more specific health conditions than whites. For African American women, many of whom are single parents, a greater portion of sick leave use may actually be a result of caring for other family members rather than because of personal illness. Perhaps Hispanic women have more backup from other adults who can stay with ill family members, enabling Hispanic women to use less sick leave.

Among prime-age workers (those under sixty-five), the youngest workers use the most sick leave (5.2 days). The use of sick leave declines through middle age, hitting a low of 3.2 days for workers between ages forty and forty-nine, and increases again for those over fifty. Among full-time workers, rates of sick leave use are particularly high for older workers. For full-time workers age sixty-five or older, the average sick leave was 16.6 days. Yet, for older part-time workers, sick leave use is relatively rare, perhaps because their participation in employment is more discretionary (older full-time workers may be more likely to work because of financial need). Part-time workers ages fifty to sixty-four average 2.6 days of sick leave, and part-time workers over age sixty-five average only 1.9 days (data not shown).

Disability

Sixteen percent of the respondents said they have disabilities, hand-icaps, or chronic diseases that keep them from participating fully in the workforce. Among full-time workers, only 7 percent reported such disability, compared with 15 percent of part-timers and one-fourth of all nonworkers. As with other health conditions, nonworkers reported having a higher rate of disabling conditions.

Disability and lack of insurance coverage are related (fig. 11.3). For all women, 16 percent of those who have health insurance reported a disability, and 19 percent of those who do not have health insurance

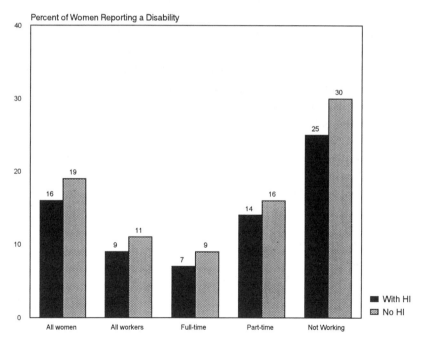

Fig. 11.3. Disability Reported by All Women, Working and Nonworking, by Health Insurance Coverage (All Ages)

Source: Analysis of The Commonwealth Fund survey on women's health, 1993.

reported a disability. Disabled women apparently have more difficulty in gaining access to health insurance; although they are likely to need medical services more, they are less likely to be covered. This relative lack of insurance holds across all employment statuses, for full-time workers, part-time workers, and nonworkers.

Among working women, minority women (African Americans and Hispanics) reported a lower incidence of being disabled, whereas they generally indicated a higher incidence of other health conditions (data not shown). Of the working minority women with health insurance, 7 percent said they have a disability, compared to 10 percent of white working women. In general, nonworkers reported a disability at over twice the rate of workers, across all racial groups. Among women who are not working, African American women have a very high incidence of disability, while Hispanic women at home reported the lowest incidence (Hispanic women are younger on average). A high of 32 percent of the insured African American nonworkers reported a disability. This finding suggests that disabled women of color have more difficulty finding employment than disabled white women.

Reported disability generally increases with age, with more older workers and nonworkers indicating disabilities than younger women. Among working-age women, reported disability rates are highest for women in their forties (11% among all workers), for both full-timers (8%) and part-timers (20%); it is likely that older disabled workers drop out of the labor market. Among nonworkers, the highest rate of disability—more than one-third—occurs in the oldest group of working-age women (fifty to sixty-four). Among postretirement-age nonworkers, the disability rate falls to 28 percent, perhaps because many disabled individuals have a shorter life expectancy.

Self-Assessment of Health

Perhaps the best single indicator of a woman's health is her own assessment of her overall health. Respondents were asked to rate their health status as excellent, very good, good, fair, or poor. Overall, working respondents rated their health status as better than nonworkers (fig. 11.4), and this difference is not due to the older age on average of the nonworking group. For parts of this analysis, we combined the "excellent" and "very good" ratings and the "fair" and "poor" ratings.

Is having health insurance related to one's self-assessment? Are healthier people more likely to have health insurance? As we have seen

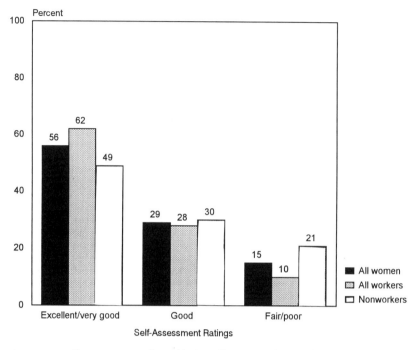

Fig. 11.4. Self-Assessment of Health for All Women, by Employment Status (All Ages)

Source: Analysis of The Commonwealth Fund survey on women's health, 1993.

for the specific diagnosed health conditions discussed above, and as we can see for self-assessment, workers with health insurance reported better health than those without. The difference is less pronounced among nonworkers, but still more of those without health insurance reported only fair or poor health. Among workers, the higher cost of covering workers with health problems possibly results in their being less likely to have health insurance, or perhaps not having access to health insurance contributes to their health problems. We cannot be certain about the direction of causation in the relationship revealed by the data. We also compared the relationship between self-assessment and employment and health insurance status for workers to that for nonworkers, with those sixty-five or older excluded. We find no significant difference for the working-age-only subsample and the full sample population.

For each race/ethnic group studied, workers reported better health status than nonworkers (tab. 11.4). In each race/ethnic group, about twice as many nonworkers as workers reported having only fair or poor health. Thus for both women of color and white women, working and good health go together.

Among workers and nonworkers, however, women of color reported substantially less good health than white women. African Americans and Hispanics are twice as likely as white women to report fair or poor health, whether working or not. White respondents are more likely than African Americans or Hispanics to give their health the highest ratings, whereas the proportions rating their health as good are approximately equal for workers and nonworkers and the different race/ethnic groups.

As above, among workers, those with health insurance reported better health than those without, but working women of color, even with health insurance, reported less good health overall than working white women. Among working women without health insurance, women of color reported substantially less excellent or good health and substantially more fair or poor health; more than one-third of working

Table 11.4. Self-Assessment of Health, by Race/Ethnicity and Employment Status (all ages)

	Excellent/ Very Good	Good	Fair/Poor
All women	56%	29%	14%
White	60	28	12
African American	44	33	23
Hispanic	48	29	23
Working women	62	28	10
White	65	27	8
African American	51	34	16
Hispanic	50	33	16
Nonworking women	49	30	21
White	52	30	18
African American	34	33	33
Hispanic	44	23	33
All working women			
Full-time	62	30	8
Part-time	63	23	13

Source: Data from The Commonwealth Fund survey on women's health, 1993.

women of color who do not have health insurance said they have fair or poor health. Thus, unfortunately, those workers who are likely to need health insurance the most are the least likely to be able to get it through employment.

About the same proportion of working women reported excellent or very good health whether they work part-time or full-time (tab. 11.4). Yet considerably more part-time workers show fair or poor health than good health, relative to full-time workers. It is likely that the health status of part-time workers inhibits their participation in work, reducing their hours of work below their preference.

For each age group, workers are more likely than nonworkers to describe their health as excellent/very good (data not shown). These women's self-assessment of their health generally declines with age for both workers and nonworkers. For example, among working women, only 8 percent of eighteen- to twenty-nine-year-olds rated their health as fair or poor, while among those sixty-five years and older, 20 percent did. Among nonworking women, only 9 percent of the eighteen- to twenty-nine-year-olds rated their own health as fair or poor, but among fifty- to sixty-four-year-olds, 32 percent did.

Summary of Employment Status and Health Outcomes

These analyses based on measures of actual health status demonstrate that workers consistently report better health ratings than non-workers. This is true across all race/ethnic and age categories. In general, older women report higher incidences of specific health conditions and disability than do younger women (depression/anxiety is an exception to this rule). Yet older workers use less sick leave than younger workers. It is generally believed that older workers with health problems tend to drop out of the labor market, accounting for the decline of sick leave use.

The connection between health insurance coverage and good health suggests that employer-based access to insurance needs to be extended to all workers. Among working women, uninsured women (compared with insured women) reported having higher rates of specific diagnosed health conditions or a disability of some kind; they also indicated a lower self-assessment of health status overall. The incidence of most specific health conditions and disability increases with age among survey respondents, but after age sixty-five nearly every woman is covered by Medicare. Therefore, the late middle-aged group is at risk for reduced employment, increased disability and other health conditions, and decreased likelihood of insurance coverage.

Although nonworking women with specific diagnosed health conditions are more likely to have health insurance (they probably purchase more because they need it more), nonworking women who reported a disability are less likely to have insurance coverage; those without insurance coverage also reported a lower self-assessment of their health. Nonworking women of color are especially likely to report a lack of health insurance.

Generally, women with health insurance give a higher self-assessment of health status, whether or not they are working. A high percentage of those without insurance reported fair/poor health; apparently those most in need of insurance coverage tend not to have it.

A CLOSER LOOK AT NONWORKING WOMEN

Nonworking women include those who do not work by choice (those who are in school or prefer family or home care to paid employment) and those who are not employed but would prefer to be (they may have been laid off, are looking for work, want work but are too discouraged to look, would like to work but have a health disability, or would like to work but lack care for family members). Half of the nonworking respondent sample reported that they would prefer to work; more than half of these said that they would work if jobs were available (tab. 11.5).

We saw above that nonworking women are generally less well-off, based on many indicators, than working women. In addition to their distinctive age distribution (they are less likely to be in the prime ages, with more nonworkers in both the younger and older age groups), nonworkers are less well educated, have lower average family incomes, and (among those under sixty-five) are less likely to have health insurance. They are less likely to be single or divorced and more likely to be widowed.

Are these disadvantages related to their work preference? Those who would prefer to work but cannot, for whatever reason, may be less healthy and more disadvantaged than both workers and those who prefer not to work (also referred to as voluntary nonworkers and the "happy at home" group). Because of these potential differences, we contrasted those who would prefer to work with those who prefer to be

Table 11.5. Characteristics of Nonworking Women: Work Preferrers and Voluntary Nonworkers (all ages)

| | All Nonworking Women[a] | | |
	Total	Work Preferrers	Voluntary Nonworkers
Age			
18–29	17%	27%	10%
30–39	15	20	9
40–49	11	13	8
50–64	20	19	19
65+	38	20	53
Total	101%	99%	99%
Race/ethnicity			
White	80%	71%	89%
African American	12	17	6
Hispanic	7	11	4
Asian and other	1	1	1
Total	100%	100%	100%
Marital status			
Single	13	20	7
Divorced/separated	9	15	4
Married	53	49	58
Widowed	25	16	31
Total	100%	100%	100%
Education			
Less than high school	33%	39%	28%
High school or GED	38	37	39
Some college	15	14	16
College+	14	11	18
Total	100%	101%	101%

(continued)

at home, examining their overall demographic profile, health insurance coverage, and health status.

Demographic Profile of Nonworking Women

Those women who prefer not to work are more likely to be white than of color, older, and married or widowed, and are more likely to have higher levels of educational attainment and higher family incomes than those who would prefer to work (tab. 11.5). Voluntary nonworkers are also substantially more likely to have health insurance.

Table 11.5.   (*Continued*)

| | All Nonworking Women[a] | | |
	Total	Work Preferrers	Voluntary Nonworkers
Family income			
<$15,000	41%	45%	36%
$15,001–$50,000	34	34	35
$50,001+	11	6	15
Don't know	15	15	13
Total	101%	100%	99%
Health insurance coverage			
With health insurance	88%	81%	94%
No health insurance	12	19	6
Total	100%	100%	100%
Sample size[b]	1,056	508	518
Percentage of total sample	100%	49.5%	50.5%

Source: Data from The Commonwealth Fund survey on women's health, 1993.

[a] Totals may not add up to 100 due to rounding.

[b] Work preference: frequency missing = 30.

African American women who would prefer to work account for more than one-quarter of all African American respondents, and nearly three-quarters (72%) of the African American nonworking pool. Among Hispanic nonworkers, 72 percent would prefer to work. In contrast, only 43 percent of nonworking white women responded that they would prefer to work (data not shown).

Only one-third of all nonworkers are under forty years old, in contrast to more than half of the working women in the sample (tab. 11.1). Of those who prefer to be at home, only one-fifth are under forty (tab. 11.5), while for those who would prefer to work, nearly half are under forty. Even when those of retirement age are excluded, work preferrers are still younger, with nearly three-fifths under age forty, compared with two-fifths for the happy-at-home group (data not shown).

Work preferrers are less well educated than any of the other groups of women. Three-fourths of the work preferrers have a high school education or less, compared with two-thirds of the voluntary nonworkers and half the working group. Among African American and Hispanic women who would prefer to work, four-fifths have a high school education or less (data not shown).

Work preferrers are less well off financially than virtually any other group of respondents. Nearly half of all work preferrers have family incomes below $15,000 per year (tab. 11.5), compared with about one-third of the happy-at-home group and less than one-fifth of the working group (see tab. 11.1). Among African American women who would prefer to work, three-fifths have family incomes under $15,000 (data not shown).

Health Insurance Coverage for Nonworking Women

Work preferrers are the least likely to have health insurance of any group of respondents, while voluntary nonworkers are the most likely to have health insurance. Nineteen percent of those women who would prefer to work do not have health insurance of any kind, in contrast to only 6 percent of those who are happy at home (tab. 11.5).

For women of color, both groups of nonworking women have higher rates of noninsurance (data not shown). Of those who would prefer to work, 24 percent lack insurance, compared to 19 percent of the voluntary nonworkers. This contrasts with the 12 percent of all nonworking women who lack insurance.

Health Outcomes for Nonworking Women

Nonworking women who would prefer to work are generally less healthy than women who are at home voluntarily. Although the two groups reveal a somewhat mixed picture of specific health diagnoses, the work preferrers are more likely to be disabled, and they also reported that they have less good health overall.

With respect to specific health diagnoses, there is no clear relationship between health outcomes and work preference among nonworking women. Voluntary nonworkers reported more hypertension and slightly more arthritis/bursitis than those who would prefer to work, while those who would prefer to work reported somewhat more heart disease and quite a bit more anxiety and depression. The voluntary nonworkers are considerably older and, thus, could be expected to have more hypertension and arthritis/bursitis as well as less anxiety/depression. That the work preferrers report more heart disease, even though they are much younger than voluntary nonworkers (and are only slightly older than the working women), suggests that health conditions may prevent substantial numbers of these women from working.

As with the group of nonworking women generally, both the voluntary nonworkers and the work preferrers who have health insurance reported a somewhat higher incidence of these specific health conditions (except for depression/anxiety). Those with poorer health likely find it more important to have insurance coverage.

Despite their younger average age, nonworking women who would prefer to work reported a higher incidence of disability (30%) than those who are voluntarily at home (21%), and reported a substantially higher incidence than those who are working (only 9%; data not shown). Nonworking women without health insurance (both work preferrers and voluntary nonworkers) indicated a higher incidence of disability than those who have insurance. This finding suggests that disabled women find it somewhat more difficult to obtain insurance coverage. As we saw for working women, even though disabled nonworking women are likely to need health insurance more, they generally have it less often.

According to the overall health assessment reported by the respondents, nonworking women who would prefer to work are in substantially worse health. Considerably fewer women who would prefer to work reported being in excellent or very good health (44%), compared with the voluntary nonworkers (54%; data not shown). In contrast to all working women, of which fully 62 percent reported being in excellent or very good health, only 49 percent of nonworkers reported being in excellent or very good health (fig. 11.4).

Health insurance coverage appears to be related to both self-assessment of health and work preference. Among the work preferrers, substantially more women who do not have health insurance reported being in only fair or poor health (39%) compared with those who do have health insurance (23%); that is, among the work preferrers those who do not have health insurance are less healthy. Among those voluntarily at home, there also exists a health gap between those who do and do not have insurance, but those who do not have insurance are much more healthy.

Summary on Nonworking Women

This comparison of women who responded that they would prefer to work with those who said they are voluntarily at home shows that the work preferrers are the most disadvantaged group of all. The work preferrers are both the least well educated and the least well off of all groups of respondents. Work preferrers are also the least likely to have health insurance. In contrast, voluntary nonworkers are the most likely to have insurance.

Those who would prefer to work are clearly at home despite their preferences. They are likely prevented from working by inadequate preparation for the labor market, reflected in their low levels of educational attainment. They may also be held back by discrimination in the labor market and/or the lack of jobs in areas where they live. Nearly three-quarters of all nonworking women of color would prefer to work, while fewer than half of the white nonworking women are work preferrers.

While there is no clear relationship between work preference and health status as measured by specific diagnoses, nonworking women who prefer to work reported markedly poorer health on other dimensions than voluntary nonworkers. Their self-assessment of health is markedly lower, and they are more likely to be disabled. Also, work preferrers without health insurance reported the lowest self-assessment and the highest incidence of disability. This finding suggests that women who are unemployed and disabled find it difficult or prohibitively costly to obtain insurance in other ways.

Those women who are involuntarily unemployed are the least healthy of all and the least likely to have health insurance overall. For some portion of these women, their inability to work or to obtain health insurance likely stems from their poor health. For other women, access to work would likely improve their health status as well as the likelihood of their obtaining health insurance.

IMPLICATIONS FOR POLICY AND RESEARCH

Our analysis of The Commonwealth Fund survey data on women's health shows a clear relationship between employment and health status. Indeed, these results confirm the finding reported in much of the literature that employed women are healthier. We find, further, that employed women with health insurance are the healthiest of all. Least healthy are those women who do not work but would like to; presumably they cannot find work they would like to do. As noted, this group of work preferrers is the most disadvantaged on nearly all indicators, having the lowest family income and the lowest levels of educational attainment. Of this group, those without health insurance are less healthy; they reported having more specifically diagnosed health conditions, a higher incidence of disability, and a lower self-assessment of overall health condition than other nonworking and working women.

We do not know whether the experience of working (and the experience of gaining access to health insurance through work) provides health benefits to women or whether only the healthier women self-select to work. The evidence reviewed here suggests that both are true. Clearly, some health conditions and disabilities are so severe that most work is precluded, especially for less well-educated persons. When work is precluded by poor health, it can be inferred that these women "choose" nonwork, while healthier women are more likely to choose work.

Yet even for women with severe health conditions, the ability to work is socially conditioned. For example, proportionately more African American and Hispanic women than white women with disabilities do not work but would prefer to; this race/ethnic differential is likely a matter of the lack of suitable employment, given their educational attainment levels, rather than a question of the severity of their disabilities. If suitable employment could be found for all who want to work, and if being employed confers health benefits (because of job satisfaction, improved self-esteem, greater opportunity for social interaction), might we not observe an improvement in the health status of these women?

With respect to policy changes, several areas stand out in the analysis undertaken here. First, older working-age women are at greater risk of health problems and of lacking insurance when working or when at home involuntarily. This finding suggests that employment should provide access to health insurance for all workers.

Second, older women with health problems seem to prefer part-time employment; perhaps it provides a way to balance the gains and losses from work. Working part-time may provide enough employment to allow women to benefit from feelings of efficacy and sociability but not so much that it contributes to stress or greater health problems. If this is the case, then part-time work, with suitable working conditions and access to health insurance, might be encouraged for older women and others who do not want full-time work.

Third, because those who would prefer to work are the worst off on so many levels, our research also suggests that, if employment could be made available to all, many women would benefit in terms of access to health insurance and self-assessment of overall health.

Fourth, because having health insurance is generally associated with better health in this study, as elsewhere, it is important to expand the availability of health insurance, for workers and nonworkers alike. Despite our observation that those who are voluntarily at home are the most likely to be insured (in this study), access to health insurance is important for those at home as well as those at work. Women who are at home involuntarily, especially women of color, have the highest likelihood of lacking health insurance. Because they are less healthy, they need health insurance more. Our study, like many others, shows that those who most need health insurance are often the ones who do not have it.

Research that would allow us to examine which aspects of the employment experience contribute to improved health and which may detract from health (job stress, exposure to health hazards) would further illuminate the potential health benefits to women of paid employment. Another research approach to the question of the benefits of employment would be to compare women with similar social and demographic characteristics, such as education, age, marital status, and externally evaluated health conditions, but whose employment status differs. Do otherwise similar employed and nonemployed women express more or less satisfaction with their health status (their own health assessment)? Yet a third approach would be to track women whose employment status changes longitudinally, comparing health status before and after the employment change.

ACKNOWLEDGMENTS

We would like to acknowledge the assistance of Jackie Chu and Gail Edie, of the Institute for Women's Policy Research, who assisted with data analysis, graphics, and editing, and of Marguerite Ro of Johns Hopkins University, who provided computer programming.

NOTES

1. Ordinarily the term *labor force participation* is used, but that concept includes unemployed persons in the labor force, whereas in the survey sample unemployed persons cannot be identified separately and are included with nonworkers.

2. Because in this sample survey the number of respondents reporting more than one source of health insurance is very large (in fact, much larger than reported in government surveys), we felt that the data on sources of insurance are most likely unreliable. However, the proportion reporting no insurance (12.4%) is close to that reported in the federal surveys (13.2% in March 1993, according to the Current Population Survey) (U.S. Bureau of the Census for women 18 or older, 1993: tab. 24). Thus, the only dimension of health insurance we consider here is whether the respondent reported having any.

3. In this sample, 314 out of 2,525.

REFERENCES

Adelmann, P. K., et al. 1989. Empty nest, cohort, and employment in the well-being of mid-life women. *Sex Roles* 20:173–89.

Anson, O., and J. Anson. 1987. Women's health and labour force status: an enquiry using a multi-point measure of labour force participation. *Social Science and Medicine* 25:57–63.

Bureau of Labor Statistics. 1994a. *Employment and Earnings* January: Table A-4.

———. 1994b. *Employment and Earnings* June 1994: Table A-13.

Herzog, A. R., J. S. House, and J. N. Morgan. 1991. Relation of work and retirement to health and well-being in older age. *Psychology and Aging* 6:202–11.

Hibbard, J. H., and C. R. Pope. 1987. Employment characteristics and health status among men and women. *Women and Health* 12:85–63.

Nathanson, C. 1980. Social roles and health status among women: the significance of employment. *Social Science and Medicine* 14:463–71.

Verbrugge, L. 1985. Gender and health: an update on hypotheses and evidence. *Journal of Health and Social Behavior* 26:156–82.

———. 1982. Work satisfaction and physical health. *Journal of Community Health* 11.

Verbrugge, L., and Madans, J. H. 1985. Social roles and health trends of American women. *Health and Society* 63:691–735.

Voydanoff, P. 1987. *Work and Family Life*. Newbury Park, Calif.: Sage Publications.

Waldron, I. 1980. Employment and women's health: an analysis of causal relationships. *International Journal of Health Services* 10:435–54.

Yoon, Y., et al. 1994. *Women's Access to Health Insurance*. Washington, D.C.: Institute for Women's Policy Research.

12

Health Insurance and Women's Access to Health Care

Anne Lenhard Reisinger, Ph.D.

In the United States, people pay for health care services through myriad health insurance plans obtained through their employers or governmental programs, or purchased directly from insurance companies. Many have no health insurance at all. Access to the various sources of health insurance depends on a number of factors, such as employment and socioeconomic status. Because benefit structures, co-payments, and deductibles differ among insurance plans, the source of health insurance can have an important effect on one's access to health care services. Having no health insurance at all is often a barrier to obtaining medical services.

The connection between health care financing and access to health care is particularly important, given recent changes in the structure of health care financing. The growth of managed care plans is changing the way many people obtain and pay for their care. The effect of managed care on people's access to care is not well understood. Even more changes in health care financing are likely to occur in the near future through state or federal reform. Because reform will build on the current system, an examination of the current system's access problems can help create a better health care financing structure.

Health insurance coverage in this country is determined largely by one's employment status. An employed person is likely, with some notable exceptions such as part-time workers and employees of very small firms, to obtain health insurance through the employer. A person who has worked, but is retired, may obtain insurance through a former employer as well as through Medicare. A person who is unemployed or underemployed may purchase insurance directly from an insurance company, may be eligible for insurance through the Medicaid program, or may have no insurance at all.

This employer-based system of health insurance coverage has resulted in different patterns of coverage for men and women, largely because of differences in their workforce participation. During childbearing years, many women cannot or choose not to work outside the home. Therefore, they are less likely to have a job with health insurance benefits, although many have such benefits through a spouse. Mothers who do not have a spouse with health insurance or a job that provides health insurance benefits may rely on public assistance programs such as Medicaid. The Medicaid program excludes most men because of its eligibility requirements. During their retirement years, most people have health insurance coverage through Medicare. Women are more likely than men to have Medicare coverage, chiefly because they live longer than men.

This broad characterization of access to health insurance masks a number of factors contributing to differential access. In addition to gender and employment status, factors such as education, age, income, race, and marital status affect health insurance coverage and, therefore, access to health care services.

This chapter examines the connection between health insurance coverage and access to health care, focusing especially on the way women obtain insurance and how insurance coverage affects their access to care. The analysis is based primarily on data from The Commonwealth Fund survey (1993) on health insurance and utilization of health care services, supplemented with findings from the research literature. The Commonwealth Fund survey is a rich source of data, allowing a detailed analysis of the connections among health insurance coverage, socioeconomic factors, and access to health care.

The results of this analysis suggest that people who are uninsured have impaired access to health care services. Therefore, to increase access to health care services, financing reform built on the current employer-based system should extend insurance coverage to those groups that fall through the cracks in such a system and that are uninsured. The results also suggest that the benefit package and costs associated with an insurance plan (co-payments, deductibles) may affect access to care. If a service is not covered in the benefit package or if the out-of-pocket costs for a service are high, one's access to that service may be impaired.

The results of this analysis also suggest that managed care plans can positively affect access to care. The current growth of managed care plans may help increase access, at least to some primary and preventive services.

Finally, the results suggest that financing reform may be only one step toward guaranteeing access to health care. Other reforms that eliminate the nonfinancial barriers to care may also be necessary.

HEALTH INSURANCE COVERAGE

Differences in Health Insurance Coverage for Men and Women

Health insurance coverage in the United States is different for women and men because women are more likely to be impoverished, less likely to be working full-time outside the home, and more likely to be elderly. Because of the way insurance coverage is provided, these characteristics affect the types of coverage that women have. While women are more likely than men to have health insurance, they are more likely to rely on public sources such as Medicare and Medicaid and less likely to be covered by their own employer-sponsored insurance.

Men are more likely than women to be uninsured. According to U.S. Census Bureau estimates, 18 percent of men and 13 percent of women over eighteen were uninsured in 1992. This pattern varies somewhat by age, however. Young adult males (under thirty-five) are much more likely than women of the same age to be uninsured. The differences diminish considerably between the ages of thirty-five and forty-five. Between the ages of forty-five and sixty-four, women are actually more likely than men to experience periods without insurance (Horton 1992; Jensen 1992; U.S. Bureau of the Census 1993a).

Part of the reason that women are more likely than men to have health insurance is that they rely more heavily on public sources of insurance, such as Medicare and Medicaid. In 1992, 5 percent of men and just under 10 percent of women age eighteen and older had Medicaid coverage. This gap exists for all age groups but, because of the structure of Medicaid eligibility, is most prominent during the childbearing years (U.S. Bureau of the Census 1993a).

Women rely more heavily on Medicaid than men, in part, because women are more likely to live in poverty. In 1992 more than 14 percent of adult women had incomes below the poverty line, as compared with just over 9 percent of men (U.S. Bureau of the Census 1993b).

While almost all elderly people are enrolled in Medicare, the program covers many more women than men because women live longer than men. In 1992 Medicare covered about 19 million women and 14 million men (U.S. Bureau of the Census 1993a).

According to The Commonwealth Fund survey, women are less likely than men to obtain insurance through their own employer. This is troubling because employer-sponsored insurance usually offers the broadest benefit coverage. Reliance on a spouse for such coverage leaves women vulnerable to loss of coverage in the event of divorce, a change in the spouse's employment, or the employer's decisions regarding coverage of dependents. Even women who work outside the home are less likely than men to have insurance through an employer. Sixty-six percent of working men and 52 percent of working women have employer-based insurance (Jensen 1992; Cooper and Johnson 1993). This may be because women are more likely to work part-time and to work for small businesses that may not provide insurance. While only 15 percent of working men are employed part-time, 30 percent of working women are (Snider 1994). Forty-one percent of employees in firms with more than five hundred employees are women, compared with 46 percent in smaller firms (Brown, Hamilton, and Medolf 1990).

Differences in Health Insurance Coverage among Women

Not all women have equal access to health insurance. We can expect socioeconomic factors such as income, ethnicity, marital status, age, and educational attainment to affect women's access to various sources of health insurance.[1] The Commonwealth Fund survey allows us to look at differences in coverage among women. For example, (1) do women with higher incomes purchase better health insurance; (2) does more education lead to better coverage associated with better jobs; (3) are married women more likely to have access to health insurance due to a spouse's employment; and (4) is there differential access to health insurance by race and ethnicity?

Poor women are more likely than other women to be uninsured or to have Medicaid, and less likely to have insurance through an employer (tab. 12.1). Twenty-one percent of women with incomes of $7,500 or less are uninsured, compared with about 6 percent of women with incomes over $50,000. Because Medicaid is structured to help poor people, reliance on Medicaid as a source of insurance is highest among

Table 12.1. Health Insurance, by Income

Insurance Source	Income (in thousands of dollars)							
	<7.5	7.5–15	15–25	25–35	35–50	50–75	75–100	100+
Own employer	11.4%	16.6%	34.9%	47.6%	53.1%	52.8%	50.7%	42.5%
Spouse's employer	3.8	6.3	15.9	24.2	27.4	23.9	32.3	28.5
Medicare	40.0	38.6	21.6	12.4	5.8	7.5	3.3	4.1
Medicaid	16.9	9.1	4.6	2.1	0.5	0.3	—	—
Direct	7.5	7.1	5.7	4.2	5.3	11.1	6.3	19.4
Uninsured	20.5	22.2	17.3	9.6	7.9	4.3	7.3	5.5
Total N	333	347	422	370	346	306	99	73

Source: Data from The Commonwealth Fund survey on women's health, 1993.

Note: Respondents to the survey may have indicated more than one insurance source. For the purposes of this analysis, respondents were assigned to a primary insurer according to the following ordering: Medicare, Medicaid, insurance through own employer, insurance through spouse's employer, insurance purchased directly by the respondent.

poor women. Seventeen percent of women with incomes below $7,500 rely on Medicaid, as do 9 percent of women with incomes between $7,500 and $15,000. Higher-income women are more likely to have insurance through an employer. The number of women covered by employer-paid insurance rises with income.

African American women are more likely than white women to be uninsured or to have Medicaid. Sixteen percent of African American women report being uninsured, compared with 13 percent of white women. Hispanic women are more likely than non-Hispanic women to be uninsured. Twenty-three percent of Hispanic women are uninsured, while only 13 percent of non-Hispanic women are. Hispanic women are also more likely than non-Hispanics to have insurance through Medicaid.

A woman's marital status can also affect her insurance coverage (tab. 12.2). Single women are almost twice as likely as any other category of women to be uninsured. Almost 30 percent of separated women rely on Medicaid—many more than women of any other marital status. More than 60 percent of married or divorced women have health insurance through an employer, compared with about 40 percent of separated and single women.

Age also affects women's access to different sources of health insurance. The number of women who have insurance through an employer rises with age until they reach their late forties, then it begins to decline. Young women (aged eighteen to twenty-four or so) and older women (over age sixty-five) are more likely than women of other ages to have Medicaid.

Increasing educational attainment among women is associated with decreases in the likelihood of having Medicaid or being uninsured and

Table 12.2. Health Insurance, by Marital Status

Insurance Source	Single	Married	Widowed	Separated	Divorced
Own employer	37.9%	36.1%	12.2%	34.6%	59.4%
Spouse's employer	0.3	29.5	3.5	8.2	2.2
Medicare	14.4	14.0	69.0	13.5	14.8
Medicaid	10.7	3.3	0.6	29.9	3.8
Direct	14.3	5.7	3.9	1.2	7.5
Uninsured	22.3	11.4	10.7	12.6	12.2
Total N	450	1,398	345	96	235

Source: Data from The Commonwealth Fund survey on women's health, 1993.

with increases in the probability of having employer-based insurance (tab. 12.3). Eleven percent of women without a high school diploma rely on Medicaid, 20 percent are uninsured, and 25 percent have insurance through an employer. This pattern changes sharply with the attainment of a high school diploma. The probability of having Medicaid or being uninsured declines with increasing educational attainment as the probability of having employer-based insurance increases.

Health Insurance and Access to Health Care

These differences in insurance coverage are especially important if coverage affects access to health care. Measuring access to care is difficult, however, because a number of possible measures of access exist. One way to measure access is to look at a person's actual use of services over a given period. Use by itself is not a good measure of access unless the person actually "needed" the service. Without reviewing the person's medical record, need is difficult to establish. One way to circumvent this problem is to look at the use of services medical experts recommend for good care. These services include preventive services such as periodic physicals and Pap smears and mammograms for women, as well as services such as timely prenatal care.

Another possible measure of access is whether an individual has a usual source of health care services. Persons who have no established relationship with a health care provider may have access to some level of care, but the adequacy of that care may be questionable. These people may end up seeking care in inappropriate settings; for example, they may use the hospital emergency room for primary care services.

Table 12.3. Health Insurance, by Education

Insurance Source	<High School	High School	Some College	College	Graduate
Own employer	13.4%	34.5%	41.0%	48.0%	65.5%
Spouse's employer	11.8	19.9	18.7	18.2	14.1
Medicare	38.0	20.9	16.1	12.6	10.7
Medicaid	11.4	5.2	4.9	1.4	0.6
Direct	5.4	5.9	7.0	11.2	6.3
Uninsured	19.9	13.7	13.2	8.5	2.8
Total N	524	938	470	463	124

Source: Data from The Commonwealth Fund survey on women's health, 1993.

While subjective, a patient's evaluation of the adequacy of care and access to care may indicate problems. Reporting either dissatisfaction with the care one receives or not receiving health care services when one feels that they were needed may likewise indicate inadequate access to services.

Previous research findings suggest an important connection between health insurance coverage and women's access to health care. Lack of health insurance coverage or cost sharing hampers women's access to a variety of needed services, such as preventive ones. A large body of research literature suggests that women with no insurance are less likely than others to receive preventive and screening services such as mammograms or Pap smears (Johnson and Murata 1988; Mamon et al. 1990; Kirkman-Liff and Kronenfeld 1992). Woolhandler and Himmelstein (1988) found that lack of insurance was a strong predictor of the failure to receive screening tests. Using data from the RAND Health Insurance Experiment, Lurie et al. (1987 found that cost sharing decreased the use of preventive care.

Furthermore, health insurance coverage affects women's use of reproductive health services. Research on a number of different groups of women suggests that uninsured women are less likely than women with insurance to get timely reproductive services (Zweig, LeFevre, and Kruse 1988; Joseph 1989; Kalmuss and Fennelly 1990). Braveman et al. (1993) found that, compared with women who have private fee-for-service insurance coverage, uninsured women initiate prenatal care too late and make too few prenatal visits.

The research literature also suggests that the type of insurance coverage a woman has may affect her use of other reproductive health services, such as cesarean sections and family planning services. Stafford (1990) and Zahnhiser et al. (1992) found that women with private insurance coverage experience higher rates of cesarean sections than women with other types of insurance. In another study, Stafford reported that women with private insurance were much less likely than indigent women to have a vaginal birth after a previous cesarean section birth (Stafford 1991). Lack of insurance also affects a woman's choice of provider for family planning services. Women without insurance are more likely than other women to seek family planning services at a clinic rather than some other setting (Radecki and Bernstein 1989).

The source of insurance affects the site of care for other types of services as well. For example, low Medicaid physician payment rates in some states cause beneficiaries to seek physician care in inappropriate settings. Low Medicaid payment rates discourage physicians from seeing beneficiaries in their private offices and, therefore, often encourage beneficiaries to seek primary care inappropriately in hospital emergency rooms (Long et al. 1986; Cohen 1989). Oberg et al. (1991) found that the insurance source affects the setting of prenatal care. Women who are privately insured are more likely to use a private physician's office for prenatal care, while Medicaid beneficiaries and uninsured women are more likely to use a public clinic.

The Commonwealth Fund survey allows us to look at a number of the previously mentioned measures of access. The results support and add breadth to the findings of prior research on the important connection between insurance and access. One measure of access to high-quality health care services is the existence of an established patient-provider relationship. Uninsured women and Medicaid beneficiaries are less likely than others to have a regular source of care, raising concerns about the adequacy of their health care services. Sixty-five percent of uninsured women and 76 percent of Medicaid beneficiaries in The Commonwealth Fund survey reported that they have a regular source of care, compared with more than 80 percent of those covered by Medicare or employer-paid insurance.

The results of The Commonwealth Fund survey also support the finding that the source of insurance affects where people get medical care. Only 48 percent of Medicaid beneficiaries and 59 percent of uninsured persons obtain regular care in a physician's office, compared with almost 80 percent of those covered by Medicare or through an employer. Fourteen percent of uninsured persons and 11 percent of Medicaid beneficiaries use emergency rooms for regular care, compared with 5 percent of Medicare beneficiaries and 3 percent to 4 percent of those with employer-sponsored insurance.

Another indication of inadequate access to health care services is the failure to secure such services when the patient perceives they are needed. Uninsured women and Medicaid beneficiaries are less likely than other women to get needed care. Thirty-six percent of uninsured persons and 19 percent of Medicaid beneficiaries reported that they did not get necessary care at some time during the past year, compared with 10 percent or less of those who are covered by employer-based plans or who are Medicare beneficiaries.

The results of The Commonwealth Fund survey support prior research findings on insurance coverage and the use of preventive services. While more than 70 percent of women with Medicaid or employer-sponsored insurance received a Pap smear in the past year, only half of women with no insurance received this service. Similarly, while 67 percent of women over fifty with insurance through an employer had a mammogram within the past year, slightly less than 40 percent of women the same age with Medicaid or who were uninsured did.[2]

In The Commonwealth Fund survey, 64 percent of the uninsured women cited cost as a reason for not getting preventive services in the past year. There is a striking differential when this is compared with 25 percent of those covered by Medicaid, and about 20 percent of those insured through an employer or through Medicare.

Health Maintenance Organizations and Access to Health Care

Managed care plans, including traditional health maintenance organizations (HMOs) and more recent variations of managed health care financing and delivery, are an increasingly important segment of the insurance market. It is important to understand how these plans affect access to care.

The Commonwealth Fund survey suggests that HMOs affect certain aspects of access to care (tab. 12.4). Insured women who belong to HMOs are approximately as likely as women in non-HMO plans to have a usual source of care. Enrollment in an HMO has only a minor effect on the site where care is received; women in non-HMO plans are slightly more likely to use the emergency room as a usual source of care than women in HMOs (5% compared with 2%). Women in HMOs are somewhat more likely than other women to report not getting needed care in the previous year.

HMO enrollment seems to make a difference in access to preventive services. Women enrolled in HMOs are more likely to have received a number of preventive services in the past year. More women in HMOs got Pap smears than did women in other plans. Likewise, more women over fifty in HMOs got mammograms in the past year than did other insured women. Women in HMOs are less likely than women in other plans to report that they went without preventive services during the previous year because of the cost of those services.

SOCIOECONOMIC BARRIERS TO ACCESS

Some of the differences in access by the type of insurance may be caused by the same socioeconomic factors that relate to the type of

Table 12.4. Access to Health Care and HMOs

	HMO Member	Not HMO Member
Have regular source	83.8%	80.0%
	(355)	(1,377)
Use doctor's office regularly	71.5%	77.4%
	(254)	(1,066)
Use ER regularly	2.3%	4.9%
	(8)	(67)
Didn't get care	13.3%	9.0%
	(56)	(155)
Had Pap smear	74.3%	65.3%
	(315)	(1,124)
Had mammogram	65.2%	55.2%
	(68)	(394)
Preventive cost too much	14.7%	23.8%
	(49)	(325)

Source: Data from The Commonwealth Fund survey on women's health, 1993.

Note: Sample sizes differ among questions because of missing data. Data on mammogram use are based on women over fifty.

coverage a person can obtain: income, ethnicity, marital status, age, and educational attainment. To determine whether to attribute differential access to the source of insurance or some other cause, we need to examine these other factors as well. The Commonwealth Fund survey allows a detailed analysis of these barriers.

An examination of the bivariate relationships between the access indicators in The Commonwealth Fund survey and the socioeconomic characteristics of respondents indicates that only marital status seems to be related to whether a woman has a usual source of care. More than 80 percent of women who are married or widowed have a regular source for medical care, compared with about 75 percent of single and divorced women (tab. 12.5).

Many socioeconomic characteristics relate to the setting where women seek regular medical care. The use of a physician's office for regular care increases as income increases. At the same time, regular use of emergency rooms declines with income. Sixteen percent of women with incomes under $7,500 and 8 percent with incomes between $7,500 and $15,000 regularly use emergency room care (see tab.

Table 12.5. Access to Health Care and Marital Status

	Single	Married	Widowed	Separated	Divorced
Have regular source	73.4%	80.5%	80.5%	83.6%	74.2%
	(331)	(1126)	(277)	(81)	(175)
Use doctor's office regularly	65.3%	77.2%	77.9%	65.5%	70.2%
	(216)	(870)	(216)	(53)	(123)
Use ER regularly	9.8%	4.2%	4.1%	5.8%	6.4%
	(32)	(47)	(11)	(5)	(11)
Didn't get care	14.1%	12.2%	8.3%	21.7%	22.5%
	(63)	(170)	(28)	(21)	(53)
Had Pap smear	64.3%	69.5%	42.8%	80.4%	59.8%
	(290)	(972)	(147)	(77)	(141)
Had mammogram	38.5%	60.3%	47.0%	75.4%	64.2%
	(18)	(272)	(148)	(13)	(54)
Preventive cost too much	32.2%	26.5%	19.8%	41.2%	40.9%
	(130)	(294)	(52)	(33)	(76)

Source: Data from The Commonwealth Fund survey on women's health, 1993.

Note: Sample sizes differ among questions because of missing data. Data on mammogram use are based on women over fifty.

12.6). Women with incomes above this level are much less likely to use an emergency room (2% to 3%). White women tend to use a physician's office regularly more than African American women, and Hispanics tend to use an office less than non-Hispanics. Married and widowed women tend to use a physician's office more than other women, as do women over age thirty-five. Education has some positive effect on the use of a physician's office for regular health care.

Several socioeconomic factors relate to whether a woman failed to get the care she felt she needed. Slightly less than 20 percent of women with incomes less than $7,500 a year reported not getting needed care at some time in the past year (tab. 12.6). This percentage generally declines with increasing income. Hispanic women are slightly more likely (17%) to go without care than non-Hispanic women (13%). Separated and divorced women were much more likely to go without care than other women. Women over sixty are slightly less likely to go without care than younger women, and the likelihood of going without needed care declines slightly with more education (tab. 12.7).

The use of preventive health care services such as mammograms and Pap smears appears to be affected by income and education. The

Table 12.6. Access to Health Care and Income

	Income (in thousands of dollars)							
	<7.5	7.5–15	15–25	25–35	35–50	50–75	75–100	100+
Have regular source	79.2%	74.8%	76.0%	76.7%	81.9%	82.9%	87.0%	86.3%
	(264)	(259)	(320)	(284)	(284)	(254)	(86)	(63)
Use doctor's office regularly	63.8%	65.8%	74.3%	76.7%	81.8%	80.0%	80.5%	84.1%
	(168)	(171)	(238)	(218)	(232)	(203)	(69)	(53)
Use ER regularly	16.0%	8.4%	2.9%	2.7%	2.6%	0.8%	3.0%	—
	(42)	(22)	(9)	(8)	(7)	(2)	(3)	—
Didn't get care	19.6%	18.7%	15.6%	11.9%	8.8%	9.2%	3.5%	9.0%
	(65)	(65)	(66)	(44)	(30)	(28)	(4)	(7)
Had Pap smear	56.2%	48.3%	63.9%	70.9%	70.8%	75.9	72.8%	83.1%
	(187)	(168)	(269)	(263)	(245)	(232)	(72)	(61)
Had mammogram	41.4%	52.1%	55.2%	60.2%	68.9%	73.1%	74.5%	77.4%
	(68)	(93)	(83)	(66)	(53)	(43)	(16)	(14)
Preventive cost too much	38.5%	36.1%	34.2%	25.3%	21.1%	19.7%	8.7%	17.9%
	(107)	(105)	(124)	(75)	(58)	(47)	(7)	(10)

Source: Data from The Commonwealth Fund survey on women's health, 1993.

Note: Sample sizes differ among questions because of missing data. Data on mammogram use are based on women over fifty.

Table 12.7. Access to Health Care and Education

	<High School	High School	Some College	College	Graduate
Have regular source	78.5%	78.2%	79.2%	78.6%	84.4%
	(411)	(733)	(372)	(364)	(104)
Use doctor's office	70.4%	75.3%	75.2%	73.5%	80.0%
regularly	(290)	(552)	(280)	(268)	(83)
Use ER regularly	10.0%	5.0%	4.3%	3.4%	0.8%
	(41)	(37)	(16)	(12)	(1)
Didn't get care	15.3%	13.2%	13.5%	12.7%	7.7%
	(80)	(124)	(64)	(59)	(9)
Had Pap smear	53.6%	61.3%	70.3%	74.3%	75.6%
	(281)	(575)	(331)	(344)	(93)
Had mammogram	43.4%	58.1%	65.2%	60.7%	67.8%
	(123)	(201)	(91)	(65)	(21)
Preventive cost too	34.8%	31.7%	25.4%	21.0%	17.2%
much	(154)	(238)	(94)	(81)	(16)

Source: Data from The Commonwealth Fund survey on women's health, 1993.

Note: Sample sizes differ among questions because of missing data. Data on mammogram use are based on women over fifty.

use of both of these services increases with increasing income levels and more education.

Lower-income women are more likely than high-income women to forgo getting preventive health care services because of the cost. Nearly 40 percent of women with incomes less than $7,500 report that cost kept them from getting preventive services in the past year. This number declines fairly steadily with rising income (see tab. 12.6). More Hispanic women than non-Hispanic women cited cost as a barrier to getting preventive services. Separated and divorced women are more likely than other women to incur a cost barrier to getting these services. While age does not seem to be related to this cost problem, increasing education diminishes it.

ACCESS TO HEALTH CARE: A MULTIVARIATE ANALYSIS

The relationships among the socioeconomic factors, health insurance, and access are complex. For example, women with more education are probably more likely than others to have higher incomes and to have insurance. Education, income, and having insurance in turn positively affect access. Multivariate analysis can separate out the individual effects of each of the factors affecting access to health insurance and health care services.

Multivariate statistical analyses show that many of the relationships detected in the bivariate analyses above remain in the multivariate analysis: access is affected by health insurance and socioeconomic factors. The results of two of these models follow. These models were chosen for discussion because their results are representative of other models.

Using Commonwealth Fund data on the number of physician visits in the past year as an indicator of access, the first regression model examines the effect on access to care of health insurance type, income, race/ethnicity, marital status, education, and health status. The use of physician visits as a measure of access has the inherent problem of using utilization to measure access. However, other studies of access have used this measure, and the results of the analysis seem to be in line with the findings of the other measures examined above.

The independent variables included in the model were chosen because the results of the bivariate analyses suggest that health insurance coverage, income, ethnicity, marital status, and education are related to at least some measures of access. The health status variable is included to adjust for differences in general health that might lead to differential need for health services. Other research has found self-reported health status to be a reliable indicator of morbidity (Idler and Angel 1990).

The regression model suggests that a number of factors affect the number of physician visits per woman.[3] Women who had a visit reported an average of six physician visits in the year before the survey.[4] Employer-based insurance (separated into those with insurance through their own employer and those with insurance through their spouse's employer), Medicare, Medicaid, and insurance purchased directly from an insurer are included as a series of categorical variables. Those with no insurance are left out of the equation and form the reference group against which the estimates should be read. Women with insurance through their spouse's employer have 1.2 more visits per year than uninsured women. Women with Medicare have more than 2 more physician visits per year, and women with Medicaid have slightly fewer than 2 more visits per year than uninsured women. Because these estimates control for differences in health status, age, marital status, and other variables, they can be interpreted as an indication of increased use of (access to) care for those with these insurance sources relative to those without insurance.

Even controlling for the source of health insurance, socioeconomic factors still affect women's access to care. The results on the income variables support the pattern of increased access at higher income levels detected in the bivariate analysis, but the effect of education is not significant. Income also relates to the number of visits. Relative to people whose income is under $15,000, people whose income is between $15,001 and $35,000 have about one more visit per year and people whose income is above $75,000 have more than one more visit.

The estimates for marital status are not statistically significant. The same is true for the estimates for the ethnic/racial groups, except for the "other" category, whose members have about 2.5 more visits per year than whites.

People aged eighteen to forty-four have 1.5 more visits per year than people aged forty-five to sixty-four. Because eighteen to forty-four is the peak childbearing time for women, this increase may be due in part to the use of reproductive services.

In addition to health insurance source and socioeconomic factors, by including a measure of health status the analysis controls for differential need for physician visits. Health status greatly affects the number of visits. Persons who rate their health as fair or poor have six more visits per year than people who rate their health as excellent or very good. People who rate their health as good have two more visits than those in excellent or very good health.

The second multivariate model examines the effect of health insurance source and the socioeconomic factors on whether a woman reported that she went without needed care at some time in the year before the survey. The independent variables in this model are the same as in the previous one, and the results also indicate that health insurance and some of the socioeconomic factors relate to access.[5] Each of the independent variables is examined to estimate the odds that a woman will not get needed care. Having any insurance decreases the odds of going without needed care, as does increasing income, being single, being older, and having better health status. For those with employer-based insurance, for example, the odds of going without needed care are about one-quarter of the odds for those without insurance.

IMPLICATIONS FOR POLICY AND RESEARCH

In the United States, women obtain insurance coverage in different ways than men. While most women are less likely than their male counterparts to be uninsured, they are more likely to rely on public sources of insurance and less likely to obtain insurance through their own employer. This reliance on public insurance affects their access to health care, particularly those services covered by Medicaid. While Medicaid coverage provides some access to health care, it appears to cause some troubling barriers. In The Commonwealth Fund survey, women with Medicaid coverage were more likely than other insured women to report going without needed care. Furthermore, Medicaid coverage seems to encourage (or at least does not discourage) the inappropriate use of emergency room settings for regular care.

Lack of insurance coverage diminishes access to health care. The Commonwealth Fund survey suggests that this means delaying the use of reproductive services, forgoing needed preventive services, being less likely to have a regular source of health care, and using the emergency room as a regular source of care at higher rates than many other women.

Enrollment in an HMO also appears to have some effect on access to health care. While HMO enrollees and nonenrollees reported similar levels of access to most services, HMO enrollees reported greater access to some preventive services. However, HMO enrollees were more likely to report that they did not get needed care in the past year.

The Commonwealth Fund survey data allow us to look in great detail at the relationship among health insurance, socioeconomic factors, and access to health care. Analysis of the survey suggests that looking at the situation of women as a group masks a number of sources of differential access to care among women. The analyses reported here suggest that, in addition to the type of insurance coverage a person has, there are also socioeconomic causes of differential access, particularly differences in income.

The results of this analysis are particularly interesting because of recent debates over health care reform. If, as is likely, reform is built on the current employer-based system of providing health insurance, special consideration should be given to providing adequate insurance for those who are often left out of such a system, such as unemployed or underemployed poor persons. Thus, extension of coverage to more people or, ideally, universal coverage is an important goal for health care reform.

Extending insurance coverage to more individuals, however, is not sufficient to ensure access. Insurance plans that do not cover certain services, such as preventive services, or that require high out-of-pocket costs for some services, may impede access to those services, particularly for those with low incomes. It is important, therefore, not only that insurance reform extend coverage but also that women have access to a benefit package that includes the basic set of services that women need and that any out-of-pocket costs associated with these basic services be affordable even to low-income women.

Many see managed care insurance plans as a means of containing costs. While managed care has well-known and much-discussed drawbacks, the survey results are mixed. On one hand, they indicate that managed care may increase women's access to some preventive services; on the other, more HMO enrollees feel they are not getting needed care. Additional research is called for on balancing the cost and access considerations in HMOs.

The results of the analysis suggest that even if health care financing initiatives succeed in extending insurance coverage to more people, some factors will still exist that create barriers to access. True "health care reform," therefore, may require more than health financing and insurance initiatives. Even when we take into account whether a person has insurance, other factors, such as health status, income, education, and age, may affect access to care.[6] This suggests the complexity of differential access. While having insurance increases access to care, it does not entirely eliminate barriers to care.

Policies to eliminate nonfinancial barriers to care will have to be tailored to the problems of different communities, and research on best practices in health care delivery in those communities will help focus resources. For example, in poor, underserved, urban communities, increasing access may require changes in the health care delivery system. Existing resources, such as hospitals, that serve these communities may have to be restructured to provide the kinds of educational and primary care services a given community needs. Additionally in poor, underserved, rural areas, the problem may be failure to attract sufficient health professionals to serve the population. While insurance reform may help solve the access problems of these communities, insurance reform alone may not be enough.

NOTES

1. While only the bivariate relationships are discussed here, multivariate analyses of the probability of having each insurance source suggest that the bivariate relationships described here remain even when controlling for other socioeconomic characteristics.

2. Note that these utilization data are self-reported and there is no way to confirm the accuracy of this information.

3. This model was estimated using an ordinary least-squares technique.

4. Note that this mean is trimmed slightly. A few respondents who reported a very large number of visits were deleted from the analysis. The mean was reported only for those who had a visit. Further, while the regression model suggests that a number of factors affect the number of physician visits, the model itself does not have a great deal of explanatory power.

5. Because the dependent variable is dichotomous, the model was estimated using a logistic procedure.

6. While it was not the central purpose of this analysis to look at the nonfinancial causes of differential access to care, these causes cannot be ignored. There is a large and growing body of literature examining nonfinancial barriers to care such as race, living in areas with shortages of health professionals (rural or urban), and living in an impoverished community (see, e.g., Goldberg et al. 1992; Blendon et al. 1989; Physician Payment Review Commission 1992).

REFERENCES

Blendon, R. J., Aiken, L. H., Freeman, H. E., and Corey, C. R. 1989. Access to medical care for black and white Americans, a matter of continuing concern. *Journal of the American Medical Association* 261:278–81.

Braveman, P., Bennett, T., Lewis, C., Egerter, S., and Showstack, J. 1993. Access to prenatal care following major Medicaid eligibility expansions. *Journal of the American Medical Association* 269:1285–89.

Brown, C., Hamilton, J., and Medolf, J. 1990. *Employers Large and Small*. Cambridge: Harvard University Press.

Cohen, J. 1989. Medicaid policy and the substitution of hospital outpatient care for physician care. *Health Services Research* 24:33–66.

Cooper, P., and Johnson, A. 1993. *Employment Related Health Insurance in 1987*. Pub. no. 93–0044, National Medical Expenditure Survey Research Findings 17. Rockville, Md.: Agency for Health Care Policy and Research.

Goldberg, K. C., Hartz, A. J., Jacobsen, S. D., Krakauer, H., and Rimm, A. A. 1992. Racial and community factors influencing coronary artery bypass graft surgery rates for all 1986 Medicare patients. *Journal of the American Medical Association* 267:1473–77.

Idler, I., and Angel, R. J. 1990. Self-rated health and mortality in the HHANES-I Epidemiologic follow-up study. *American Journal of Public Health* 80:446–52.

Horton, J. A., ed. 1992. *The Women's Health Data Book: A Profile of Women's Health in the United States.* Washington, D.C.: Jacobs Institute on Women's Health.

Jensen, G. A. 1992. The dynamics of health insurance among the near elderly. *Medical Care* 30:598–614.

Johnson, R. A., and Murata, P. J. 1988. Demographic, clinical, and financial factors relating to the completion rate of screening mammography. *Cancer Detection Prevention* 11:259–66.

Joseph, C. L. 1989. Identification of factors associated with delayed antenatal care. *Journal of the National Medical Association* 81:57–63.

Kalmuss, D., and Fennelly, K. 1990. Barriers to prenatal care among low-income women in New York City. *Family Planning Perspective* 22:215–18, 231.

Kirkman-Liff, B., and Kronenfeld, J. J. 1992. Access to cancer screening services for women. *American Journal of Public Health* 82:733–35.

Long, S. H., et al. 1986. Reimbursement and access to physician services under Medicaid. *Journal of Health Economics* 5:235–51.

Lurie, N., Manning, W. G., Peterson, C., Goldberg, G. A., Phelps, C. E., and Lillard, L. 1987. Preventive care: do we practice what we preach? *American Journal of Public Health* 77:801–4.

Mamon, J. A., Shediac, M. C., Crosby, C. B., Sanders, B., Matanoski, G. M., and Celentano, D. D. 1990. Inner-city women at risk for cervical cancer: behavioral and utilization factors related to inadequate screening. *Preventive Medicine* 19:363–76.

Oberg, C. N., Lia-Hoagberg, B., Skovholt, C., Hodkinson, E., and Vanman, R. 1991. Prenatal care use and health insurance status. *Journal of Health Care for the Poor and Underserved* 2:270–92.

Physician Payment Review Commission. 1992. *Monitoring Access of Medicare Beneficiaries: Report to Congress.* No. 92–5. Washington, D.C.

Radecki, S. E., and Bernstein, G. S. 1989. Use of clinic versus private family planning care by low-income women: access, cost, and patient satisfaction. *American Journal of Public Health* 79:692–97.

Snider, S. 1994. Part-time work: characteristics of the part-time workforce: analysis of the March 1993 current population survey. *EBRI Issue Brief.* Washington, D.C.: Employee Benefits Research Institute.

Stafford, R. S. 1990. Cesarean section use and source of payment: an analysis of California hospital discharge abstracts. *American Journal of Public Health* 80:313–15.

———. 1991. The impact of nonclinical factors on repeat cesarean section. *Journal of the American Medical Association* 265:59–63.

U.S. Bureau of the Census. 1993a. Health Insurance Coverage Status by Age and Sex, 1992. Data from the March 1993 Current Population Survey (unpublished).

———. 1993b. *Poverty in the United States, 1992.* Current Population Reports, Consumer Income, series P60–185.

Woolhandler, S., and Himmelstein, D. U. 1988. Reverse targeting of preventive care due to lack of health insurance. *Journal of the American Medical Association* 259:2872–74.

Zahnhiser, S. C., Kendrick, J. S., Franks, A. L., and Saftlas, A. F. 1992. Trends in obstetric operative procedures, 1980–1987. *American Journal of Public Health* 82:1340–44.

Zweig, S., LeFevre, M., and Kruse, J. 1988. The health belief model and attendance for prenatal care. *Family Practice Research Journal* 8:32–41.

Conclusion: Moving Forward—Evolving an Agenda on Women's Health

Karen Scott Collins, M.D., M.P.H.
Joan M. Leiman, Ph.D.

There is significant information and experience on which to build the next phase of a women's health agenda. Taken as a whole, the chapters of this book provide a rich definition of women's health through understanding women's experiences. Such understanding should assist all concerned with women's health and well-being, in developing responses that promote greater health and well-being for health care providers, policy makers, employers, family members, and patients.

This book defines women's health broadly, through analysis of how women experience health care services, their knowledge of health issues, their mental and physical health, and the impact of environment, including violence, on health. The information contributes to identifying the health care and information needs of women at different ages, especially women at risk. The authors use this knowledge to suggest policies and programs, as well as to identify needed research. It is therefore a firm base on which to build an evolving agenda on women's health, with components of communication, public policy, and research.

This agenda for moving forward in women's health proposes action in five strategic areas: expanding economic and educational opportunities, assuring adequate financial coverage and access to health care, training health care professionals in women's health issues, building women's awareness of their health needs, and, finally, continuing research on women's health.

EXPANDING ECONOMIC AND EDUCATIONAL OPPORTUNITIES

It is striking that so many of the authors in this book, while approaching the data in different ways, wind up highlighting the roles of education and employment in health. The experiences of the women in The Commonwealth Fund survey, as presented in this volume's expert analysis, make evident the social and economic factors that influence health.

A low level of education or low income places women at greater risk for not receiving care, limits the choice of health care providers, and limits resources when women are victims of violence. Less-educated and low-income women receive less preventive care and have less knowledge of services such as hormone therapy. They are also less likely to practice healthy behaviors that are increasingly linked with reduced mortality and morbidity, such as exercise.

In addition to facilitating financial access to health care, employment and education help increase self-esteem, which can contribute to an ability to play an active role in taking care of oneself and in communicating with health care providers. This positive environment for receiving health care is an important aspect of the quality of care. It can determine whether patients seek needed care or follow through on prescribed treatments, thereby influencing health outcomes. Recent Commonwealth Fund surveys have highlighted that patients' satisfaction with health care depends in part on having a choice of providers, lack of language barriers, and whether they feel welcome (Louis Harris and Associates 1995a, 1995b). Employment and education contribute significantly to giving women the tools they need to gain access to health care, make choices, and develop relationships with providers that can lead to satisfactory care and better health outcomes.

Nationally and internationally, it is increasingly being recognized that women's health is influenced by their roles in society and their opportunities. Opportunities to obtain employment and advance education provide women with options, choices, and self-esteem, which can be the starting point of improving health outcomes. Internationally, a broadened approach to achieving improvements in women's health is also being pursued. Programs in developing nations are moving from a condition-specific focus, such as family planning, to a recognition that employment and education must come first.

Expanding economic and educational opportunities will have a positive impact on health. It is also clear that further improvement of women's health and well-being will require a combined focus on health care delivery and increasing attention to the full range of factors that have an impact on women's health, based on their experiences. The lesson that public programs play an important role in providing access to health care comes through in this volume—but equally striking is the lesson that public programs in child care, family support, job training, and, most of all, education, have a strong impact on women's health and well-being. Proponents of women's health, therefore, must also be proponents of women's employment, women's education, and programs that strengthen families and communities, thereby providing social support.

ASSURING ADEQUATE FINANCIAL COVERAGE AND ACCESS TO HEALTH CARE

The positive influence of health insurance and access to a regular source of health care on the use of preventive health services and the receipt of needed care is strong and common across all ages and races. There have been some important gains in women's access to health care over the past few years. Expanded Medicaid coverage in the late 1980s gave thousands of pregnant women access to health care (Kaiser Commission on the Future of Medicaid 1993). Medicare's coverage of mammography and Pap smears in the early 1990s increased access to these services for many elderly women (Blustein 1995).

Despite this progress, the changing health care environment presents several challenges: the potential for the erosion of insurance coverage, potential restructuring of publicly funded programs (including Medicaid and Medicare), and unanswered questions about managed care. Recent trends in private insurance coverage show fewer employers offering insurance, employers offering coverage with greater costs to employees, and employers not offering dependent coverage (Thorpe 1995).

For women, who rely disproportionately on Medicaid and Medicare, the potential restructuring of these programs and constraints on financing them may have an impact on the ability to gain access to health care or on the quality of the care received. These changes in public programs and declining employer coverage will place women at increased risk for being uninsured.

For women with health insurance, that insurance is increasingly likely to be through a managed care plan. The experiences of women in managed care, and the access and quality of services women need, will require continued research and observation.

The Commonwealth Fund's 1994 survey of patient experiences with managed care found patients in managed care to be less satisfied with aspects of services (such as choice of physicians, access to specialty care, and access to emergency care), whereas they more often rated highly the access to preventive services and lower out-of-pocket costs (Louis Harris and Associates 1995b). Such findings highlight the need for monitoring various aspects of care. For women's health, developing measures of quality in health care is critical and timely.

An environment of competitive health plans and limited public funding may be counter to an expanding definition of women's health. For example, will health care-based programs in the prevention and treatment of violence continue to be developed? Will greater screening and appropriate treatment for mental illness, particularly depression, be available? Will health plans be responsive to women's preferences and needs regarding interaction with physicians? Will health plans contribute to expanding access to preventive care?

TRAINING HEALTH CARE PROFESSIONALS IN WOMEN'S HEALTH ISSUES

Making sure that physicians, scientists, and other health care professionals are well trained in biomedical and psychosocial issues of women's health is a major strategy in moving forward on women's health. The medical profession is increasingly recognizing the necessity for a specific focus on women's health. The *Journal of the American Medical Association*, for example, devoted issues to women's health (1992, vol. 268, no. 14) and to domestic violence (1992, vol. 267, no. 23). The American Medical Association initiated a campaign against family violence, helping physicians recognize this entity as a medical and public health problem. The internal medicine boards now include a section on women's health. Further, as the demand for primary care practitioners increases, some obstetrician-gynecologists are expressing interest in nonreproductive health issues, such as depression. Most important, women themselves are increasingly demanding attention and information from researchers and health care providers about their health.

Yet, as the survey findings demonstrate, communication between physicians and women patients often fails. The second most common reason given for the failure to receive clinical preventive services was the physician's failure to refer. Women with a history of abuse, violence, or mental health problems have particular difficulty discussing their concerns and getting help from their physicians.

All physicians should receive a thorough grounding in women's health. This education should begin in medical school, then continue in residency training and practice. Primary care providers should be trained to recognize and treat depression and to counsel women on a full range of preventive health care. Training to identify and help women who have been—or are being—abused is also needed. There are initiatives in domestic violence training for emergency room care providers and for some primary care providers. Such initiatives will make an even greater impact as training is disseminated to a growing number of providers in different health care settings and is incorporated into professional education.

BUILDING WOMEN'S AWARENESS OF THEIR HEALTH NEEDS

Women of all ages need to know the importance of health-related behaviors. The Commonwealth Fund survey data indicate a wide divergence of awareness, with higher-income, better-educated women more informed about risks to their health such as osteoporosis and heart disease. Targeted endeavors should reach all women with the message that they can, and should, take measures to protect their health.

Such endeavors also have to provide women with the information and tools they need to make decisions about their health. Often, such decision making is done in partnership with health professionals and family members. One barrier that persists in making health care decisions is the uncertain or contradictory information available on some aspects of care. Recommendations on mammography for women under age fifty and on hormone therapy are two important points of confusion for women. Some of this confusion will be resolved only as biomedical research continues. In the interim, it is necessary to develop strategies for assessing and making decisions based on available information.

Interactive video programs, such as those developed by the Foundation for Shared Decision Making, are one example of an innovative approach to facilitating the dissemination of information and decision making on serious health concerns (Kasper, Mulley, and Wennberg 1992). These programs provide disease-specific information, display treatment options, and interview patients who have made treatment decisions. The interactive program allows the patient viewing the video to tailor the information to her own risk factors and clinical situation.

Women also get a significant amount of health information through women's magazines, the press, and other media. These communication vehicles can play an important role in providing valuable information.

CONTINUING RESEARCH ON WOMEN'S HEALTH

The issue of women's health has been blurred by the assumption that, except for reproductive health, there is no need to distinguish between men and women when looking at diseases or health service issues common to both sexes. Until the recent National Institutes of Health's women's health initiative, there has been little focused research on problems specific to women. There is, therefore, a great deal of catching up to do. Continued research on women's health is required in several major areas: health, psychosocial, and biomedical services.

To intervene effectively to improve health services, one must understand the fragmentation of health care experienced by many women, the type of services and providers preferred by women, and reasons for not receiving preventive care. Research is needed on the effectiveness and outcomes of different health care providers (such as women's health centers, primary care, and specialty care) in addressing these issues. Experiences with managed care have been found to vary by type of plan and geographic location (Louis Harris and Associates 1995b). Tracking access to specialty services and the quality of women's health care in different types of managed care arrangements is therefore also needed.

The impact of psychosocial factors on women's health, such as the interactions between women's social and economic roles and their health, requires greater understanding. Similarly, the consequences of traumatic experiences of abuse and violence on physical and mental health demand further attention.

Many of the concerns addressed throughout this book point to the need for more biological and clinical research to provide the basis for treating women appropriately. This requires a greater understanding of gender differences in diseases common to both men and women, and, in particular, the role of hormones. For conditions that are specific to women or that disproportionately affect women, much more information is needed. The effects of hormone therapy, recommendations for mammography for women under age fifty, and effectively identifying and treating depression are some examples. Finally, the developing field of monitoring the quality of care represents a further area where work is needed, bringing together findings from health services, behavior, and biomedical research to define quality in women's health care.

THE COMMONWEALTH FUND COMMISSION ON WOMEN'S HEALTH

The Commonwealth Fund has used the findings from the women's health survey to develop a program agenda in women's health that includes access to health care, preventive health services, psychological well-being, violence against women, and health care decision making. Through this program, The Commonwealth Fund is actively identifying programs and information that can lead to improving the health of women.

Individual projects under the program include surveys and analyses to continue building knowledge, case studies and best-practice studies to identify what works and what is effective, and the development and testing of new interventions such as training health professionals in domestic violence and interactive videos.

Audiences for the findings and products of this work include health care providers, women patients, policy makers, and researchers in women's health. Information is developed and presented to each of these audiences in formats useful to them. For example, Commonwealth Fund-supported work has been included in the national press, women's magazines, national policy documents, and professional journals.

The commission's first policy report provided goals for health care reform for women's health (Leiman et al. 1994). While the direction of health reform has changed since this publication, the goals remain critical to building a women's health agenda that can achieve improved health for all women. These goals are:

- Affordable health coverage for all Americans. This goal is particularly important for low-income women who are more frequently unable to obtain affordable coverage for themselves and their families.
- Benefits should include services essential to women's health: preventive care, mental health care, long-term care, and the full range of reproductive health services.
- Financing should assure affordable health care for women and their families, whatever their economic circumstances.
- The availability of primary care and other essential providers, particularly in underserved communities, and of the support services that women need to be able to use health care services should be supported.
- Funding for public programs should not jeopardize access to care for women who are covered through Medicare and Medicaid.
- Health plans and providers should be required to collect and make public information on performance, quality, consumer satisfaction, and cost.
- Support for medical innovation and research is needed to assure continuing progress in the prevention of disease and the promotion and maintenance of health and quality of life.

In retrospect, it is clear that The Commonwealth Fund survey of women's health was undertaken at a propitious moment in American history, when a number of forces converged to give recognition to the need to pay attention to women's health issues. We would like to think that the survey itself made a major contribution to this awareness, as will the studies in this book.

It is also clear that this book will be published in a different climate. A few short years are seeing dramatic changes in American health care policy and the American health care marketplace. It is important that in the midst of change we continue the efforts to advance women's health and well-being to meet the goals highlighted by the commission. The knowledge in this book, and other work that we hope will follow, provides a platform on which to build future advances in women's health.

REFERENCES

Blustein, Jan. 1995. Medicare coverage, supplemental insurance, and the use of mammography by older women. *New England Journal of Medicine* 332:1138–43.

Kaiser Commission on the Future of Medicaid. 1993. *The Medicaid Cost Explosion: Causes and Consequences*. Baltimore: Frunek Design Associates, Inc.

Louis Harris and Associates, Inc. 1995a. Commonwealth Fund National Comparative Survey on Minority Health. March.

————. 1995b. Commonwealth Fund Survey of Patient Experiences with Managed Care. July.

Kasper, Joseph F., Mulley, Albert G., Jr., and Wennberg, John E. 1992. Developing shared decision-making programs to improve the quality of health care. *Journal of Quality Improvement* 18:182–90.

Leiman, Joan M., Reisinger, Anne, Collins, Karen Scott, Davis, Karen, et al. 1994. "Health Care Reform: What Is at Stake for Women?" July.

Thorpe, Kenneth. 1995. Tulane University Analysis of 1994 Current Population Survey.

Index

Library of Congress Cataloging-in-Publication Data

Women's health : the Commonwealth Fund survey / edited by Marilyn M.
  Falik and Karen Scott Collins.
     p.   cm.
   Includes index.
   ISBN 0-8018-5353-2 (hc : alk. paper). — ISBN 0-8018-5354-0 (pbk.
: alk. paper)
    1. Women—Health and hygiene—United States—Sociological aspects.
2. Women's health services—Utilization—United States.   3. Women—
Health and hygiene—United States—Psychological aspects.
   I. Falik, Marilyn.   II. Collins, Karen Scott.   III. Commonwealth
Fund.
  RA408.W65W665   1996
  362.1'98—dc20   95-46435
                                               CIP